Mosby's Color Atlas and Text of

Diabetes
and
Endocrinology

This book is dedicated to Gill, Amy, Leo, Rebecca and Ruth, from Paul, for unfailing love and patience and keeping me sane (hopefully); and to Kate, Ned, Will and Millie for your enduring and unstinting love, support and encouragement, from Peter.

Commissioning Editor: Michael Parkinson
Project Development Manager: Fiona Conn
Project Managers: Ailsa Laing/Frances Affleck
Designer: Erik Bigland
Illustrations Manager: Bruce Hogarth

Mosby's Color Atlas and Text of

Diabetes and Endocrinology

Dr Paul Belchetz
Consultant Physician/Endocrinologist,
Department of Endocrinology,
The General Infirmary,
Leeds, UK

Dr Peter J Hammond
Consultant Physician,
Department of Medicine,
Harrogate District Hospital,
Harrogate, UK

Mosby

EDINBURGH   LONDON   NEW YORK   OXFORD   PHILADELPHIA   ST LOUIS   SYDNEY   TORONTO   2003

MOSBY
An affiliate of Elsevier Science Limited

First published 2003

ISBN 0-7234-3104-3

British Library Cataloguing in Publication Data
A catalogue record for this book is available from the British Library

Library of Congress Cataloging in Publication Data
A catalog record for this book is available from the Library of Congress

Notice
Medical knowledge is constantly changing. Standard safety precautions must be followed, but as new research and clinical experience broaden our knowledge, changes in treatment and drug therapy may become necessary or appropriate. Readers are advised to check the most current product information provided by the manufacturer of each drug to be administered to verify the recommended dose, the method and duration of administration, and contraindications. It is the responsibility of the practitioner, relying on experience and knowledge of the patient, to determine dosages and the best treatment for each individual patient. Neither the Publisher nor the authors assumes any liability for any injury and/or damage to persons or property arising from this publication.

The Publisher

Printed in Spain

Contents

Contents

Preface

The chance of writing this book immediately attracted us, but we recognized the great demands it would place on us, both being involved in very busy medical practice. Why should we have bothered and what were our goals?

An early and enduring attraction was the possibility, provided by recent technical advances, to write an authentic textbook focused on clinical practice, but founded on a sound scientific and pathological base, which could use almost unlimited colour illustrations, photographs, diagrams and summary tables to reinforce the written text vividly and memorably.

A further incentive was to write the two parts essentially as solo efforts, yet working closely together and not simply having one person write one section and the other write the second section. In the conventional multi-author tome, editorial rigour can achieve high levels of consistency and minimize duplication. We hoped, as two longstanding colleagues, we would optimize this element. We also share backgrounds in academic units dedicated to high-level basic and clinical research, which have indelibly imprinted on us an appreciation of the scientific background to our specialities. Both of us, however, have chosen to pursue largely clinical careers, in which we see large numbers of patients spanning the entirety of our respective areas of interest.

We hope our book blends the lessons of science, medical literature and perhaps above all our own personal clinical experiences, and will be of value to medical students, doctors in training and practising specialists alike.

September 2002

Paul Belchetz and Peter Hammond
Leeds and Harrogate

Acknowledgements

Our thanks and appreciation to Dr Bob Bury (Consultant Radiologist), Dr Gary Butler (Consultant Paediatric Endocrinologist), Dr Steve Gilbey (Consultant Endocrinologist), Dr Mark Liddington (Consultant Plastic Surgeon), Dr Rod Mawhinney (Consultant Radiologist), Mr Mitch Ménage (Consultant Ophthalmologist), Dr Mike Nelson (Consultant Neuroradiologist), Dr David Scullion (Consultant Radiologist) and Miss Gillian Shepherd (Associate Specialist in Ophthalmology), for their contributions to the photographs/illustrations, and to Mrs Marilyn Saville and Ms Lisa Grylls for secretarial assistance.

chapter 1

Diabetes – Introduction

Diabetes mellitus is a disease characterized by elevated blood glucose levels. It is the result of defective insulin secretion or action, or both. The resulting chronic hyperglycaemia is associated with damage to and subsequent dysfunction of various organs, especially the eyes, kidneys, nerves, heart, and blood vessels.

A condition characterized by a polyuric state resembling diabetes mellitus was described in the Ebers papyrus, which dates from the 15th century BC. Aretaeus of Cappadocia first used the term diabetes, from the Greek word meaning 'to pass through', in the 2nd century AD, describing the disease as a dreadful affliction resulting in a short life. The sweetness of the urine in this disease was first recorded in Sanskrit literature of the 5th–6th centuries, and the great Arabian physician Avicenna, in the 10th century, described the clinical characteristics and noted the complications of gangrene and 'collapse of sexual function'.

Thomas Willis, physician to Charles II, repeated the observation that this polyuric state was characterized by sweet urine. However, it was not until the late 17th century that the adjective 'mellitus', derived from the Latin for honey, was applied to distinguish this disease from those polyuric states in which the urine is tasteless – 'insipidus'.

Experimental physiology in the 19th century implicated dysfunction of the pancreas as the probable cause of diabetes, but effective treatment remained elusive. Patients with insulin-dependent diabetes still faced a short life, and death usually resulted from ketoacidosis (**Fig. 1.1**). A starvation diet could briefly normalize blood glucose levels, but malnutrition was inevitable and, in those patients who opted for such a diet, life was prolonged for only a few months.

In 1921, Frederick Banting, a physician surgeon, working at the University of Toronto in Ontario, Canada with a student assistant, Charles Best, demonstrated that extracts of chilled

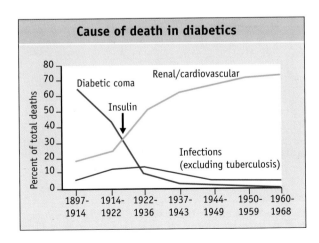

Fig. 1.1 *Causes of death in patients with diabetes over the last century (from Marble 1972 Diabetes 21: 632–636, with permission from* **The American Diabetes Association**).

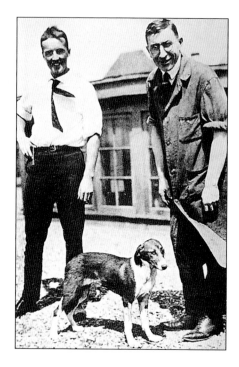

Fig. 1.2 *Banting (right) and Best with one of the dogs used in their experiments. From Professor Michael Bliss, University of Toronto, Canada, with permission.*

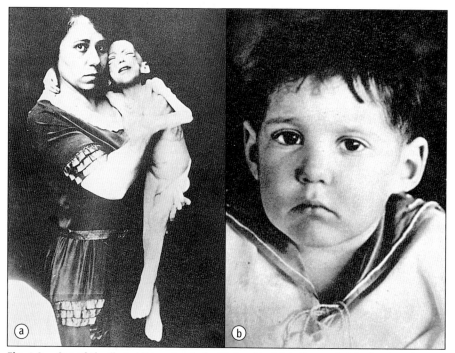

Fig. 1.3 *One of the first children treated with insulin (a) before and (b) after insulin treatment. From Professor Michael Bliss, University of Toronto, Canada, with permission.*

whole pancreas could reduce blood glucose levels in pancreatectomized dogs (**Fig. 1.2**). Insulin was isolated using an extraction and purification process developed by James Collip, and, after further refinement of this process, injected into a 14-year-old boy, Leonard Thompson. The first injection, on 1 January 1922, was ineffective, but injection of a further extract 3 weeks later normalized his blood glucose levels and abolished ketonuria. In collaboration with Eli Lilly and Co. of Indiana, insulin was then produced commercially, and was widely available in Europe and North America by October 1923. The impact on morbidity (**Fig. 1.3**) and mortality (**Fig. 1.1**) from insulin-dependent diabetes was immediate.

Over the remaining years of the century, advances have been made in the delivery and design of insulin, the development of drugs for type 2 diabetes and in our understanding of the physiology and pathophysiology related to diabetes (**Fig. 1.4**). The impact of these developments on patients with diabetes has been ensured, worldwide, by diabetic associations. The first of these was founded in Portugal in 1926 to ensure the availability of insulin for poor diabetic patients. The British Diabetic Association (BDA, now called Diabetes UK) was founded in 1934 as a result of the work of R. D. Lawrence, a physician at King's College Hospital, London, whose life had been saved by insulin and one of his diabetic patients, the author H. G. Wells. Its aims are as follows:

- To provide an organization for the benefit of and service to the diabetic community, and those interested in the disease
- To act as an authoritative and advisory body to safeguard the social and economic interests of patients with diabetes
- To publish educational material and to promote lectures and discussions for the information and benefit of diabetic people and their relatives, of their medical advisors and involved paramedical personnel, and the general public
- To promote the study of the causes and treatment of diabetes mellitus and the diffusion of information about this amongst all those concerned with the care of diabetic people at home or in hospital

The impact of diabetes on healthcare worldwide emphasizes the importance of these organizations. In developed countries, diabetes care is responsible for up to 5% of total healthcare costs. The estimated direct and indirect cost of diabetes care in the USA is almost

Fig. 1.4 Milestones in the understanding and treatment of diabetes

1930 Sulfonamides shown to cause hypoglycaemia
1936 Protamine–zinc prolonged-action insulins manufactured
1942 First sulfonylurea developed
1955 Insulin sequenced
1956 Tolbutamide used to treat diabetes
1957 Phenformin used to treat diabetes
1959 Insulin measured by radioimmunoassay
1967 Proinsulin identified
1969 Three-dimensional structure of insulin defined
1991 St Vincent Declaration
1993 Diabetes control and complications trial (DCCT) published

$100 billion, comprising $44 billion on medical expenditure, $17 billion from premature mortality and $37 billion from disability. In the UK the direct medical expenditure on diabetes is over $1 billion. Most of the above costs are related to treating its complications; in the USA these account for $12 billion of the expenditure.

In England the prevalence of diagnosed diabetes ranges from about 1.05 to 1.35%. Type 1 (insulin-dependent) diabetes accounts for 10–15% of cases, whilst up to 40% of patients will be treated with insulin. The prevalence is higher in the elderly and in certain ethnic groups, such as Afro-Caribbeans and Asians, owing to an excess of type 2 diabetes. Furthermore, up to 50% of people with diabetes are undiagnosed, given existing criteria, and these individuals are at particularly high risk of ischaemic heart disease (IHD) and cerebrovascular disease (CVD).

The prevalence of type 2 diabetes will continue to increase as a result of the ageing of the population, if for no other reason. This increase is likely to be of the order of 5% over the next decade. New guidelines for the diagnosis of diabetes, endorsed by the American Diabetes Association are expected to 'create' 2 million new diabetic patients in the USA, and would have a similar impact in the UK. There is also a rise in the number of cases of type 1 diabetes, particularly in northern European countries, which could result in a doubling of the prevalence in the next 30 years.

These trends indicate that the burden of diabetes on individuals and on healthcare systems is likely to increase. Future initiatives are likely to aim for the following.

- Earlier diagnosis, possibly through screening programmes
- Improvements in insulin delivery, through the development of insulin analogues and different delivery systems, to minimize the impact on lifestyle
- Novel therapies for type 2 diabetes, to address the underlying pathophysiology
- Prevention and early detection of complications, as a result of the above measures, combined with improved glycaemic control and better education of patients and their relatives

chapter 2

Clinical Presentation of Diabetes

CLINICAL CLASSIFICATION

Diabetes mellitus may be classified into two types:
- **Type 1 diabetes** Absolute insulin deficiency, where insulin treatment is necessary for survival
- **Type 2 diabetes** Insulin resistance or relative insulin deficiency, where control of blood glucose levels may be achieved by lifestyle changes or oral therapy, although insulin may also be used to improve control

This distinction is the basis for all clinical classifications of diabetes, such as those proposed by the American Diabetes Association in 1997 (**Fig. 2.1**).

There are a number of rare causes of diabetes, which were formerly defined as secondary causes, but are now classified as specific types of diabetes (**Fig. 2.2**). Such a classification reflects the disease aetiology, rather than the therapy. The latter was the basis of the previous distinction between insulin-dependent (IDDM) and non-insulin-dependent diabetes (NIDDM), which resulted in the cumbersome concept of insulin-treated non-insulin-dependent diabetes!

Fig. 2.1 Classification of diabetes mellitus according to aetiology

Type 1 diabetes Autoimmune
Idiopathic

Type 2 diabetes

Other specific types Genetic defects of β-cell function
— maturity onset diabetes of the young
— mitochondrial diabetes
Genetic defects in insulin action
— type A insulin resistance
— insulin receptor mutations
— lipodystrophies
Diseases of the exocrine pancreas
Endocrine disease
Drug or chemical induced
Infections
Rare immune-mediated forms
Other genetic syndromes associated with diabetes
Gestational diabetes mellitus

Fig. 2.2   Rare causes of diabetes

Diseases of the exocrine pancreas	Pancreatitis
	Trauma
	Neoplasia
	Cystic fibrosis
	Haemochromatosis
	Fibrocalculous pancreatopathy
Endocrine disease	Acromegaly
	Cushing's syndrome
	Glucagonoma
	Phaeochromocytoma
	Primary hyperaldosteronism (Conn's syndrome)
	Thyrotoxicosis
	Somatostatinoma
Drug or chemical induced	Thiazides
	Glucocorticoids
	Diazoxide
	β_2-adrenoreceptor agonists (e.g. salbutamol)
	Pentamidine
	Nicotinic acid
	α interferon
	Vacor
Infections	Congenital rubella
	Cytomegalovirus
	Mumps
Rare immune-mediated forms	Stiff-man syndrome
	Anti-insulin receptor antibodies (type B insulin resistance)
Genetic syndromes associated with diabetes	Down's
	Klinefelter's
	Turner's
	Wolfram's: DIDMOAD (diabetes insipidus, diabetes mellitus, optic atrophy, deafness)
	Laurence–Moon–Biedl
	Myotonic dystrophy
	Prader–Willi
	Friedreich's ataxia

DIAGNOSTIC CRITERIA

The patient with type 1 diabetes, who presents with classical symptoms associated with hyperglycaemia or ketoacidosis, does not present a diagnostic problem. Individuals with type 2 diabetes, in contrast, often do not present with classical symptoms, but are identified when asymptomatic (**Fig. 2.3**). In 1985 the World Health Organization (WHO) agreed the criteria on which the diagnosis of diabetes should be made in such patients. In 1997 these criteria were revised by the American Diabetes Association, and endorsed by WHO – the main change being that the level of fasting glucose above which the diagnosis should be made was reduced from 7.8 mmol/L down to 7.0 mmol/L (**Fig. 2.4**). This was done because the latter figure is more consistent with the threshold blood glucose level of 11.1 mmol/L 2 hours after a glucose load of 75 g. These values define an approximate threshold for the potential

Fig. 2.3   Presenting features of patients with newly diagnosed type 2 diabetes

	%
Classical symptoms	50
Infections – usually skin, urinary tract or perineal	15
Complications – usually retinopathy or macrovascular disease	5
Incidental findings	30

Fig. 2.4   Criteria for the diagnosis of diabetes mellitus

1 Random plasma glucose > 11.1 mmol/L (200 mg/dl) in association with symptoms of hyperglycaemia
2 Fasting plasma glucose > 7.0 mmol/L (126 mg/dl): no calorific intake for previous 8 hours
The diagnosis should be confirmed by repeat testing on a different day unless there is overt metabolic decompensation

development of microvascular complications, and for a significant increase in mortality from ischaemic heart disease. The revised guidelines also advise that the diagnosis should be based on two plasma glucose estimations performed on two different days whilst the patient is fasting, since this is more practical, more reproducible and less expensive than the oral glucose tolerance test (OGTT). The latter should be reserved for research studies, and for defining impaired glucose tolerance particularly in relation to pregnancy. In patients with type 2 diabetes who present with classical symptoms, a random glucose level of more than 11.1 mmol/L is sufficient for the diagnosis. These new diagnostic criteria and guidelines have been accepted by the WHO and Diabetes UK. However, there remains some concern that basing the diagnosis on a fasting glucose will still miss some patients who would have had a blood glucose level of greater than 11.1 mmol/L 2 hours after a glucose load of 75 g, and who may be at particularly high risk of macrovascular disease. It has therefore been suggested that those people with impaired fasting glycaemia (defined as a glucose level of 6.1–7.0 mmol/L) should have an OGTT performed.

Screening for type 2 diabetes remains a controversial issue. Up to 50% of individuals may remain undiagnosed, and many individuals are diagnosed only when the disease has been present for some years. However the economic implications of population screening argue for limited screening in the following higher risk groups:

- All patients over 45 years of age, repeated every 3 years if normal
- Younger individuals with:
  — Obesity, defined as a body mass index (BMI) greater than 27 kg/m^2
  — A first-degree relative with diabetes
  — High risk ethnicity, particularly Afro-Caribbean or Asian
  — A previous diagnosis of gestational diabetes or an offspring weighing more than 9 lb (4 kg) at birth
  — Syndrome-X-type risk factor profile (see below)

EPIDEMIOLOGY

Type 1 diabetes

There is considerable geographical variation in the incidence of type 1 diabetes. The incidence is particularly high in countries in more northerly latitudes, such as Scotland and Scandinavia. There are also surprising and unexplained areas of high incidence, such as Sardinia. In the UK and USA the annual incidence rate is between 10 and 15 in 100 000 children and adolescents under the age of 19, although the rates are lower in non-Caucasian populations. This incidence appears to be increasing and it is estimated that it will double over the next 20 to 30 years.

The peak age of onset of type 1 diabetes is 12 years, but the diagnosis should not be overlooked in older age groups (see below); 10% of those diagnosed with diabetes over the age of 65 are insulin dependent (**Fig. 2.5**).

Type 2 diabetes

The variability in the incidence of type 2 diabetes is largely determined by ethnicity. Much higher rates are seen in Afro-Caribbean and Asian communities. This pattern was initially observed in migrant groups exposed to 'westernized' cultures, but a similar prevalence has since been found in urban areas where these ethnic groups are the indigenous population. In the UK the age-adjusted prevalence of clinically diagnosed type 2 diabetes is between 1 and 1.5% of the population, but may be up to five times greater in these ethnic subgroups. Furthermore, up to 50% of individuals with type 2 diabetes remain undiagnosed.

In developing, largely rural, societies the prevalence of type 2 diabetes is usually considerably less than 1%. The effect of a move from a predominantly rural existence to an urbanized lifestyle was most dramatically demonstrated in Nauru, in the South Pacific. The impact of extreme wealth from phosphate mining resulted in an increase in the prevalence rate of type 2 diabetes to greater than 40% of the population. However, the highest prevalence of type 2 diabetes in the world is amongst the Pima Indians of Arizona, a largely sedentary and overweight population, where over 50% of individuals are affected.

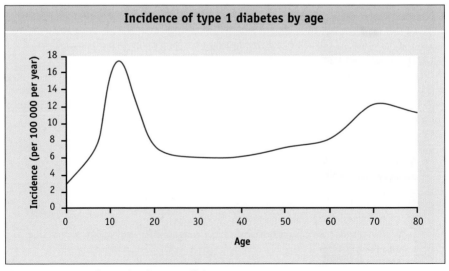

Fig. 2.5   Age at diagnosis of type 1 diabetes.

The peak age at diagnosis of type 2 diabetes is about 60, but in populations at high risk this age is significantly lower.

PATHOPHYSIOLOGY

Type 1 diabetes

Type 1 diabetes is usually an autoimmune disease characterized by cell-mediated destruction of the insulin-producing β cells in the pancreatic islets (**Fig. 2.6**). The trigger for the cell-mediated destruction appears to be a combination of genetic susceptibility and environmental factors. Family studies have shown that a sibling of an individual with type 1

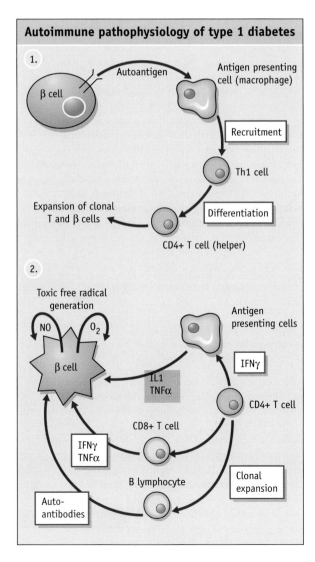

Fig. 2.6 *The cell-mediated autoimmune destruction of β cells in type 1 diabetes (IL-1 = interleukin 1, TNFα = tumour necrosis factor alpha, IFNγ = interferon gamma, NO = nitric oxide, O$_2$ = superoxide radical).*

Fig. 2.7   Possible environmental triggers for autoimmune β-cell destruction

Viruses	Coxsackie, particularly the B_4 strain, which has homology with GAD
	Mumps
	Cytomegalovirus (CMV)
	Rubella
Nutrients	Cow's milk protein
	Nitrosamines/nitrites
Stressful life-events	

diabetes has about a 10% chance of developing the disease, rising to about 25% for dizygotic twins, and 50% for monozygotic twins.

The strongest predictor of the development of type 1 diabetes is human leukocyte antigen (HLA) linkage: inheritance of the DR_3 locus increases the risk fivefold, the DR_4 locus eightfold and both loci 15-fold. In contrast, inheritance of HLA-DR_2 protects against type 1 diabetes, reducing the risk by 80%. These haplotypes are not the true susceptibility genes but are linked to and almost invariably transmitted with them. Other loci that may be candidates for increased susceptibility to type 1 diabetes, which include the insulin gene region itself, have been identified by techniques such as linkage analysis of deoxyribonucleic acid (DNA) using microsatellite markers.

There are probably also different environmental triggers, which may include viruses and toxins (**Fig. 2.7**), although there has been no convincing evidence for any one factor. The rate of development of type 1 diabetes once autoimmune destruction of the β cells has commenced varies between individuals, which may influence the clinical presentation.

The destruction of β cells exposes a variety of antigens and, in consequence, a number of autoantibodies can be identified:

- Islet cell antibodies (ICA)
- Glutamic acid decarboxylase (GAD)
- Insulin autoantibodies (IAA)
- IA_2

Islet cell antibodies are present at diagnosis in 80% of patients with type 1 diabetes, and GAD (glutamic acid decarboxylase) antibodies may be present in even more affected individuals. These autoantibodies are also useful in identifying high risk individuals who are likely to develop diabetes and who may be helped by strategies to prevent progression of the autoimmune process, which are currently being studied (**Fig. 2.8**).

Some individuals with type 1 diabetes have a personal or family history of other autoimmune endocrine disease, particularly thyroid dysfunction, and occasionally may suffer from a rare, inherited polyglandular autoimmune syndrome, of which there are two types (**Fig. 2.9**).

A small subset of individuals, who are usually African or Asian in origin, have an absolute requirement for insulin therapy but do not have evidence for autoimmune destruction of β cells; these are classed as having idiopathic type 1 diabetes.

Fig. 2.8   Strategies for the prevention of type 1 diabetes in high risk individuals

Nicotinamide*
Insulin prophylaxis*
Induction of tolerance   Antigen specific
                             Monoclonal antibodies

* Trials ongoing in humans; other strategies successfully applied in animal models.

Fig. 2.9   Features of the polyglandular autoimmune syndromes

	Type 1	Type 2 (HLA-B$_8$ associated)
Peak age of onset (years)	12	30
Adrenal insufficiency	+	+
Hypoparathyroidism	+	–
Candidiasis	+	–
Pernicious anaemia	+	–
Hypogonadism	+	–
Thyroid dysfunction	+	+
Diabetes mellitus (type 1)	–	+

Type 2 diabetes

Type 2 diabetes results from a combination of resistance to insulin action and an inadequate compensatory increase in insulin secretion. There is a strong genetic tendency to type 2 diabetes, which is much greater than in type 1 diabetes. However, in the majority of affected individuals the genetic abnormalities responsible have not yet been elucidated. In most cases it is a polygenic disorder, although a few monogenetic disorders have been identified that result in defects in insulin secretion – notably those causing maturity onset diabetes of the young (MODY) (**Fig. 2.10**).

Fig. 2.10   Mutations identified in families with MODY

	MODY-1 (HNF-4α)	MODY-2 (glucokinase)	MODY-3 (HNF-1α)
Frequency in UK	5%	10%	70%
Hyperglycaemia	Progresses to severe	Mild	Progresses to severe
Microvascular complications	Frequent	Rare	Frequent
Defect	Maximal insulin secretion	Glucose sensing	Maximal insulin secretion

Features of MODY

- Diagnosis of diabetes mellitus at age < 25 years in at least one family member
- Not requiring insulin therapy or measurable C peptide if on insulin
- Autosomal dominant pattern of inheritance

Disorders due to defects in mitochondrial DNA have also been identified (**Fig. 2.11**). These have been reclassified as specific types of diabetes mellitus (see **Fig. 2.2**, p.6) and are responsible for a very small proportion of cases diagnosed as having type 2 diabetes. Factors associated with the development of type 2 diabetes include:

- Obesity, particularly truncal
- Increasing age
- Sedentary lifestyle
- Use of drugs, especially glucocorticoids and thiazides

The major environmental factor predisposing to type 2 diabetes is obesity. Most individuals with type 2 diabetes are obese and this is, at least in part, responsible for their resistance to insulin action. An individual with a BMI of more than 35 kg/m^2 has a 40-fold increased risk of developing type 2 diabetes, compared with a non-obese person.

The distribution of body fat also appears to be an important factor in determining the risk of developing diabetes. An excess of visceral fat mass, which predominates in those with android (central or truncal) (**Fig. 2.12**) rather than gynoid (gluteofemoral) obesity, is associated with insulin resistance, hypertension, dyslipidaemia and coagulation abnormalities, and, in consequence, a greatly increased risk of atherosclerotic cardiovascular disease. This constellation of risk factors for coronary heart disease (CHD) has been termed 'syndrome X' or 'Reaven's syndrome' (**Fig. 2.13**; see also Ch. 7).

Fig. 2.11   Genetic defects in mitochondrial DNA in diabetes – invariably transmitted maternally

Defect	Associated features
Deletion/duplication	
10.4 kb	Deafness
Variable	Kearns–Sayre syndrome
	Pearson's syndrome
Mutation	
A3243G	MELAS (mitochondrial encephalopathy, lactic acidosis)
	Diabetes and deafness
T14709C	Myopathy, mental retardation
C12258A	

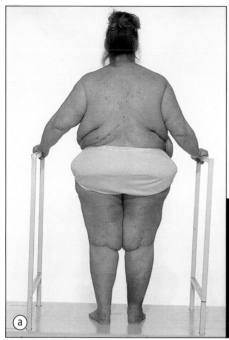
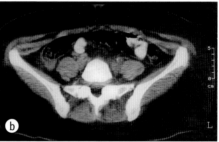

Fig. 2.12 *(a) Android pattern of obesity with (b) computerized tomography (CT) scan showing large amounts of intra-abdominal fat but little subcutaneous fat (fat appears grey-black on the scan).*

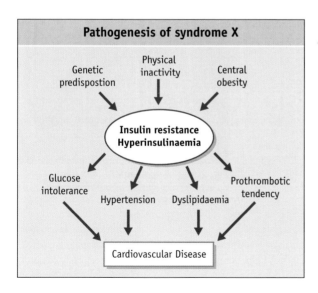

Fig. 2.13 *The probable pathogenesis of syndrome X.*

Non-esterified fatty acids, released into the portal circulation following lipolysis in visceral fat stores, may be the cause of this metabolic syndrome (**Fig. 2.14**). Their effects on hepatic glucose production and insulin extraction, and peripheral glucose utilization, may result in hyperglycaemia, hyperinsulinaemia and insulin resistance, all of which possibly contribute to the macrovascular and microvascular complications of type 2 diabetes.

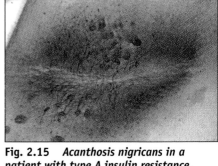

Fig. 2.15   Acanthosis nigricans in a patient with type A insulin resistance.

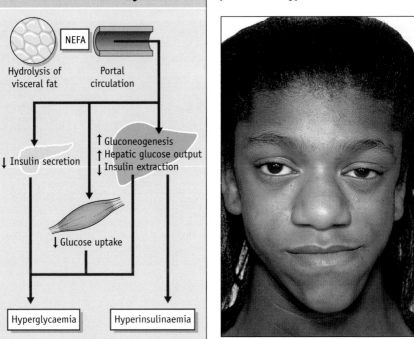

Non-esterified fatty acids

NEFA

Hydrolysis of visceral fat

Portal circulation

↓ Insulin secretion

↑ Gluconeogenesis
↑ Hepatic glucose output
↓ Insulin extraction

↓ Glucose uptake

Hyperglycaemia

Hyperinsulinaemia

Fig. 2.14   The metabolic effects of NEFA in the portal circulation.

Fig. 2.16   Acromegaloid features (pseudoacromegaly) in a patient with type A insulin resistance.

Other causes

Endocrine diseases associated with an excess of counter-regulatory hormones, particularly growth hormone (GH) (acromegaly) and glucocorticoid (Cushing's syndrome), may cause impaired glucose tolerance.

Diseases of the exocrine pancreas, such as cystic fibrosis, haemochromatosis and rarely pancreatic carcinoma, may involve the endocrine pancreas, so affecting insulin secretion. In tropical countries a frequent cause of diabetes is fibrocalculous pancreatopathy, which was previously termed 'malnutrition-related diabetes'.

Defects in the insulin receptor and insulin action may be congenital or acquired, and cause insulin resistance. The resultant hyperinsulinaemia is characterized clinically by acanthosis nigricans (**Fig. 2.15**) and acromegaloid features (**Fig. 2.16**).

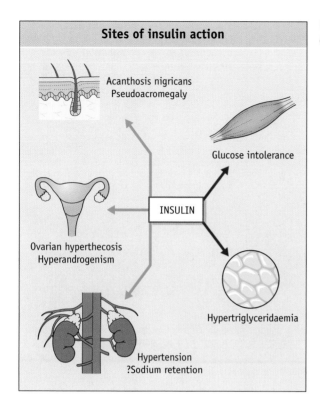

Fig. 2.17 *Sites of insulin action.*

A number of other organs may be affected by the elevated insulin levels (**Fig. 2.17**). Insulin stimulates ovarian testosterone synthesis resulting in hyperandrogenism, which causes hirsutism, menstrual disturbance and variable virilization. A similar pathological process explains at least part of the polycystic ovary syndrome (PCOS), and affected individuals have an increased incidence of type 2 diabetes and coronary heart disease.

Type A insulin resistance is a genetically determined syndrome invariably affecting women, but without obesity or lipoatrophy. Type B insulin resistance is caused by autoantibodies against the insulin receptor. Lipodystrophies may be congenital or acquired, and probably result from defects in the postreceptor insulin-signalling pathway. In congenital total lipoatrophy (Berardinelli–Seip syndrome) there is virtually no adipose tissue (**Fig. 2.18**) and instead of hyperglycaemia the major metabolic abnormality is hypertriglyceridaemia, which may cause acute pancreatitis and fatty liver with later cirrhosis. Acquired total lipodystrophy usually occurs after a viral illness. Lipoatrophy may be confined to specific areas of the body, such as face-sparing, where lipohypertrophy of the face and extremities may occur, and cephalo-thoracic, where fat is lost from the face and trunk and there may be associated type II mesangio-proliferative glomerulonephritis.

METABOLIC CONSEQUENCES OF INSULIN DEFICIENCY

Insulin synthesis and secretion

Insulin is secreted by the β cells in the islets of Langerhans, the endocrine unit of the pancreas (**Fig. 2.19**). The precursor molecule for insulin is preproinsulin, encoded by a gene on chromosome 11. This is cleaved to proinsulin, which is then converted to insulin by

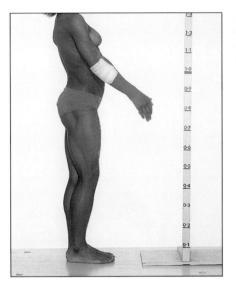

Fig. 2.18 *A 14-year-old girl with congenital total lipoatrophy showing a lean body habitus with no apparent adipose tissue.*

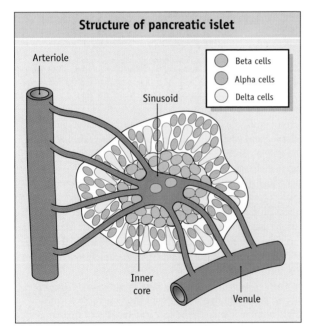

Structure of pancreatic islet

Arteriole

Beta cells
Alpha cells
Delta cells

Sinusoid

Inner
core

Venule

Fig. 2.19 *Structure of a pancreatic islet.*

proteolytic removal of the connecting peptide (C peptide) (**Fig. 2.20**). Insulin and C-peptide are cosecreted by the β cell, and so C-peptide secretion is a marker for β-cell function.

The major stimulant to insulin secretion is the ambient blood glucose concentration. Phosphorylation of glucose by the enzyme glucokinase is the rate-limiting step in glucose metabolism within the β cell. It is this phosphorylation of glucose that triggers insulin release, and so glucokinase acts as the β-cell glucose sensor. Inactivating mutations of the

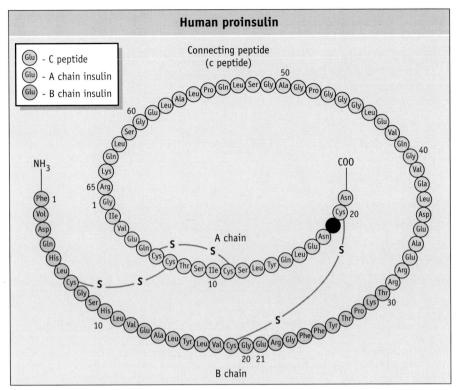

Fig. 2.20 *Amino acid sequence of insulin and C peptide, which are the peptide products of the enzymatic cleavage of proinsulin.*

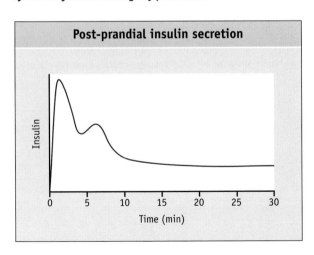

Fig. 2.21 *The biphasic secretion of insulin in response to glucose.*

gene for glucokinase, which are found in a subset of patients with MODY (see above), result in impaired insulin secretion.

Glucose-stimulated insulin secretion is biphasic (**Fig. 2.21**), and a similar pattern is seen in response to a mixed meal. The initial 'cephalic' phase of secretion occurs before glucose

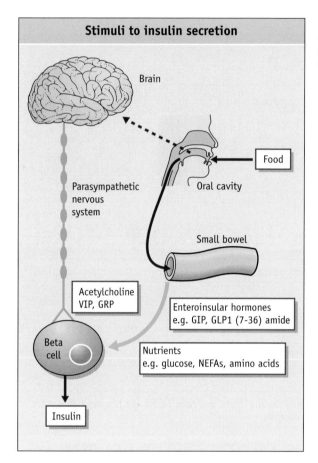

Fig. 2.22 *The interaction of stimuli to insulin secretion following ingestion of a mixed meal.*

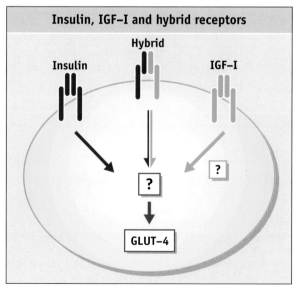

Fig. 2.23 *The hypothetical relationship between insulin and the hybrid insulin–IGF-I receptors.*

levels are elevated in the portal circulation; this phase appears to be mediated by neural stimuli in response to feeding. The subsequent release of incretins, such as glucose-stimulated insulinotropic peptide (GIP) and two glucagon-like peptides (GLP-1 and -2), in response to a meal, augments the effect of the nutrients themselves during the sustained second phase of insulin secretion (**Fig. 2.22**).

Insulin action

Insulin exerts its cellular effects by binding to a dimeric tyrosine kinase receptor. The postreceptor signalling pathway remains unclear, but it is likely that abnormalities in this pathway play a part in the development of insulin resistance. The insulin receptor shares considerable homology with the receptor for insulin-like growth factor I (IGF-I), and hybrid dimeric receptors comprising one of each receptor subunit have been found (**Fig. 2.23**). This discovery has led to the study of IGF-I therapy as a possible means of overcoming the insulin resistance of puberty and of ketoacidosis. Mutations of the insulin receptor are a rare cause of diabetes, but are associated with characteristic clinical syndromes (**Fig. 2.24**).

Insulin is important in the regulation, not only of carbohydrate metabolism, but also that of fat and protein. Normally the blood glucose levels are tightly regulated, the entry of glucose into the bloodstream being balanced by its uptake into peripheral tissues. Insulin suppresses hepatic glucose production, by inhibiting gluconeogenesis and glycogenolysis, and stimulates peripheral glucose uptake, mainly by skeletal muscle but also by fat. The glucose transporter GLUT-4 mediates insulin-stimulated glucose transport.

The major energy store in the body is adipose tissue triglyceride (**Fig. 2.25**). Insulin stimulates triglyceride synthesis from non-esterified fatty acids (NEFA), called lipogenesis, and inhibits the breakdown of triglyceride, called lipolysis. It also inhibits protein breakdown and may play a role in enhancing protein synthesis.

The differences between the metabolic consequences of type 1 and type 2 diabetes are largely attributable to the degree of insulin deficiency (**Fig. 2.26**). In both conditions the alteration in glucose metabolism is due to two processes:

- *Increased* hepatic glucose production in the fasted state
- Decreased (insulin-stimulated) peripheral uptake postprandially – although hyperglycaemia is accompanied by increased uptake in the fasted state by the non insulin-dependent glucose transporters GLUT-1 and GLUT-3

Fig. 2.24 Syndromes resulting from mutations in the insulin receptor

Leprechaunism
- Intrauterine growth retardation
- Acanthosis nigricans
- Hypertrichosis
- Phallic enlargement
- Hyperglycaemia with fasting hypoglycaemia
- Death usually within first year of life

Rabson–Mendenhall syndrome
- Pineal hyperlasia
- Dental dysplasia
- Acanthosis nigricans
- Accelerated growth
- Pseudoprecocious puberty
- Poorly controlled diabetes with severe microvascular complications and early death

Fig. 2.25   Human body energy stores in a 70 kg man

Triglycerides (adipose tissue)	110 000 kcal
Protein (muscle)	24 000 kcal
Glycogen (muscle)	1 600 kcal
(liver)	320 kcal

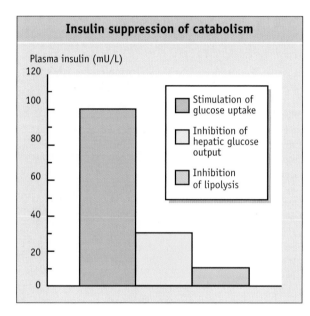

Fig. 2.26 *Insulin concentration required for suppression of catabolic processes.*

The relative insulin deficiency in type 2 diabetes results in a diabetic dyslipidaemia (see Ch. 7). However, the stimulus to lipolysis is not great enough to result in the ketogenesis that may accompany type 1 diabetes. Type 2 diabetes is not associated with abnormal protein metabolism, in contrast to type 1 diabetes where the insulin deficiency is sufficient to stimulate protein catabolism, which results in weight loss through muscle wasting.

CLINICAL PRESENTATION

Type 1 diabetes

Most patients with type 1 diabetes will present with a trio of classical symptoms:

Symptoms of type 1 diabetes

- Polyuria and polydipsia
- Weight loss
- Blurred vision

Once the threshold for renal glucose excretion is exceeded the hyperglycaemia is accompanied by glycosuria, and this results in an osmotic diuresis – hence the polyuria. The thirst is a homeostatic mechanism activated by the subsequent volume depletion and it results in polydipsia. The weight loss reflects the increased catabolism that occurs with insulin deficiency (see above). The blurred vision is a result of the osmotic movement of water, which distorts the shape of the lens.

The duration of these symptoms will depend on the rate at which β-cell function has been declining. In some individuals the destruction of β cells may have been going on for as long as 5 years, and symptoms become apparent only when the residual insulin secretion is insufficient to control blood glucose levels – usually when about 90% have been destroyed. Where the onset of the disease has been more insidious other symptoms may be apparent, such as growth failure in children, and an increased susceptibility to certain infectious conditions such as candidiasis.

In the UK and USA, only 10% of patients with type 1 diabetes now present with acute, life-threatening ketoacidosis (see Ch. 6).

Type 2 diabetes

In type 2 diabetes, where resistance to insulin action is the initial abnormality, the failure of the β cell to compensate with a sufficient increase in insulin secretion is usually a slowly developing process. An elevated blood glucose level may therefore be present for many years before diagnosis, and result in damage to various target tissues before clinical symptoms become apparent. During this asymptomatic period, individuals with type 2 diabetes may be identified by finding an elevated plasma glucose level (as defined in the diagnostic criteria on p.7). Despite this, 50% of patients with type 2 diabetes are identified when they present either with some of the classical symptoms (polyuria, polydipsia, blurred vision), or recurrent infections, or with more non-specific symptoms of fatigue and malaise. Others are identified when they present with the consequences of glucose intolerance; these are usually macrovascular complications, such as myocardial infarction, but may rarely be microvascular complications, such as retinopathy.

Differentiation between type 1 and type 2 diabetes

There is usually no problem in differentiating between those with type 1 and type 2 diabetes, but it should be remembered that although type 1 diabetes is most common in the young it can present at any age, and occasionally in obese individuals. The distinction is important to make, since the patient with type 1 diabetes who is treated with oral hypoglycaemic agents rather than insulin may not lapse into ketoacidosis because the small residual pancreatic insulin secretion is stimulated further, but will usually remain symptomatic for many months before insulin therapy is commenced. In patients where uncertainty exists a number of features may help in distinguishing between the two types of diabetes:

Clinical features suggestive of type 1 diabetes

- Rapid onset of symptomatic hyperglycaemia
- Significant, sustained ketonuria
- Weight loss
- Absence of family history or family history of type 1 diabetes

Features such as the speed of onset and severity of symptoms are very suggestive; however, the only absolute discriminators between the two types are the presence of diagnostic autoantibodies or the absence of C-peptide secretion.

chapter 3

Living with Diabetes

INTRODUCTION

One of the principles underlying the management of all patients with diabetes is to allow them to live as normally as possible, given the impact of blood glucose monitoring and insulin injections. However there are a number of areas where diabetes has an impact on routine aspects of living. These include:

- Diet, including alcohol intake
- Exercise
- Sexual function
- Employment
- Travel, including driving
- Insurance

An understanding of the implications of diabetes for these activities is important to allow the patient with diabetes to lead a life approaching normality.

DIET

Changes in dietary recommendations over recent years have made it easier for patients with newly diagnosed diabetes to adapt their diet without a major impact on lifestyle. Indeed the 'diabetic diet' could be regarded as the model for a healthy diet to which the population as a whole should adhere. Various diets for diabetes have previously included:

- 10 g carbohydrate exchanges, which are still favoured by a few patients with type 1 diabetes
- Low carbohydrate diets, which produced good glycaemic control, but encouraged increased saturated fat intake

  However, current dietary recommendations (**Fig. 3.1**) for all patients emphasize the following:
- *Increased* consumption of complex carbohydrates, optimally by using high fibre options. Foods such as pasta that are particularly slowly absorbed may be preferable because they cause less of a fluctuation in the blood glucose level, and so are said to have a 'low glycaemic index'
- Sparing use of refined carbohydrates, such as sucrose, with preferential use of artificial sweeteners such as aspartame where necessary to sweeten food
- Avoidance of diabetic food products, which have no metabolic advantage over refined sugars, are expensive and often cause diarrhoea

Fig. 3.1   Dietary recommendations for people with diabetes

Nutrient	Proportion of total energy intake (%)
Carbohydrate	>50
● Complex – high fibre, low glycaemic index	
● Limit simple sugars: <25 g/day added, <50 g/day total	
Fat	<35
● Saturated fats <10% of the total energy intake	
● Increase monounsaturates, e.g. olive oil	
Protein	10–15
Others	
● Salt <6 g/day	
● Recommended moderate alcohol intake	
● Avoid 'diabetic' foodstuffs	

- Reduction and alteration of fat intake – in particular, limitation of saturated (animal) fats and increased consumption of unsaturated fats (vegetable and fish), particularly the monounsaturated types (e.g. olive oil, rapeseed oil). One portion of oily fish is recommended per week, which lowers triglyceride levels, but if taken in excess may elevate blood glucose levels
- Consumption of five portions daily of fruit, vegetables or pulses
- Limited salt intake, particularly in patients with hypertension
- Moderate intake of alcohol

Obese patients (BMI > 30 kg/m^2) should have a calorie-restricted diet, with a calorie deficit of about 500 kcal daily. Very low calorie diets may be considered in those patients with morbid obesity (BMI > 40 kg/m^2) or those with lesser degrees of severity who fail to respond to the above calorie restriction.

It is helpful to be able to put these dietary recommendations into practical terms for patients (**Fig. 3.2**), although, where possible, all patients should have the benefit of at least one discussion with an approved dietitian, preferably with an annual review. The following is an example of some simple advice that can be given by the doctor:

- Make foods such as pasta, bread, potato or cereals the main component of each meal and use high fibre foods as much as possible
- Have a helping of fruit or vegetables, or both, with each meal, and at least five helpings of these per day
- Restrict consumption of animal fat – trim fat off meat, and use low fat dairy produce
- Grill rather than fry food and, if oils are needed, use olive or rapeseed
- Make meat a small part of the meal, and eat fish or vegetables rather than red meat or eggs
- For snacks avoid convenience foods, eating fruit in preference
- Avoid added sugar, but there is no need to exclude sugar completely from the diet
- Avoid added salt and restrict its use if hypertension is evident
- Adhere to recommended guidelines for alcohol intake

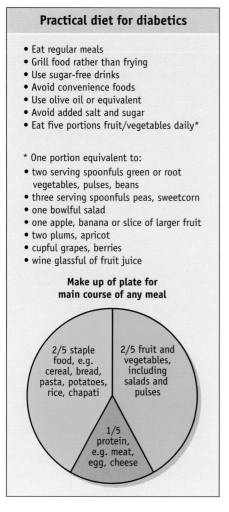

Practical diet for diabetics

- Eat regular meals
- Grill food rather than frying
- Use sugar-free drinks
- Avoid convenience foods
- Use olive oil or equivalent
- Avoid added salt and sugar
- Eat five portions fruit/vegetables daily*

* One portion equivalent to:
- two serving spoonfuls green or root vegetables, pulses, beans
- three serving spoonfuls peas, sweetcorn
- one bowlful salad
- one apple, banana or slice of larger fruit
- two plums, apricot
- cupful grapes, berries
- wine glassful of fruit juice

Make up of plate for main course of any meal

2/5 staple food, e.g. cereal, bread, pasta, potatoes, rice, chapati

2/5 fruit and vegetables, including salads and pulses

1/5 protein, e.g. meat, egg, cheese

Fig. 3.2 *Practical dietary advice for people with diabetes.*

Type 1 diabetes

Patients with type 1 diabetes will also need advice about meal frequency and having snacks to avoid hypoglycaemia, although the type of insulin regimen used will determine the specific recommendations. Many patients will need to eat a snack containing complex carbohydrate, usually a sandwich, before going to bed so as to avoid nocturnal hypoglycaemia. This is particularly important if the blood glucose level is less than 7 mmol/L on retiring. Patients taking insulin or sulfonylureas also need advice about dietary action to take in the event of hypoglycaemia (see Ch. 6).

Type 2 diabetes

In patients with type 2 diabetes the diet is the mainstay of treatment, and most patients will be given a trial of diet therapy alone for the first 3 months. Good education with practical advice enabling patients to continue eating a varied, satisfying diet aids compliance and improves the chances of diet therapy being successful.

Alcohol

Sensible alcohol consumption is important because an excess intake may have a number of adverse effects in patients with diabetes:

- Acutely it may aggravate hypoglycaemia
- Alcohol contains 56 kcal per unit, and other constituents, particularly in beer, may increase carbohydrate content further, worsening obesity and glycaemic control
- Hypertension and hypertriglyceridaemia may be exacerbated
- Alcohol-related damage may contribute to neuropathy

EXERCISE

Exercise is beneficial to all patients with diabetes and particularly to those with type 2, where the improvement in insulin sensitivity and reduction in body fat contribute to improved glycaemic control and lipid profiles, and lowering of blood pressure (BP). These benefits include:

- Improved insulin sensitivity
- Lowering of blood pressure
- Reduction in triglyceride levels
- Improved fibrinolysis
- Weight reduction – e.g. intra-abdominal
- Improved psychological well-being

One-third of men and almost half the women with type 2 diabetes over the age of 55 would be classed as sedentary – that is, taking less than 30 minutes exercise, such as brisk walking, five times per week. Thus improving uptake of exercise programmes may benefit a large number of patients with diabetes. Indeed exercise may be important in preventing or delaying the onset of type 2 diabetes.

Exercise does not seem to have the same benefit on glycaemic control in type 1 diabetes. Nevertheless it is an important part of normal living and should be encouraged in those with type 1 diabetes. More flexible guidelines with regard to pre-exercise carbohydrate ingestion and insulin administration may be beneficial. Guidelines should include the following advice:

- Monitor before and after exercise to:
  — Assess the response to a particular type and length of exercise
  — Identify any changes needed to the insulin dose or food intake
- Keep fast-acting carbohydrate-based foods readily available, to ingest if the blood glucose drops below 5.5 mmol/L before exercise and as needed to avoid hypoglycaemia
- Avoid exercise if the blood glucose is over 15 mmol/L

Hypoglycaemia after exercise is of particular concern, and may occur not only immediately afterwards but sometimes many hours later, and even the following morning. Patients need to be prepared for this and to adjust their food intake and insulin doses as appropriate once a clear pattern has been established.

Fig. 3.3 Exercise choices for diabetic patients with complications

Retinopathy
- Moderate to severe non-proliferative retinopathy
  — *avoid* activities causing BP increase or jarring
- Proliferative retinopathy
  — *use* low-impact cardiovascular conditioning
  — *avoid* strenuous activity

Neuropathy with loss of protective sensation
- *Avoid* treadmill, walking, jogging and steps
- *Use* non-weight-bearing exercise

Caution is needed when recommending exercise to those patients with complications, particularly vascular disease, significant retinopathy or neuropathic feet, and they may need to be advised to restrict themselves to certain types of exercise (**Fig. 3.3**). However, those patients at increased risk of progressive vascular disease may gain particular benefit from exercise. In patients at risk of ischaemic heart disease it may be prudent to arrange for an exercise test first before advising a particular exercise programme.

Controversy surrounds the best way of approaching the subject of exercise with the diabetic patient. The benefits of exercise should certainly be included in any patient education programme and can be stressed at review visits. However, studies suggest that the best way of encouraging uptake of exercise programmes is to provide:
- An initial supervised, graded exercise programme
- An individualized home exercise programme
- A follow-up assessment

SEXUAL FUNCTION

MALE SEXUAL FUNCTION

Aetiology
Penile erection requires integrated nerve and blood vessel function (**Fig. 3.4**). Erectile dysfunction affects up to 40% of men with diabetes, with a multifactorial aetiology (**Fig. 3.5**), resulting in failure of these integrated actions. Although organic causes are more likely in men with diabetes, it should be remembered that psychogenic erectile dysfunction may be at least a component of the problem, particularly in the absence of other diabetic complications.

Clinical assessment
Clinical assessment of the patient (**Fig. 3.6**) should particularly focus on:

- Drug history
- Exclusion of endocrine disorders, which usually also cause loss of libido
- Relationship difficulties, since these are unlikely to be overcome by treating erectile problems
- Evidence of neuropathy or peripheral vascular disease
- Penile anatomy

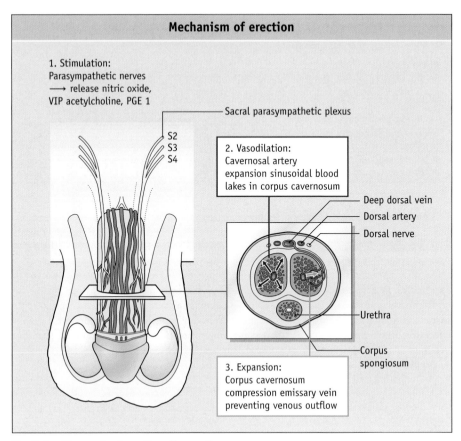

Mechanism of erection

1. Stimulation:
Parasympathetic nerves
⟶ release nitric oxide,
VIP acetylcholine, PGE 1

Sacral parasympathetic plexus

S2
S3
S4

2. Vasodilation:
Cavernosal artery
expansion sinusoidal blood
lakes in corpus cavernosum

Deep dorsal vein
Dorsal artery
Dorsal nerve

Urethra

Corpus
spongiosum

3. Expansion:
Corpus cavernosum
compression emissary vein
preventing venous outflow

Fig. 3.4 *The mechanism of penile erection.*

Fig. 3.5 Aetiology of erectile dysfunction

Vascular
- Peripheral vascular disease*
- Venous leakage

Neurogenic
- Autonomic neuropathy*

Hypertension*

Iatrogenic
- Drugs
  — antihypertensives, particularly β blockers and thiazides*
  — antiandrogens
  — cimetidine
  — antipsychotics
  — alcohol
- Pelvic surgery

Psychogenic

*Particularly common in patients with diabetes.

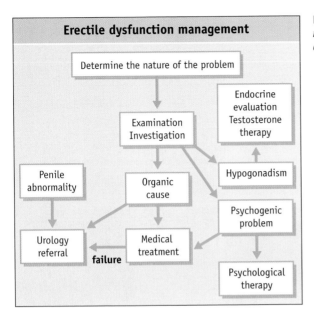

Erectile dysfunction management

Determine the nature of the problem

Examination
Investigation

Endocrine
evaluation
Testosterone
therapy

Penile
abnormality

Organic
cause

Hypogonadism

Psychogenic
problem

Urology
referral

failure

Medical
treatment

Psychological
therapy

Fig. 3.6 *Algorithm for the management of erectile dysfunction.*

Fig. 3.7 Treatment options in erectile dysfunction

Medical treatment
- Oral agents
  — sildanefil (Viagra)
  — yohimbine
- Intracavernosal therapy
  — alprostadil
  — papaverine
  — phentolamine
  — moxisylyte
- Transurethral therapy
  — alprostadil
- Vacuum device

Surgical treatment
- Arterial reconstruction
- Venous reconstruction
- Penile implants

Psychosexual counselling

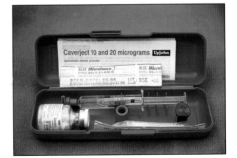

Fig. 3.8 *Intracavernosal injection therapy – alprostadil.*

Management

Treatment options (**Fig. 3.7**) include:

- Oral therapy: the novel phosphodiesterase inhibitor, sildanefil (Viagra), which augments levels of cyclic guanosine monophosphate (cGMP), appears to be as effective as more invasive therapies, although may cause headache and hypotension, and should be used with caution in those with ischaemic heart disease, avoiding co-administration with

29

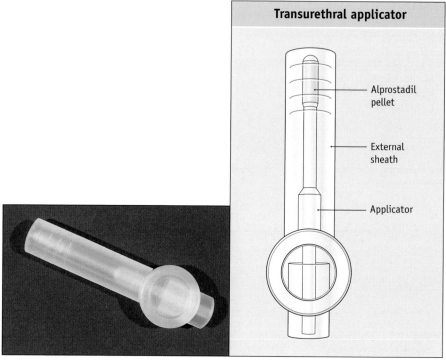

Fig. 3.9   *Transurethral alprostadil delivery system.*

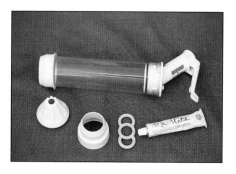

Fig. 3.10   *A vacuum device.*

nitrates; it has largely superseded the α_2-adrenergic receptor antagonist, yohimbine, which is much less effective in improving erectile function, although often useful in those with partial failure. Sublingual apomorphine (Uprima) is a newer alternative to sildenafil

- Intracavernosal injection therapy (**Fig. 3.8**), with alprostadil, moxisylyte, or papaverine
- Transurethral alprostadil administration (**Fig. 3.9**)
- Vacuum assist device (**Fig. 3.10**)
- Surgical treatment, including arterial or venous reconstruction and penile implants
- Psychosexual counselling

The most commonly used pharmacological agent is alprostadil. This is a formulation of prostaglandin E_1 that causes engorgement of the corpora cavernosum, and, if administered transurethrally, the corpus spongiosum if an adequate arterial supply is present. The main potential side-effect of intracavernosal injection therapy is prolonged erection (priapism). Patients therefore need to be advised what to do in the event of an erection lasting more than 4 hours, and should preferably be given written instructions.

Many clinics provide an erectile dysfunction service for patients with diabetes. The uptake for such a service depends on whether patients are facilitated to bring up the problem themselves or asked directly whether they have a problem. Only about 5% of men will self-report, although this number is probably increasing, but this group accepts therapy more often than other patients.

Clinical features

There are also other much less common problems with sexual function in diabetic men. They include:

Uncommon clinical features of male sexual dysfunction

- Loss of libido, which may be a psychological consequence of any chronic disease
- Retrograde ejaculation, which is due to impaired sympathetic nerve function, and may result in subfertility
- Recurrent balanitis (**Fig. 3.11**), which may interfere with sexual function

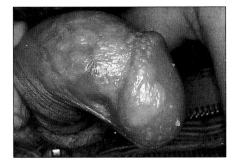

Fig. 3.11 *Balanitis.*

FEMALE SEXUAL FUNCTION

Clinical features

Abnormalities in female sexual function are less overt than in men, but the following problems affecting female sexuality are seen:

Clinical features of female sexual dysfunction

- Diminished vaginal lubrication due to lack of engorgement, which is the result of autonomic neuropathy – the corollary of erectile failure in males
- Anorgasmia, although its relationship with diabetes is disputed
- Altered psychosexuality
- Vaginal infection

Fig. 3.12   Contraceptive alternatives for the diabetic woman

Method	Recommended?	Pros/cons
Natural family planning	No	Not effective enough
Barrier methods	Yes	Reduced risk of pelvic inflammatory disease ? Sufficiently effective
Intrauterine contraceptive device (IUCD), including Mirena	Yes	Use if low risk of sexually transmitted disease (STD) ?Cover insertion with antibiotics
Combined oral contraceptive	Yes	Use if good control and minimal complications
Progestagen only contraceptive	Yes	Avoid if severe vascular complications exist
Depot progestagen	Yes	
Norplant	Yes	Unreliable return of fertility on stopping

Contraception

The other important aspect of female sexual function is contraception. This needs to be effective, as diabetic pregnancy is associated with particular risks and requirements and should be planned as far as possible. Unexpected pregnancy is likely to be harder to cope with, and, if prior glycaemic control has been poor, associated with increased risks to the fetus (see Ch. 12).

Most forms of contraception are suitable for diabetic women (**Fig. 3.12**). However, natural family planning is associated with too high a failure rate to be used safely, given the concerns about unplanned pregnancy. In the past combined oral contraceptive pills (OCP) were avoided because they increased the risk of stroke and myocardial infarction, greatly adding to the increased risk of these events from the diabetes itself. In reality, though, the risk of these remains very small in diabetic women, particularly if they are using low dose estrogen (e.g. 30 or 35 μg ethinylestradiol plus low dose levonorgestrol or norethisterone) or third-generation OCPs such as Cilest, and for most women requiring maximal safety this is the contraception of choice. However, if the diabetic woman also suffers from hypertension an OCP should not be used, unless all other options are contraindicated, and a progesterone-only pill is probably the preferred option.

EMPLOYMENT

Diabetic patients should not be discriminated against when seeking employment and if they experience discrimination they should contact their patient support organization. However, there are some occupations where the risk of even occasional hypoglycaemia is too great for an insulin-treated diabetic to be employed, or impracticalities that for some other reason argue against employment of individuals with diabetes (**Fig. 3.13**).

BENEFITS

Diabetic patients who are unable to seek employment because of a related disability, or who require the support of a carer, should be advised about the benefits to which they are entitled. Research has indicated that many patients fail to claim such benefits, however. Possible benefits to which patients may be entitled include:

Fig. 3.13 Employment considerations for the diabetic patient

Occupation	Restriction
Airline pilot	Not if on insulin or sulfonylureas
Air traffic controller	Not if on insulin or sulfonylureas
Armed forces*	No recruitment of individuals with diabetes
Diplomatic service*	No recruitment of individuals with diabetes
Docks worker*	Unlikely to be recruited if on insulin
	If on insulin cannot control vehicles or lifting apparatus
Firefighter*	No recruitment of individuals with diabetes
Oil and gas industries*	If on insulin cannot work offshore
Police service*	No recruitment of individuals with diabetes
Prison service*	No recruitment of individuals on insulin
Railways, including underground*	Many jobs not available for those on insulin
Shipping, including navy*	No recruitment of individuals with diabetes
	Those in employment needing insulin considered permanently unfit for seafaring
Jobs involving driving	If on insulin cannot drive if PCV or LGV licence is required
Hazardous occupations	Must:
	• Have stable control and self-monitor
	• Avoid disabling hypolycaemia
	• Not have significant complications
	• Be under regular specialist review

*For those already employed or not falling into the category mentioned, or both, an individual assessment will usually be made.

- Disability living allowance
  — Mobility
  — Care
- Attendance allowance
- Inability to work
  — Unemployment benefit
  — Income support
  — Incapacity benefit
  — Severe disablement allowance
- Disability working allowance
- Invalid care allowance (for the carer)

TRAVEL

DRIVING

The main area in which diabetes impacts on travel is with regard to driving regulations. In most countries all diabetic drivers are required by law to inform the national licensing authority, and insulin-treated drivers are precluded from holding vocational driving licences. In the UK, diabetic patients treated with insulin have not been allowed to obtain a large goods vehicle (LGV) licence since 1991. They had previously also been prohibited from holding a passenger-carrying vehicle (PCV, or public service vehicle) licence, which includes driving minibuses and all vehicles in excess of 3 tonnes weight, so as to bring the UK into line with mainland Europe. However, they may now, at the discretion of the DVLA, be allowed to drive vehicles up to 7.5 tonnes. In the USA, insulin-treated drivers cannot drive a commercial vehicle across a state border, but the rules within each state are highly variable.

Hypoglycaemia is clearly a major hazard for the diabetic driver. The reported rates of hypoglycaemia-related accidents are low. However, hypoglycaemia can cause erratic driving of which the driver is often unaware. Unawareness of the hypoglycaemia will compound the problem further, and may lead to withdrawal of the licence, and prosecution if the driver is involved in an accident.

The diabetic driver should therefore be given this advice for preventing and dealing with hypoglycaemia:

- Check your blood glucose level before starting any journey and continue to monitor it on long journeys
- Stop driving *as soon as* you become aware of imminent hypoglycaemia
- Keep a supply of short-acting carbohydrate in the car
- Ensure that regular meals and rest stops are taken

The other diabetes-related problem that may affect driving ability and lead to loss of a driving licence is visual impairment. Severe retinal ischaemia can affect visual acuity, while panretinal photocoagulation may cause restriction of visual field that is sufficient to prevent safe driving. A cataract will accentuate headlamp glare, affecting night driving.

Despite these concerns there have been studies showing diabetic drivers to have better safety records than non-diabetic drivers.

AIR TRAVEL

Air travel poses problems with regard to:
- Insulin storage
- Rapid transport across time zones affecting timing of insulin doses
- Travel insurance
- Immunization

Immunization and insurance requirements are the same as for non-diabetic individuals, although the choice of travel insurance may be more restricted.

Insulin can be safely kept at room temperature for up to a month, but will denature if frozen, and therefore should not be put in baggage destined for the aircraft hold. In hot climates, it is not imperative to refrigerate insulin, but it should be kept in a cool, shaded place. Soluble insulin that becomes cloudy or insulin suspensions (i.e. longer-acting insulin) that becomes granular should be discarded. Wherever possible sufficient insulin should be taken for the whole trip as this avoids problems arising from the use of different formulations (see Ch. 4) or lack of availability of insulin.

Changes to insulin regimens whilst flying are dependent on the time difference between zones and the type of regimen. Patients on basal-bolus regimens (see Ch.4) can take longer-acting insulin as usual and simply take short-acting insulin with each meal. Those on other regimens should not need to make any changes unless the time difference is greater than

6 hours. In this case one or more small additional insulin doses may be required, usually with meals, if travelling from east to west, whereas it may be necessary to reduce or omit a dose when travelling in the opposite direction.

INSURANCE

Patients with diabetes must declare this fact to potential insurers. Unfortunately, despite recent significant improvements in life expectancy – to the extent that one recent study suggested that diabetic patients without significant complications may live longer than non-diabetics – life insurance is likely to be weighted by 10 to 50%. However, national patients' organizations have often negotiated the best deals and should be contacted for advice.

This situation also occurs with motor insurance, where weighting against diabetic drivers seems even more unjustified.

chapter 4

Management of Diabetes

INTRODUCTION

The management of the patient with diabetes has four components:

- Control of blood glucose levels
- Monitoring of blood glucose levels
- Education about living with diabetes (see Ch. 3)
- Prevention and detection of complications (see Chs 5–11)

This is usually achieved through the coordinated efforts of a diabetes team, with involvement of a variety of health professionals depending on the individual's needs. There are a number of approaches to therapy in type 1 and type 2 diabetes. The therapeutic options will be considered first and then their place in management.

DRUG THERAPY

SULFONYLUREAS

The major action of sulfonylureas is to close adenosine triphosphate (ATP)-sensitive potassium channels in the β–cell membrane, which results in an influx of calcium that in turn stimulates insulin release. It is this augmentation of insulin secretion that explains the drugs' hypoglycaemic action and in humans it seems unlikely that they have significant extrapancreatic actions.

There are a number of sulfonylureas available (**Fig. 4.1**). The second-generation drugs, gliclazide, glipizide and glibenclamide, are more potent, whereas the longer-acting drugs are

Fig. 4.1 Sulfonylurea drugs and their characteristics

Drug	Duration of action (h)	Dosage range (mg)	Route of excretion
Tolbutamide	6–8	500–3000	Renal
Chlorpropamide	24–72	100–500	Renal
Glibenclamide	18–30	1.25–20	Renal 50%, biliary 50%
Gliclazide	10–15	40–320	Renal 70%, biliary 30%
Glipizide	12–14	2.5–40	Renal 80%, biliary 20%
Gliquidone	18–24	45–180	Renal 5%, biliary 95%
Glimepiride	24	1–6	Renal 40%, biliary 60%

more likely to cause hypoglycaemia, particularly in the elderly. These features tend to influence the choice of agent, favouring gliclazide and glipizide. These are usually given twice daily. Gliclazide is particularly favoured in the elderly and patients with renal impairment, since only 5% of the drug is excreted unaltered by the kidney, and so it does not accumulate in these patients. Chlorpropamide, which is more frequently associated with side-effects, particularly severe hypoglycaemia, is no longer recommended.

Side-effects
These include:

- Rash – this is more common with first-generation agents
- Dyspepsia and nausea
- Alcohol-induced flushing – this is almost exclusively from chlorpropamide
- Weight gain – this is a result of the anabolic effects associated with increased circulating insulin
- Hypoglycaemia – this is a particular concern in the elderly; severe hypoglycaemia, which is almost always due to chlorpropamide or glibenclamide, carries a 10% mortality rate; drugs augmenting the hypoglycaemic action of sulfonylureas (**Fig. 4.2**) should be avoided
- Cholestatic jaundice and marrow suppression – these are rare

There have been concerns about a possible deleterious effect of sulfonylureas in patients with ischaemic heart disease, because these drugs also close cardiac ATP-sensitive potassium channels, which some regard as important in ischaemic preconditioning. However, there is little evidence to support this and it remains a controversial issue.

BIGUANIDES
Biguanides were first introduced in the 1950s, but phenformin was widely withdrawn in the 1970s because of the risk of lactic acidosis. There is a tenfold lower risk of this complication

Fig. 4.2   Drugs which may exacerbate hypoglycaemia in patients on sulfonylureas

- Non-steroidal anti-inflammatory drugs
- Salicylates
- Antibiotics/antifungals
  — tetracyclines
  — sulfonamides
  — chloramphenicol
  — quinolones
  — miconazole
- Coumarins
- Monoamine oxidase (MAO) inhibitors
- Clofibrate
- Disopyramide
- Cimetidine
- β blockers

with metformin. Metformin has therefore remained in widespread use, except, notably, in the USA, where it received FDA approval only recently.

The mechanism of action of metformin is not fully understood, but it appears to improve insulin sensitivity, causing suppression of hepatic glucose output and enhancing insulin-stimulated glucose uptake into muscle. It is particularly effective at reducing postprandial blood glucose levels, and, because circulating insulin levels are not increased, its use is not associated with weight gain or hypoglycaemia. It has a dosage range of 500 to 2000 mg daily taken in two or three divided doses with meals.

Side-effects

The major side-effect of metformin therapy is gastrointestinal upset. This affects at least 20% of patients, with nausea and diarrhoea prominent, and often proving intolerable. If the drug is taken with meals and started at a low dose these side-effects may be minimized.

The other rare side-effect associated with metformin is lactic acidosis (see Ch. 6). This can largely be avoided, however, if metformin is not given to high risk patients such as those with:

- Severe cardiac failure
- Renal failure
- Hepatic cirrhosis
- Respiratory failure
- Alcoholism

  For added efficacy metformin can also be used in combination with sulfonylureas.

ALPHA-GLUCOSIDASE INHIBITORS

Alpha-glucosidase inhibitors, such as acarbose, act by inhibiting disaccharidases in the small bowel. This delays enzymatic digestion of complex carbohydrates, which in turn delays their absorption and hence results in a more gradual flux in glucose concentrations in the portal vessels. They are effective in reducing postprandial hyperglycaemia, and are probably best used at the time of diagnosis of type 2 diabetes, when β-cell dysfunction results in abnormal postprandial insulin release.

Side-effects

Unfortunately, as a consequence of the mode of action, significant carbohydrate malabsorption occurs, causing flatulence, abdominal bloating and diarrhoea. This may be reduced by starting at a low dosage of 50 mg daily, and building up to a maintenance dose of 50–100 mg with each meal. Even so, many patients remain intolerant of the drug because of the gastrointestinal side-effects, and in consequence its use has been limited.

NEW DRUGS

A number of targets are being used to design drugs that lower blood glucose levels (**Fig. 4.3**).

Thiazolinedione

Thiazolinediones are peroxisome proliferator activating receptor (PPAR) γ agonists, which act on adipose tissue, liver and muscle as insulin sensitizers, potentiating the actions of insulin. These agents initially appeared attractive because they addressed the underlying pathophysiology of insulin resistance, rather than responding to it by increasing insulin secretion.

The first of this class of drug introduced was troglitazone. Preliminary studies suggested that it not only improved glycaemic control but also had beneficial effects on lipid profiles, BP and microalbuminuria. Unfortunately it was subsequently reported rarely to cause

Fig. 4.3 Potential targets for novel drugs to treat type 2 diabetes

Site of action	Drug
Augmentation of insulin secretion	Insulin secretagogues • Glimepiride • Repaglinide Amylin antagonists
Enhancement of insulin action	Insulin potentiators • Thiazolinediones
Insulin receptor agonists	Insulin analogues Insulin mimetics • Vanadate
Increased glucose disposal	β_3-adrenoreceptor agonists

hepatic failure, with several fatalities, and was thus withdrawn from the UK market soon after launch, and later from the US market.

The introduction of other drugs in this class has consequently been more cautious, although structural differences from troglitazone seem to protect against hepatotoxicity. Rosiglitazone and pioglitazone have been licensed for add-on therapy to sulfonylureas or metformin, with a marked improvement in glycaemic control and insulin sensitivity when used in these combinations.

Prandial glucose regulators

Repaglinide is similar to the non-sulfonylurea part of the glibenclamide molecule and acts at the β-cell surface to transiently stimulate insulin release. It is therefore ideal for control of high postprandial glucose levels when fasting levels are not elevated. Nateglinide is a d-phenylanine derivative which augments non-glucose stimulated insulin release and fulfils a similar purpose.

INSULIN

Insulin preparations (**Fig. 4.4**) can be classified according to:

- *Species*　　　　— Human
　　　　　　　　— Pork
　　　　　　　　— Beef
- *Duration of action*　— Short acting (soluble)
　　　　　　　　— Intermediate acting (isophane)
　　　　　　　　— Long acting (lente)

Most insulin worldwide is now U100, with an insulin concentration of 100 IU/ml, but a few countries, particularly on mainland Europe, use U40, with 40 IU/ml.

Species

Most patients now use human insulin, which is largely manufactured by recombinant DNA technology. Animal insulin is obtained by isolation from the bovine or porcine pancreas.

Duration of action

In solution, unmodified insulin associates into hexamers, comprising a zinc atom and three identical insulin dimers (**Fig. 4.5**). After injection these hexamers diffuse through the

Fig. 4.4   Insulin preparations

Duration of action	Insulin type/brand	Species
Rapid-acting, 2–5 h	Humalog Novorapid	Analogue (Lispro) Analogue (Aspart)
Short-acting, 6–8 h	Soluble: • Humulin S • Actrapid • Hypurin bovine neutral • Hypurin pork neutral • Pork velosulin	 • Human • Human • Beef • Pork • Pork
Medium-acting, 18–24 h	Isophane: • Humulin I • Insulatard • Hypurin bovine isophane • Hypurin pork isophane • Pork insulatard Mixed insulin-Zn suspensions: • Humulin lente • Monotard • Lentard	 • Human • Human • Beef • Pork • Pork • Human • Human • Pork/beef
Long-acting, 24–36 h	Crystalline insulin–Zn suspensions: • Humulin Zn • Ultratard	 • Human • Human
Premixed	Variable proportions of soluble and isophane: e.g. Humulin M1–M5, Mixtard 10–50; M3 = Mixtard 30 = 30% soluble, 70% isophane	• Human or pork

subcutaneous tissues, so creating a concentration gradient. As the concentration decreases the hexamers dissociate into dimers, then into monomers, which are absorbed much more rapidly into the circulation (**Fig. 4.6**).

Modification of insulin makes it less soluble and retards its absorption. The combination of insulin with protamine or zinc produces intermediate-acting insulins, and its combination with zinc only produces long-acting insulins. The resulting preparations are cloudy, being suspensions of insulin with protamine or zinc in crystalline form.

Short-acting insulin can also be combined with intermediate-acting, and probably long-acting, insulin without altering its absorption profile. There is a range of fixed mixtures available, containing different ratios of short-acting to longer-acting insulin. The most widely used is a 30:70 combination.

Administration

Insulin is commonly administered by subcutaneous injection, usually into fatty areas in the thighs, buttocks, upper arms or lower abdomen (**Fig. 4.7**). The skin should be pinched up and the needle introduced vertically or at a slight angle.

A variety of factors may alter the rate of absorption. These include:

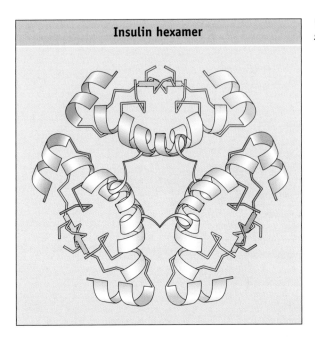

Insulin hexamer

Fig. 4.5   *The structure of soluble insulin.*

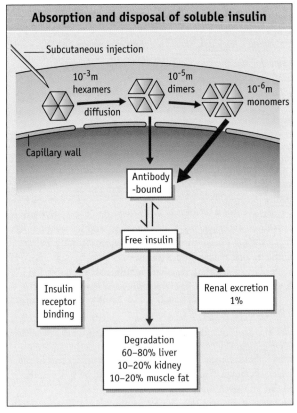

Absorption and disposal of soluble insulin

Subcutaneous injection

10^{-3}m hexamers

10^{-5}m dimers

10^{-6}m monomers

diffusion

Capillary wall

Antibody -bound

Free insulin

Insulin receptor binding

Renal excretion 1%

Degradation
60–80% liver
10–20% kidney
10–20% muscle fat

Fig. 4.6   *Absorption of soluble insulin following subcutaneous injection.*

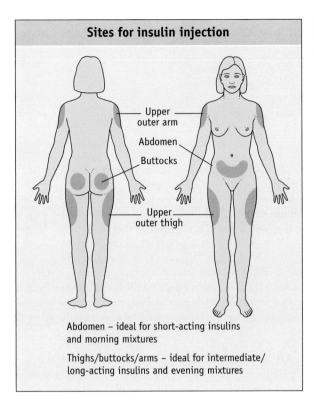

Fig. 4.7 *Recommended sites for subcutaneous insulin injection.*

Within the figure:

Sites for insulin injection

Upper outer arm
Abdomen
Buttocks
Upper outer thigh

Abdomen – ideal for short-acting insulins and morning mixtures

Thighs/buttocks/arms – ideal for intermediate/ long-acting insulins and evening mixtures

- Insulin preparation
- Mode of administration
- Site:
  — region
  — lipoatrophy/lipohypertrophy
- Temperature
- Exercise
- Massage
- Vasoactive drugs

In addition, most patients have insulin antibodies, which reversibly bind free insulin following absorption. Insulin is released unpredictably from these antibodies.

Insulin is degraded in the:

- Liver – 60–80%
- Kidney – 10–20%

Insulin accumulation may, therefore, occur in renal or hepatic impairment and doses may need reducing.

Side-effects

Side-effects of insulin therapy are unusual, with the exception of hypoglycaemia (see Ch. 6). They include the following reactions:

- An allergic, urticarial reaction occurs rarely with highly purified and human insulins
- Peripheral oedema, which is thought to be due to increased sodium retention, may be an acute and usually transient complaint

INSULIN ANALOGUES

The unpredictability of insulin availability following subcutaneous injection and of its absorption into the systemic circulation, in contrast to endogenous insulin secretion into the portal circulation, are just two examples of the ways in which insulin therapy fails to match physiological insulin secretion. Another is the failure of preprandial short-acting insulin injection to match the normal postprandial insulin profile (**Fig. 4.8**). Modification of the insulin molecule to inhibit formation of dimers and hexamers, so that monomeric insulin is injected, would allow much more rapid absorption, more closely mimicking the normal profile (**Fig. 4.8**). One way of achieving this has been to switch the lysine and proline residues at positions 29 and 28 on the B chain of the insulin molecule (see Ch. 2). This results in a flatter three-dimensional structure that is less likely to dimerize, and this short-acting insulin analogue has recently been marketed as Lispro. It is particularly effective at reducing postprandial hyperglycaemia and preprandial hypoglycaemia.

However, use of a much shorter-acting insulin analogue merits a better basal insulin than those currently available. Such insulins are in development using different modifications of the insulin molecule to retard its absorption. Insulin glargine, the first of these longer-acting analogues, has recently been marketed in some parts of the world.

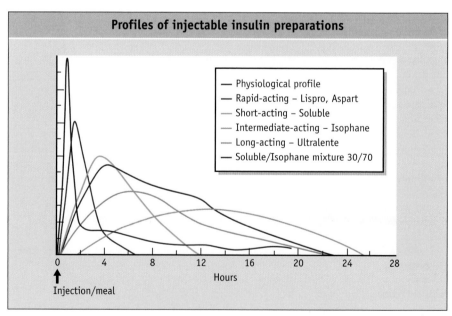

Fig. 4.8   *Physiological insulin release and profiles of injectable insulin.*

MANAGEMENT

MANAGEMENT OF TYPE 1 DIABETES

Insulin therapy

Patients with type 1 diabetes need insulin for survival. Subcutaneous insulin injection is conventionally given in one of two regimens:

- **A bd regimen** A twice-daily mixture (self-mixed or a fixed mixture) of short- and longer-acting insulin
- **A basal bolus regimen** Short-acting insulin preprandially with a longer-acting insulin at night

The basal-bolus regimen more closely mirrors physiological insulin profiles, particularly if the insulin analogue Lispro is used as the short-acting insulin. In practice, though, most patients achieve reasonable control using conventional short-acting insulin, and Lispro is reserved for patients with particular problems (**Fig. 4.9**).

The basal-bolus regimen offers patients greater flexibility and is the preferred regimen for younger patients, especially pregnant women (see Ch. 12). The DCCT demonstrated that these intensive insulin regimens probably improve glycaemic control. Basal-bolus regimens allow dosage adjustment depending on anticipated carbohydrate intake, and place less emphasis on snacks between meals (see Ch. 3), which are an important part of twice-daily regimens because of the injection of longer-acting insulin before breakfast. However patients on basal-bolus regimens should still be encouraged to eat regular meals. One advantage of Lispro is that, with its rapid absorption, it can be injected immediately before, or even with, a meal rather than 20–30 minutes before eating, as with conventional short-acting insulins.

Subcutaneous insulin injection can be given by syringe (**Fig. 4.10**), insulin being drawn up from a vial (**Fig. 4.11**), or can be administered using a pen containing an insulin cartridge, either reusable (**Fig. 4.12**) or disposable (**Fig. 4.13**). Pen delivery systems are increasingly popular, being more discreet and dispensing with the need to draw up insulin. Patients need to have a method for safe disposal of needles (**Fig. 4.14**).

Continuous subcutaneous insulin infusion   Better, more physiological methods of insulin delivery are constantly being sought. The only other method in routine clinical practice is continuous subcutaneous insulin infusion (CSII) using a small pump attached to a plastic cannula in the abdominal wall (**Fig. 4.15**). This is in common usage in the USA and some

Fig. 4.9   Indications for Lispro therapy

Control problems due to:
- Frequent hypoglycaemia
- Significant postprandial hyperglycaemia

Lifestyle:
- Active life
- More convenient injection timing

Improved control in patients on CSII

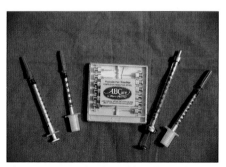

Fig. 4.10   A selection of insulin syringes.

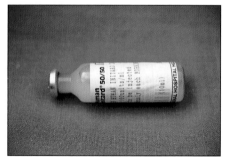

Fig. 4.11   Insulin vial for use with insulin syringe.

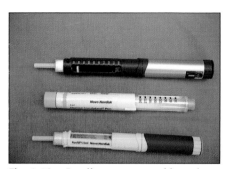

Fig. 4.12   Insulin pens – reusable and disposable.

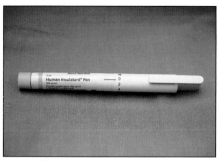

Fig. 4.13   A disposable insulin pen.

Fig. 4.14   Safe disposal of insulin injection needles: (a) sharps box and (b) safeclip for needle removal.

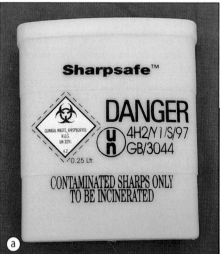

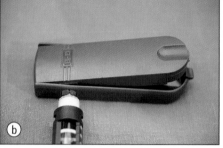

areas of mainland Europe, but has not been favoured in the UK because of concerns particularly related to pump failure and the risk of ketoacidosis and the risk of infection at the cannula site. However, these fears can be largely allayed with use of current pumps

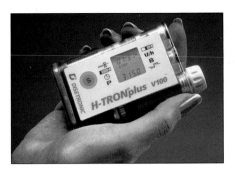

Fig. 4.15 *CSII pump.*

provided patients are properly educated. Usage of CSII is likely to increase but probably for selected patients only.

Indications for CSII include:

- Inadequate control on optimized conventional regimen
- Frequent hypoglycaemia or loss of hypoglycaemia awareness
- Erratic lifestyle needing greater mealtime flexibility
- Patient preference
- Pregnancy

Other methods   Other methods of insulin delivery that are either currently, but rarely, available, or in development include:

- Implantable insulin pumps
- Aerosol delivery
- Oral insulin
- Nasal insulin
- Transdermal insulin
- Insulin implants

Monitoring glycaemic control

Blood glucose monitoring   There is no place for urine glucose monitoring (see below) in patients with type 1 diabetes, because it is too insensitive and is unable to detect imminent hypoglycaemia. These patients need to be taught home blood glucose monitoring. Capillary blood is obtained from the finger pulp using a lancet, and applied to a test strip. The change in colour of the test strip can be compared to a chart on the bottle to obtain an estimate of blood glucose concentration, but a more accurate reading is obtained by inserting the test strip into a meter (**Fig. 4.16**). All meters are very accurate between 3 and 18 mmol/L, providing they are used correctly, but there are varying degrees of inaccuracy outside this range.

Frequency of testing will depend on the individual's control and commitment. Ideally at least one test performed at a different time each day (**Fig. 4.17**) is the minimum to allow a satisfactory profile to be obtained. However, the glycaemic control in patients with type 1 diabetes is more erratic because of the vagaries of insulin absorption and availability in

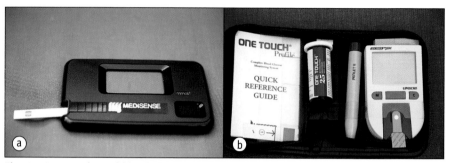

Fig. 4.16   *A variety of blood glucose meters, with an automatic lancet device for obtaining a capillary sample (b, centre).*

Fig. 4.17   Suggested routine for daily blood glucose monitoring

Time	Before breakfast	After breakfast	Before lunch	After lunch	Before supper	After supper	Before bed	03.00–04.00
Target (mmol/L)	4–7	4–10	4–7	4–10	4–7	4–10	7–10	3.5–7
Type 1; unstable type 2	x		x		x	x		
Stable type 2	x Day 1		x Day 2		x Day 3	x Day 4		
Pregnancy, intensive control	x	x	x	x	x	x	x	
Nocturnal hypos; high waking glucose								x

people not producing any insulin of their own, and so more frequent testing in these patients will give a truer representation of control.

Insulin doses should preferably be adjusted when a pattern is observed, except in acute illness (see Ch. 6). In most cases a high blood glucose will be corrected by increasing the preceding insulin dose, and a low blood glucose by decreasing the same dose. The possible exception to this is morning hyperglycaemia following a normal blood glucose on going to bed. This is termed the Somogyi effect, after the physician who first described this phenomenon. He found that the explanation for it was rebound hyperglycaemia following hypoglycaemia at around 3.00 a.m. He corrected the problem by additional insulin in the middle of the night, rather than decreasing the night-time insulin dose, which is the common response. However the importance of this phenomenon in most patients with type 1 diabetes is hotly disputed.

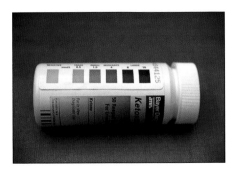

Fig. 4.18 *Ketostix for monitoring urine ketones.*

Fig. 4.19   Assays for glycosylated haemoglobin and potential interference

	Electrophoresis	HPLC	Immunoassay
Analyte	HbA$_1$c HbA$_1$	HbA$_1$	HbA$_1$c
Hb variant interference:			
HbF – elevates value	Y	N	Y
HbS/C – lower value	N	Y	N
Other interference:	Uraemia, alcoholism		

Decreased mean red cell age lowers value on all assays; causes include: haemolysis, acute or chronic blood loss, pregnancy

Monitoring of urinary ketones   Monitoring of urinary ketones (**Fig. 4.18**) should be encouraged when blood glucose levels are greater than 18 mmol/L to warn of incipient ketoacidosis (see Ch. 6).

Assessment of glycosylated haemoglobin   Glycaemic control over the preceding 6–8 weeks can be assessed using an estimation of glycosylated haemoglobin. Glucose binds irreversibly to the *N*-terminal valine of haemoglobin, and the percentage of bound haemoglobin (Hb) can therefore be used as a measure of overall glycaemic control. HbA$_1$ or, more commonly, HbA$_{1c}$ may be assayed (**Fig. 4.19**). Reference ranges vary between laboratories, but a target of within 2 σ above the upper limit of the normal range is regarded as defining optimal glycaemic control.

Cure of type 1 diabetes

Immunosuppressive therapy   In 70% of patients with newly diagnosed type 1 diabetes, near metabolic normality can be achieved on less than 0.5 U/kg per day of insulin, with a nadir in insulin requirements at 3–4 months. A few patients are able to come off insulin, and may remain off it for up to 2 years. This 'honeymoon phase' reflects a functional recovery of the remaining β cells, raising the possibility that the disease could be stabilized or even that there could be a recovery. Thus there have been trials of immunosuppressive therapy, notably with cyclosporin, in an attempt to modify the disease process. This did increase the rates of clinical remission, but virtually all treated individuals will need insulin after, at most, 2 years of treatment and so, given the toxicity of cyclosporin, such an approach has not been widely pursued.

Transplantation   The other option that would allow cure is transplantation, either of whole pancreas or isolated pancreatic islets. Most pancreas transplants have been performed in patients undergoing simultaneous renal transplantation for end-stage diabetic nephropathy as these patients already require immunosuppression for their renal graft. Pancreatic transplantation is also more successful in these patients than when performed alone, with the pancreatic graft surviving for 5 years in over two-thirds of patients.

Islet transplantation has been performed in a few individuals, by direct injection of islets into the portal vein, but survival of the graft is usually not prolonged. It is hoped that islets could be modified to be non-immunogenic, so that patients would not require immunosuppression. However, the major obstacle to widespread use of this technique is the number of whole pancreata that would be needed to obtain sufficient islets for transplantation.

MANAGEMENT OF TYPE 2 DIABETES
The management of type 2 diabetes consists of three components:

- Lifestyle advice, particularly with regard to diet and exercise
- Achievement of good glycaemic control
- Modification of risk factors for vascular disease (see Ch. 7)

Treatment targets should be determined (**Fig. 4.20**) but will need modifying for each individual. Obviously the elderly patient may require control of blood glucose only to achieve symptom relief, rather than aggressive pursuit of vascular risk factors (see Ch. 12).

Diet
Diet is the mainstay of treatment (see Ch. 3) and newly diagnosed patients should have a 3 month trial of diet therapy alone unless:
- They are severely symptomatic
- Their blood glucose level is consistently greater than 20 mmol/L

Over 75 % of patients with type 2 diabetes are obese and will also need calorie restriction.

Fig. 4.20   Standard treatment targets for patients with type 2 diabetes

	Optimal	Acceptable
BMI (kg/m^2)	< 25 M	< 27 M
	< 24 F	< 26 F
Fasting glucose (mmol/L)	4.5–6.5	< 8
HbA$_1$c (σ from normal mean)	< +2	< +4
Total cholesterol (mmol/L)	< 5.2	< 6.2
High density lipoprotein (HDL) cholesterol	> 1.1	> 0.9
Fasting triglycerides	< 1.7	< 2.2
BP	< 140/80	< 160/90

Oral medication

Unfortunately about 50% of patients will fail the initial trial of diet therapy and will require oral medication (**Fig. 4.21**). Sulfonylureas are usually the first-line treatment in non-obese patients and metformin in the obese. Roughly two-thirds of patients on sulfonylureas and one-third of those on metformin will achieve their metabolic targets, but about 10% per year will lose control thereafter. Combination therapy may then be tried, with an initial response rate of up to 50%. However, for morbidly obese patients, in whom weight gain on sulfonylureas (or insulin) will aggravate insulin resistance, very low calorie diets may be a better alternative.

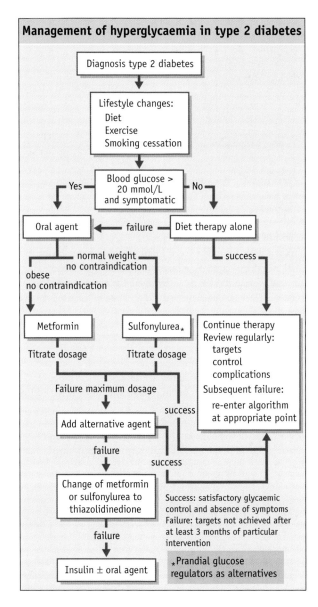

Fig. 4.21 *Algorithm for management of type 2 diabetes.*

Insulin therapy

Once combined oral hypoglycaemic therapy has proved ineffective then insulin should be introduced. This step is often delayed because of reluctance on the part of physician or patient, but most patients when started on insulin notice a substantial improvement in their well-being. Patients who do not have symptoms of hyperglycaemia, which may simply be fatigue or malaise, and are reluctant to take insulin on the basis of failing to meet metabolic targets, may be persuaded to have a trial of insulin therapy. Some patients may also experience a temporary need for insulin therapy. Temporary insulin therapy should be considered in:

- Myocardial infarction
- Infection
- Surgery
- Pregnancy
- Steroid therapy
- Acute neuropathy
- Hyperosmolar non-ketotic coma

Most patients with type 2 diabetes will be started on one of the following regimens:
- Once-daily insulin
- Once-daily insulin with oral hypoglycaemic agent
- Twice-daily mixed insulin

A few patients will opt for a basal-bolus regimen for flexibility.

Once-daily insulin therapy combined with sulfonylurea or metformin has been shown to be as effective as other regimens with respect to control, whilst causing less increase in circulating insulin levels and less weight gain, particularly if the insulin is given at night to suppress hepatic glucose output (**Fig. 4.22**). A few patients with severe insulin resistance may require doses of insulin as great as 1000 U/day.

Monitoring glycaemic control

Urinary monitoring   Glucose can be detected in the urine when blood glucose levels rise above the threshold for renal glucose excretion, which is about 10 mmol/L in most people. Urine monitoring (**Fig. 4.23**) is therefore not particularly accurate and should be reserved for patients on diet or tablets whose control is very stable.

Blood glucose monitoring   Blood glucose monitoring is a better indicator of glycaemic control, and can be performed once a week if levels are stable. Blood glucose levels tend to be much more stable in patients with type 2 diabetes, even if insulin treated, and fasting blood glucose correlates very well with glycosylated haemoglobin.

ORGANIZATION OF DIABETES CARE

Many patients with diabetes can be looked after in primary care, if screening processes are put in place, with secondary care provided for patients with more complicated problems. These shared care arrangements work very well when all parties are well motivated. Hospital care is often centred on diabetes centres, where a number of interested professionals such as

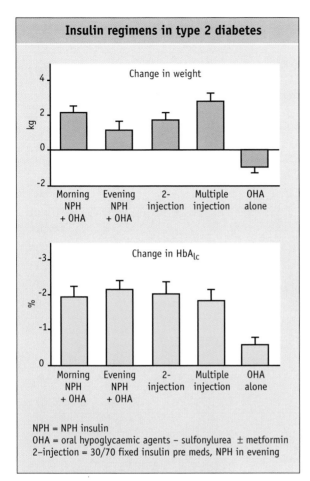

Fig. 4.22 *Effect of different insulin regimens in type 2 diabetes (from Yki-Jarvinen et al. 1992 New England Journal Of Medicine 327: 1426–1433, with permission).*

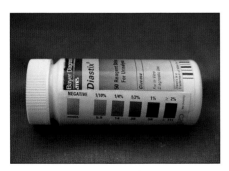

Fig. 4.23 *Diastix for urine glucose monitoring.*

diabetologists, diabetes specialist nurses, chiropodists and dietitians can provide an integrated service.

Whatever system is put in place the important aspect of diabetes care is that all patients receive appropriate education, have regular assessments of metabolic control, are regularly screened for complications and have access to other healthcare professionals as required.

chapter 5

Complications of Diabetes

INTRODUCTION

Complications of diabetes can be classified into three categories:

Classification of diabetic complications

- Acute metabolic
- Microvascular
- Macrovascular

In addition there are a number of skin and soft tissue problems, and infections that are particularly associated with diabetes.

Type 1 diabetes

Patients with type 1 diabetes are most susceptible to microvascular complications. These are rarely seen within 5 years of diagnosis and virtually never before puberty. It has been recognized for decades that poor glycaemic control is associated with an increased risk of microvascular complications. The DCCT and the United Kingdom Prospective Diabetes Study (UKPDS) confirmed, for type 1 and type 2 diabetes respectively, that good glycaemic control reduces the risk of development and progression of complications (**Fig. 5.1**). Other factors, such as hypertension, hyperlipidaemia and genetic factors, also determine the natural history of complications.

Type 2 diabetes

Patients with type 2 diabetes can also develop microvascular complications, which may be present at diagnosis, reflecting the fact that many patients will have had significant

Fig. 5.1 The impact of good glycaemic control on diabetic complications

	DCCT (type 1 diabetes)		UKPDS (type 2 diabetes)	
Retinopathy	76%	$P < 0.001$	21%	$P = 0.015$
Nephropathy	54%	$P = 0.01$	33%	$P < 0.001$
Neuropathy	57%	$P < 0.001$		
Myocardial infarction			16%	$P = 0.052$

Fig. 5.2   The annual incidence of cardiovascular disease per 1000 population

	Male Diabetic	Non-diabetic	Female Diabetic	Non-diabetic
Cardiovascular disease	4.7	1.9	6.2	1.7
Peripheral vascular disease	12.6	3.3	8.4	1.3
Ischaemic heart disease	24.5	14.9	17.8	6.9

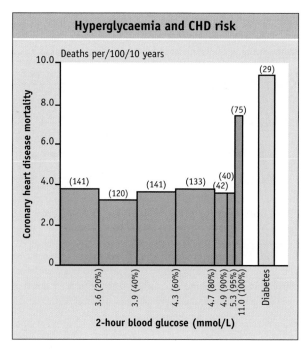

Fig. 5.3   *The effect of impaired glucose tolerance on ischaemic heart disease risk (from Fuller et al. 1983 British Medical Journal 287 (6396): 867–870, with permission).*

hyperglycaemia for many years before the diagnosis is made. However, these patients are most at risk of macrovascular complications, which are the major cause of mortality in type 2 diabetes (**Fig. 5.2**). The increased risk of vascular disease is seen even with apparently mild degrees of impaired glucose tolerance (**Fig. 5.3**). The impact of improved glycaemic control on complications has not been fully established in type 2 diabetes, however. Long-standing undiagnosed hyperglycaemia may diminish the effect of improved control on microvascular complications. The DCCT did not look at a population at high risk of developing macrovascular disease during the study, although there was a trend to reduced levels in the intensively treated patients, and so there are no data to extrapolate to this higher risk population. The most important aspect of management in type 2 diabetes may be addressing other vascular risk factors, as much as improving glycaemic control.

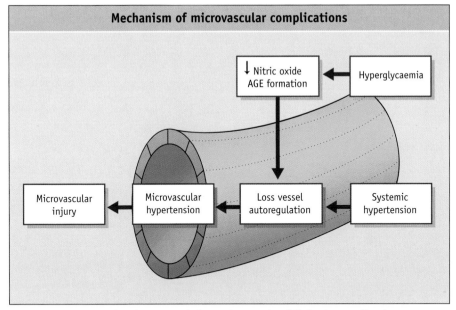

Mechanism of microvascular complications

↓ Nitric oxide AGE formation

Hyperglycaemia

Microvascular injury

Microvascular hypertension

Loss vessel autoregulation

Systemic hypertension

Fig. 5.4 *Microvascular changes and the pathogenesis of diabetic complications.*

PATHOPHYSIOLOGY

The pathophysiology of diabetic complications is not fully understood. Hypertension plays an important part in the development of microvascular and probably macrovascular complications. One mechanism for this effect may be increased capillary pressure, which damages the endothelium and causes extravasation of proteins. Loss of autoregulation within the microvasculature compounds this effect (**Fig. 5.4**).

The glycation of proteins and other molecules is closely linked with this damaging process. Acute glycation of proteins reflects ambient blood glucose concentrations, and is utilized in glycated haemoglobin assays. Some long-lived molecules, such as collagen and DNA, undergo a series of chemical modifications once glycated to produce advanced glycation end-products (AGEs). These AGEs can cause a cascade of events that are potentially damaging to the endothelium, exacerbating the effects of increased capillary pressure (**Fig. 5.5**). Cross-linking of AGEs derived from matrix proteins affects their function, such as the elasticity of collagen.

The possible role of glucose metabolism via the polyol pathway in the genesis of complications is considered under the pathophysiology of diabetic neuropathy (see Ch. 11).

MANAGEMENT

Therapy aimed at treating or preventing complications by targeting the above pathways is not yet available for use in humans. Aminoguanidine retards AGE formation and prevents the development of microvascular complications in diabetic animal models. Trials of aminoguanidine are ongoing in humans and this substance may prove a useful adjunct to tight glycaemic control by reducing the morbidity associated with complications.

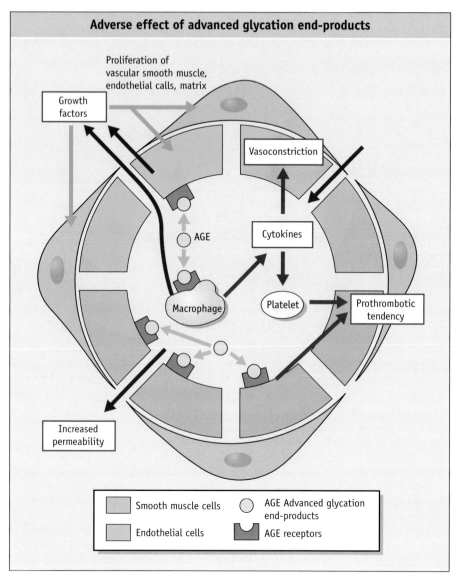

Fig. 5.5 *Adverse effects of AGEs.*

Aldose reductase inhibitors, which block metabolism of glucose via the polyol pathway, are similarly effective in animals. However, they have not as yet been shown to benefit patients with established diabetic complications.

chapter 6

Acute Diabetic Complications

INTRODUCTION

The acute metabolic complications of diabetes are characterized by hyperglycaemia with or without acidosis. Hypoglycaemia, which is by far the most common acute complication, is iatrogenic, resulting from the failure of insulin or sulfonylurea therapy to reproduce a physiological insulin profile. Lactic acidosis may occur in association with ketoacidosis, but can also be caused by biguanide therapy. Coma is often the presenting feature of these acute complications and it is important to make the correct differential diagnosis (**Fig. 6.1**).

DIABETIC KETOACIDOSIS

EPIDEMIOLOGY AND PATHOPHYSIOLOGY

Diabetic ketoacidosis (DKA) occurs as a result of marked insulin deficiency associated with an increase in circulating levels of counter-regulatory hormones in type 1 diabetes. Prior to the advent of insulin therapy in the 1920s it was almost invariably fatal and the usual cause of death in type 1 diabetes. The mortality rate fell to 10% by the 1960s but has remained unchanged since then, and is particularly high in children – accounting for over 60% of the deaths in diabetic children. The annual incidence of DKA is about 1 per 100 patients, although many of these are recurrent episodes in the same patient, the recurrence rate being up to 10% in one year.

In 10% of cases DKA is the presenting feature of type 1 diabetes, but more usually it occurs in patients with established disease. A number of factors may precipitate DKA, including the following:

- New onset type 1 diabetes
- Infection
- Other acute illness, e.g. myocardial infarction
- Trauma, surgery
- Management errors:
  - Inappropriate reduction or omission of insulin dose
  - CSII pump failure
- Emotional disturbance, especially in adolescence
- Drugs
  - Glucocorticoids
  - β_2 agonists
- Pregnancy ketosis

Fig. 6.1   Causes of coma in patients with diabetes

- Ketoacidosis
- Hyperosmolar non-ketotic coma
- Hypoglycaemia
- Lactic acidosis
- Cerebrovascular event:
  — arterial
  — venous: sinus thrombosis may complicate acute metabolic disturbances
- Postictal*
- Head trauma*
- Ethanol intoxication – promotes hypoglycaemia
- Drug overdose

* May be precipitated by hypoglycaemia.

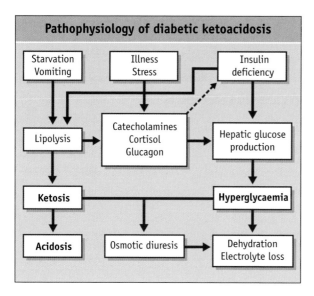

Fig. 6.2   *Pathophysiology of DKA.*

However, often no obvious cause is identified. A frequent problem is that patients often fail to increase insulin doses appropriately, or omit injections completely, during stressful illnesses, hastening the onset of ketoacidosis. Non-compliance with insulin therapy leading to DKA is a particular problem in adolescent diabetics.

The physiological response to the fasted state is to ensure an adequate substrate for brain metabolism; initially glucose is used and later on ketone bodies. In the diabetic patient a similar response occurs as a result of the increased secretion of counter-regulatory hormones in response to stress, but the relative lack of insulin leads to a loss of physiological control and the development of ketoacidosis (**Fig. 6.2**).

The increased excretion of glucose accompanying the hyperglycaemia stimulates an osmotic diuresis, with a decrease in water and sodium reabsorption in the proximal tubule. Potassium loss occurs because of two mechanisms:

Fig. 6.3 Typical fluid and electrolyte losses in DKA

Water	5–10 litres
Sodium	500 mmol
Chloride	300–600 mmol
Potassium	300–1000 mmol
Magnesium	30–60 mmol
Phosphate	50–100 mmol
Calcium	50–100 mmol

- Loss of the gradient for sodium reabsorption
- Coexcretion with ketoacids

Other cations are depleted – notably magnesium, which also accompanies ketoacids, and phosphate – owing to inhibition of proximal tubular reabsorption by glucose (**Fig. 6.3**).

CLINICAL FEATURES

Patients often describe symptoms of hyperglycaemia. Clinical signs of DKA include Kussmaul respirations as a result of the acidosis, a characteristic sweet-smelling fetor due to ketonaemia and an acute abdomen.

Clinical features of DKA

- Thirst, polyuria
- Weakness
- Blurred vision
- Kussmaul respiration
- Ketotic fetor
- Dehydration
- Abdominal pain
- Leg cramps
- Nausea and vomiting
- Mild hypothermia
- Confusion, drowsiness
- Coma

There may also be clinical features of an antecedent infection or other precipitating illness. Up to 30% of patients present in coma. Peripheral vasodilatation secondary to the acidaemia may lead to mild hypothermia, masking the anticipated pyrexia from a precipitating infection.

Investigations reveal hyperglycaemia, acidosis and ketonuria. Other routine investigations to determine the precipitants or consequences of the metabolic disturbance may need to be interpreted with caution (**Fig. 6.4**). Patients may rarely have relatively low glucose levels if there is a much greater degree of ketogenesis than gluconeogenesis.

Hyponatraemia is usually dilutional, with the hyperglycaemia drawing extracellular water into the vascular compartment. However, there is also the possibility that it may be

Fig. 6.4 Interpretation of laboratory investigations in diabetic ketoacidosis	
Analyte	**Caution**
White blood cell (leukocyte) count Cardiac enzymes Amylase	Non-specific elevations: do not necessarily reflect infection, myocardial infarction or pancreatitis
Creatinine	Spurious elevation may occur as a result of ketones cross-reaction assay
Sodium	Hyponatraemia may be spurious owing to elevated glucose or triglyceride levels

spurious as a result of hypertriglyceridaemia; if severe, this can result in plasma sodium estimations less than 120 mmol/L. Despite the total body potassium losses there is usually also initial hyperkalaemia as a result of the acidosis and insulin deficiency, which promote transport of potassium out of cells. Plasma creatinine levels may be increased because of hypotension causing renal failure, but can also be raised spuriously by ketones cross-reacting with the assay.

MANAGEMENT

The management of DKA is threefold, consisting of:

- Rehydration
- Administration of insulin
- Correction of electrolyte disturbances

This promotes a restoration of normal metabolism (**Fig. 6.5**).

Fluid replacement

Fluid replacement is the most important initial management, the correction of hyperglycaemia being a secondary consideration. The increase in urine output and enhanced perfusion of liver and skeletal muscle as a result of rehydration will contribute to a fall in blood glucose. The usual fluid deficit is about 6 litres. If the patient is cardiovascularly shocked then colloid can be used initially until an adequate BP has been achieved.

The usual rate of rehydration may need to be adjusted in children, who are more likely to develop cerebral oedema, and in the elderly or those with impaired myocardial function or renal failure. In children the rate of fluid administration should be less than 4 L/m^2 of body surface area per day. Careful monitoring of central venous pressure, or pulmonary artery wedge pressure, especially in patients who have suffered a myocardial infarct, should allow adequate fluid replacement while avoiding precipitation of pulmonary oedema in those at risk.

Correction of electrolyte disturbance

Initial crystalloid replacement should be with normal saline, unless there is marked hypernatraemia (which is rare in ketoacidosis), when half-normal saline may be used.

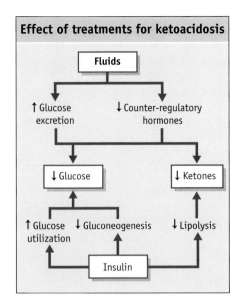

Effect of treatments for ketoacidosis

Fig. 6.5 *The effect of therapy on the metabolic disturbances in DKA.*

Dextrose should be used instead of saline once the glucose concentration falls below 15 mmol/L, probably as a 10% solution to promote more rapid disposal of ketones. Potassium should not be added to the initial fluid therapy, but replacement should be started once the plasma potassium concentration is known (**Fig. 6.6**). Glucose and electrolyte concentrations should be monitored every 1 to 2 hours depending on the clinical response, and the replacement adjusted appropriately.

The use of sodium bicarbonate to correct acidosis remains controversial because of the following possible deleterious effects:
- Central nervous system (CNS) acidosis due to diffusion of carbon dioxide, but not bicarbonate, across the blood–brain barrier
- Tissue hypoxia and lactic acidosis due to impaired oxygen dissociation as the pH rises

Use of sodium bicarbonate is usually avoided unless the acidosis is sufficiently severe to impair myocardial contractility and cause shock – usually when there is a pH of less than 6.9 and bicarbonate level of less than 5 mmol/L.

Phosphate depletion in ketoacidosis may result in tissue hypoxia due to 2,3-diphosphoglycerate (2,3-DPG) depletion. However, trials of phosphate replacement have shown no effect on morbidity or mortality. Hypomagnesaemia may occur but does not appear to result in an adverse outcome.

Insulin administration

Insulin is usually administered either by low dose intravenous infusion via a pump or by coadministration with fluid therapy. High dose insulin replacement at up to 100 U per hour was used in the past, but is unnecessary and may be associated with rapid falls in osmolality. If insulin cannot be administered intravenously it may be given intramuscularly, but not subcutaneously because absorption is too unreliable by this route, particularly in hypotensive patients. Insulin infusion is usually continued until the patient has recovered sufficiently to start eating.

Any precipitating illness should be treated and broad-spectrum antibiotics are widely given as routine.

63

Fig. 6.6 Example of a treatment protocol for DKA/HONK

Initial investigations
Metabolic assessment:
Glucose (laboratory, U&E, HCO_3^-, blood gases (may be deferred if $HCO_3^- < 10$), urinalysis for ketones
?Osmolality

Identify precipitant:
FBC, Chest X-ray, ECG, cardiac enzymes, MSU, blood cultures
?Sputum culture, ?throat swab, ?CSF culture

Fluid replacement
1 litre Normal saline given intravenously:
- stat (i.e. about $\frac{1}{2}$ hour)
- over 2 hours
- × 2 over 4 hours
- then 8 hourly

Monitor replacement with measurements of urine output 1 hourly and venous pressure, using central venous pressure (CVP) when appropriate
If Na > 155 mmol/L consider $\frac{1}{2}$ normal saline

Reduce infusion rate and use CVP measurements if:
elderly; cardiac or renal impairment; signs of ARDS or cerebral oedema;

In children the infusion rate should not exceed 4 L/m^2 per day

Once blood glucose < 15 mmol/L change to 5% or 10% dextrose (10% may correct ketosis more rapidly)

Potassium replacement
Total body losses of 300–600 mEq
Do not add potassium to the first litre of saline/fluid
If plasma potassium is not yet known add 20 mmol KCl to the second litre
Once plasma potassium is known then:
- < 3.5 mmol/L   add   40 mmol KCl per litre fluid
- 3.5–5 mmol/L   add   20
- 5 mmol/L   add   0

Insulin replacement
Give via intravenous infusion pump: make up 50 U Actrapid in 50 ml N/saline
If pump is not immediately available give 10 U bolus i.v. or im
Aim to reduce glucose by about 5 mmol/L per hour sliding scale (example below):

Bm's (checked 1 hourly)	Insulin infusion rate (ml/h = U/h)
0–2	0
2.1–4.5	0.5
4.6–6.5	1
6.6–9	2
9.1–11	3
11.1–17	4
17.1–22	6
> 22	8 and inform doctor

Fig. 6.6 (Cont'd)

Bicarbonate
Theoretical reasons for avoiding bicarbonate include paradoxical CNS acidosis, exacerbation tissue hypoxia

Administer if pH < 6.9 with persistent hypotension after initial fluid replacement; give isotonic bicarbonate, 500–1000 ml in place of normal saline in fluid regimen

Other considerations
Treat precipitating cause: give intravenous broad-spectrum antibiotics
If comatose pass nasogastric tube because of gastric dilatation
If severely dehydrated or hyperosmolar then anticoagulate with heparin

Monitoring

$\frac{1}{2}$ hourly	pulse and BP
1 hourly	glucose (can use meter once < 20 mmol/L); urine output, CVP; review by doctor
0, 2, 4, 8 hours (more frequently if necessary)	Urea and electrolytes, arterial blood gases
4 hourly	urinalysis for ketones

Continue intravenous insulin and fluids until eating and drinking normally

Comatose patients should have a nasogastric tube on suction to prevent aspiration, since gastric dilatation is a common complication of DKA. Shocked or unconscious patients should have a urinary catheter to monitor urine output.

COMPLICATIONS

There are a few, rare complications attributable to DKA itself rather than the precipitating illness, including:

- Cerebral oedema
- ARDS
- Thromboembolism – venous, arterial
- Rhabdomyolysis

Thrombosis

There is an increased risk of both venous and arterial thromboses, although these occur more commonly in hyperosmolar coma (see below), owing to:
- Dehydration
- Low cardiac output
- Hypercoagulability as a result of increased clotting factors and deranged platelet function

Routine anticoagulation therapy is not recommended although prophylactic subcutaneous heparin may be of benefit in patients with predisposing factors to thrombosis.

Cerebral oedema

Cerebral oedema is an uncommon complication of ketoacidosis but carries a particularly poor prognosis, with a mortality of up to 90%. Clinically apparent oedema occurs almost exclusively in children, affecting up to 10% of patients under the age of 20 admitted with ketoacidosis. The aetiology remains unclear, but it may reflect too rapid a decline in serum osmolality, possibly coupled with the effect of acidosis or insulin on fluid and electrolyte transport in brain cells.

Presenting features include:

Presenting features of cerebral oedema

- Worsening headache
- Incontinence
- Behavioural change
- Abrupt neurological deterioration
- Respiratory arrest

Cerebral oedema occurs after several hours of treatment, when the patient appears to be improving biochemically. Infusion of mannitol, up to 1 g/kg may be beneficial particularly if the condition is recognized early.

Adult respiratory distress syndrome (ARDS)

Adult respiratory distress syndrome is probably the result of non-cardiac pulmonary oedema forming in a similar way to cerebral oedema. It is characterized by a number of features:

Clinical features of ARDS

- Sudden dyspnoea
- Hypoxaemia
- Low pulmonary artery wedge pressure
- Radiological signs consistent with pulmonary oedema

Despite treatment with positive end-expiratory pressure ventilation, the prognosis is poor.

Mortality from DKA is usually the result of the precipitating illness, particularly if this is septicaemia or myocardial infarction, but more rarely due to complications such as intestinal infarction, cerebral oedema and cerebral haemorrhage.

PREVENTION

Recurrent episodes of DKA account for 10% of cases each year. Education is vital to reduce this recurrence rate and patients should be given appropriate illness advice, such as:

In the event of illness:
- Increase the insulin dose
- Maintain a good intake of fluid and glucose
- Closely monitor blood glucose levels and adjust insulin dose accordingly
- Monitor urinary ketones

Seek medical help promptly if:
- There is intercurrent illness
- Urine ketones are consistently moderate or greater
- Blood glucose levels are uncontrollable

Fig. 6.7 Biochemical features of HONK: comparison with DKA

	DKA	HONK
Ketosis	++ to ++++	– to +
Bicarbonate	< 18 mmol/L	> 18 mmol/L
Plasma osmolality	< 340 mosmol/L	340 mosmol/L
Urea	↑	↑↑ to ↑↑↑↑
Glucose	> 15 mmol/L	> 60 mmol/L

HYPEROSMOLAR NON-KETOTIC SYNDROME

EPIDEMIOLOGY AND PATHOPHYSIOLOGY

Hyperosmolar non-ketotic syndrome (HONK) occurs exclusively in patients with type 2 diabetes. It shares many features in common with DKA, the major exception being the absence of ketosis and acidosis (**Fig. 6.7**). This may reflect residual insulin secretion in type 2 diabetes, which suppresses lipolysis sufficiently to avert ketone body formation. However, rarely patients with type 2 diabetes develop ketoacidosis and it may be the magnitude of the counter-regulatory hormone response that determines the metabolic features.

The precipitants of the syndrome are similar to those causing DKA (see p. **59**), although, as would be expected with an older population, infections, acute vascular events and drugs, notably glucocorticoids, are most commonly implicated. The hyperosmolar non-ketotic state accounts for between 10 and 30% of hyperglycaemic emergencies. Up to two thirds of those affected have not previously been diagnosed as having diabetes.

CLINICAL FEATURES

The clinical and biochemical features are not dissimilar to those seen in patients with DKA (see above), the major differences being the absence of Kussmaul respiration, since acidosis does not occur, and the lower frequency of vomiting, which is often precipitated by ketosis. Clinical features include:

Clinical features of HONK

- Polyuria and polydipsia
- Severe dehydration
- Marked hyperglycaemia and hypernatraemia
- Acidosis
- Plasma osmolality > 340 mosmol/L

Fig. 6.8   Formula for calculating plasma osmolality

Plasma osmolality = 2 ([Na$^+$] + [K$^+$]) + [glucose] + [urea]

[ ] is the plasma concentration of the substance

Symptoms of polyuria and polydipsia may have been developing over some weeks and often there has been a deterioration in conscious level preceding admission.

Severe dehydration with circulatory collapse is a common feature. The biochemical hallmarks are marked hyperglycaemia and hypernatraemia, frequently accompanied by hypotension-related renal impairment. Acidosis occurs rarely as a result of tissue hypoperfusion but ketosis is never observed. Plasma osmolality is invariably greater than 340 mosmol/L and can be calculated using other biochemical parameters if necessary (**Fig. 6.8**).

MANAGEMENT

Management of the metabolic derangement is the same as for DKA, although hypotonic (0.45%) saline is more frequently indicated (**Fig. 6.6**). Mortality may be as high as 50% in patients with hyperosmolar non-ketotic syndrome. The cause is often the precipitating illness, but other potentially fatal complications include arterial thrombosis, which usually affects the circulation in the lower limbs or cerebrum, and venous thrombosis, which may affect the cerebral venous sinuses. Despite the frequency of thrombotic complications the benefits of anticoagulation therapy are not proven, although there should probably be a low threshold for therapeutic heparin administration. If patients recover they often need to be maintained on subcutaneous insulin initially, although may be transferred to oral hypoglycaemic agents at a later date.

LACTIC ACIDOSIS

EPIDEMIOLOGY AND PATHOPHYSIOLOGY

Lactic acidosis occurs in two situations in patients with diabetes:
- In diabetic ketoacidosis, with a frequency of 10–15%
- In patients on biguanide therapy

The cause of lactic acidosis in diabetic ketoacidosis is probably multifactorial. It responds to conventional therapy for ketoacidosis, although administration of insulin inhibits gluconeogenesis and so decreases hepatic uptake of lactate. If significant acidosis is prolonged despite evidence of recovery then lactate levels should be measured.

The biguanide phenformin was withdrawn because of the frequency with which it caused lactic acidosis. It is seen much less frequently in patients taking metformin and almost exclusively when the drug should be contraindicated.

Contraindications to metformin therapy include:

- Renal impairment
- Chronic liver disease
- Cardiac failure
- Alcoholism
- Respiratory failure
- ?Acute myocardial infarction

CLINICAL FEATURES

Clinical features are those of severe metabolic acidosis:

Clinical features of lactic acidosis

- Kussmaul respiration
- Decreased level of consciousness
- Abdominal pain
- Vomiting

MANAGEMENT

The standard therapy is intravenous bicarbonate administration, although dialysis may be useful for managing fluid and electrolyte disturbances and removing metformin, and ventilation may be used to assist correction of the acidosis. The mortality rate is still about 30% and therefore the best policy is to ensure safe usage of metformin.

HYPOGLYCAEMIA

EPIDEMIOLOGY AND PATHOPHYSIOLOGY

Hypoglycaemia is an iatrogenic complication of diabetes. It occurs when there is an inappropriate excess of circulating insulin, as a result of either sulfonylurea or insulin therapy, and reflects the inadequacy of therapy in reproducing physiological insulin profiles.

Up to 30% of patients with type 1 diabetes experience at least one severe episode of hypoglycaemia each year. The tighter the degree of glycaemic control, the more frequent are the episodes of mild and severe hypoglycaemia (**Fig. 6.9**).

SYMPTOMS

Patients are usually aware of impending hypoglycaemia due to the presence of autonomic warning symptoms:

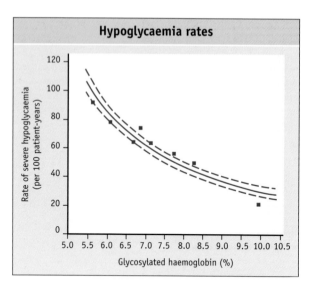

Fig. 6.9 *The incidence of severe hypoglycaemia compared with the level of glycaemic control, as measured by glycosylated haemoglobin, in the DCCT.*

Symptoms associated with hypoglycaemia and typical blood glucose concentrations at their onset

Blood glucose level 3.2–2.8 mmol/L:
- Autonomic symptoms
- Sweating
- Palpitations
- Tremor
- Hunger
- Nausea
- Early neuroglycopenic symptoms
- Difficulty in thinking
- Odd behaviour
- Headache

Blood glucose level <2.8 mmol/L:
- Later neuroglycopenic symptoms
- Drowsiness
- Confusion
- Speech difficulties

Blood glucose level <1.5 mmol/L:
- Severe neuroglycopenia
- Coma
- Convulsions

The danger is when the speed of onset does not allow patients to act in time to avert some degree of impairment of consciousness owing to neuroglycopenia. Alternatively, warning signs may become lost over time (called 'hypoglycaemia unawareness') and severe hypoglycaemia ensues, necessitating assistance from family, friends, colleagues or healthcare professionals.

MANAGEMENT

Patients need to be aware of the above symptoms of hypoglycaemia in order to be able to avert severe hypoglycaemic episodes. They should also ensure that anyone who may be called upon to intervene when they are unable to take appropriate action themselves is also educated about both the clinical signs and management (**Fig. 6.10**).

If the hypoglycaemic person is conscious and able to take the appropriate action, or is cooperative, 10–20 g of oral glucose should be taken, for example in the form of a glucose drink or tablet (**Fig. 6.11**). The response occurs within minutes. Then a longer-acting carbohydrate should be consumed, for example a sandwich, to ensure a gradual restoration and maintenance of normal blood glucose levels.

The semiconscious, uncooperative patient can be given glucose gel (**Fig. 6.11**) by direct administration to the gums and cheek, since it is rapidly absorbed through the buccal

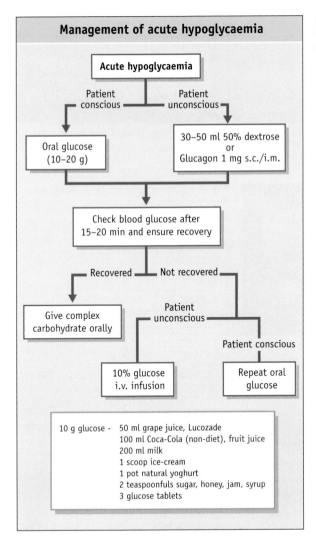

Fig. 6.10 *Example of a treatment algorithm for acute hypoglycaemia.*

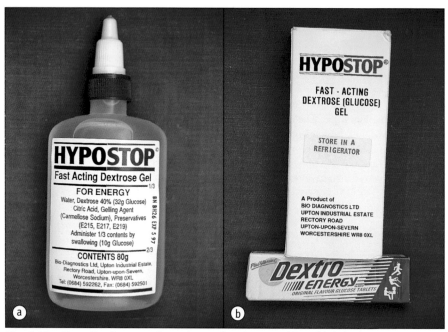

(a) (b)

Fig. 6.11   *Remedies for acute hypoglycaemia: glucose tablets (right) and glucose gel (both).*

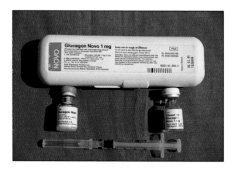

Fig. 6.12   *Glucagon kit for reversal of hypoglycaemia by injection.*

mucosa. If this is not possible or the patient is unconscious then glucagon, 1 mg, can be administered by intramuscular or subcutaneous injection (**Fig. 6.12**).

- Glucagon should probably *not* be used in patients with sulfonylurea-induced hypoglycaemia (see Ch. 4), since it stimulates insulin secretion from the β cell

If these measures are ineffective or unavailable then the obtunded patient should be transferred to hospital, where a 50% dextrose solution can be administered. Adults usually respond rapidly to about 50 ml, and children to much smaller doses. Any failure to respond should raise the possibility of accidental or deliberate insulin overdose, and a continuous infusion of 10% dextrose may be required to restore normal blood glucose levels. In this case it is, of course, important to consider whether there may be another cause for prolonged coma (see **Fig. 6.1**, p. 60).

COMPLICATIONS

The morbidity, both acute and chronic, associated with hypoglycaemia should not be underestimated (**Fig. 6.13**). The body's response to incipient hypoglycaemia is to divert the blood flow to increase cerebral perfusion, and to mount a counter-regulatory response to maintain blood glucose levels, thereby providing sufficient glucose for the brain's energy requirements. Neuroglycopenia represents a failure of this homeostatic mechanism and most acute consequences of hypoglycaemia reflect this. The commonest complication of hypoglycaemia is convulsion, which occurs in up to 7% of patients with type 1 diabetes. Protracted hypoglycaemia, albeit rare, may have devastating neurological consequences.

The long-term impact of hypoglycaemia also gives cause for concern, with increasing evidence for intellectual impairment leading to advice that patients should not only attempt to avoid hyperglycaemia but should also try to keep blood glucose levels consistently above 4 mmol/L.

Furthermore there may be social consequences of hypoglycaemia (see Ch. 3). It has been implicated in fatal road traffic accidents and frequent, severe hypoglycaemia will result in withdrawal of a driving licence. It may also affect employment, particularly where heavy machinery is involved. It has also been used as a defence for criminal actions, and hypoglycaemia-related automatism has occasionally been accepted as the reason for such actions.

PREVENTION

Patient education is crucial to avoidance of hypoglycaemia. Mild hypoglycaemia occurring up to twice per week may be an acceptable consequence of good glycaemic control. Precipitating factors should be sought either when hypoglycaemia occurs more frequently or following an episode of severe hypoglycaemia, and either avoided or measures introduced to counter their effects. Possible precipitants of acute hypoglycaemia include:

Fig. 6.13

Acute	Chronic
Convulsions	Permanent neurological deficit
Focal neurological deficits	Intellectual impairment
Accidental injury	Behavioural changes
Arrhythmias	
Acute vascular events	
Fatal hypoglycaemia coma	
? Unexplained diabetes-related deaths	

Morbidity associated with hypoglycaemia – acute and chronic complications.

- Increased circulating insulin levels
  - Inappropriate insulin dose
  - Intentional overdose insulin or sulfonylurea
  - Rapid absorption e.g. exercise, heat
- Missed meal
- Exercise
- Alcohol
- Drugs
  - Salicylates – augment sulfonylurea action
  - β blockers – diminished counter-regulatory response
- Menstrual cycle variation
- Breast feeding

Extra carbohydrate may be needed, for example, prior to exercise or in breast-feeding mothers. Injection into the thighs may need to be avoided prior to exercise if the resulting increase in blood flow results in more rapid absorption of insulin.

COUNTER-REGULATORY MECHANISMS

If nothing is done to avert hypoglycaemia then the body's counter-regulatory mechanisms (**Fig. 6.14**) will restore normal blood glucose levels by two mechanisms:

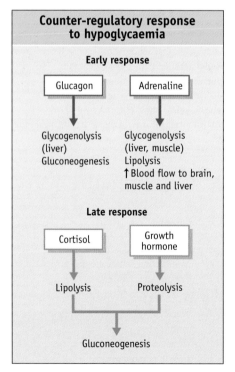

Fig. 6.14 *The counter-regulatory hormone response to acute hypoglycaemia.*

- Stimulation of hepatic glucose output by activation of the sympathetic nervous system
- Release of counter-regulatory hormones

Patients can thus be reassured that even if they lapse into coma this counter-regulatory system will restore normal blood glucose levels. This advice is particularly important to patients who suffer from nocturnal hypoglycaemia, which is a common problem. The diabetic person sweating profusely, becoming restless or suffering a convulsion often wakens partners. However there is evidence that nocturnal hypoglycaemia can persist for some hours and it has been implicated in a few cases of sudden death in young diabetics, in whom it has been presumed to cause cardiac arrhythmia.

HYPOGLYCAEMIA UNAWARENESS

Some patients lose their awareness of hypoglycaemia, either acutely or chronically. Acute loss occurs when tight control is instituted, and chronic loss occurs in most patients with type 1 diabetes after about 15 years. It was thought that the latter reflected impaired autonomic function with loss of the counter-regulatory hormone response. However, it now seems likely that both causes of loss of awareness result from neuroglycopenic symptoms occurring in close proximity to autonomic symptoms. In the acute situation this happens because the glycaemic threshold for the counter-regulatory hormone response is lowered, and in the chronic situation because this response is delayed.

In both situations, allowing blood glucose levels to run at a higher level reduces the problem of loss of awareness. In the acute situation the autonomic symptoms then occur at a higher blood glucose threshold, and in the chronic situation episodes of hypoglycaemia then occur less frequently. It has been suggested that the use of human insulin is the cause of chronic hypoglycaemia unawareness. There is little evidence to support this assertion. However, if a patient feels that this may have been the cause of the problem, converting to animal insulin would seem reasonable, particularly since there is no evidence that there is any advantage in the use of human insulin.

chapter 7

Macrovascular Diseases and Hypertension in Diabetes

EPIDEMIOLOGY AND PATHOPHYSIOLOGY

Macrovascular disease, which includes ischaemic heart disease, cerebrovascular disease and peripheral vascular disease, is a common cause of morbidity and mortality in patients with diabetes (**Fig. 7.1**). Indeed lesser degrees of glucose intolerance are associated with an increased risk of ischaemic heart disease (see **Fig. 5.3**, p. 56).

Type 1 diabetes

Patients with type 1 diabetes are at increased risk of macrovascular disease when they develop nephropathy, possibly because the same factors that result in endothelial damage within the glomerulus can cause damage to the vascular endothelium in larger arteries. This will predispose to accelerated atherosclerosis, which will be aggravated by the hypercholesterolaemia and hypertension that are associated with increasing proteinuria.

Type 2 diabetes

All patients with type 2 diabetes have a greater predisposition to macrovascular disease, often having a constellation of risk factors, which has been termed syndrome X, or Reaven's syndrome (see below and **Fig. 7.2**). Cardiovascular and cerebrovascular disease account for up to 70% of deaths in patients with type 2 diabetes. Microalbuminuria (see Ch. 9) correlates with vascular disease risk in these patients, probably reflecting widespread endothelial dysfunction. It is associated with clotting abnormalities and dyslipidaemia.

Women are affected to the same extent as men (**Fig. 7.1**). Also, premenopausal women appear to lose the protective effect of estrogen, which in non-diabetic women is responsible

Fig. 7.1 The increased risk of macrovascular complications associated with type 2 diabetes

	Estimated prevalence	Cause of mortality
Ischaemic heart disease	20%	50%
Cerebrovascular disease	15%	10%

Fig. 7.2 Estimated prevalence of risk factors in type 2 diabetes

Hypertension	40–65%
Micro/macroalbuminuria	40%
Obesity: BMI > 25 kg/m²	75%
Cholesterol > 6.5 mmol/L	40%
Triglycerides > 2.3 mmol/L	65%

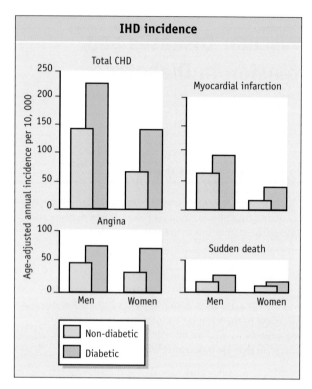

Fig. 7.3   *Prevalence of ischaemic heart disease by age and sex (from Pyörälä 1989 Diabetes and heart disease. In: Mogensen and Standl (eds) Prevention and Treatment of Diabetic Late Complications. Walter de Gruyter, with permission).*

for the very low incidence of vascular disease under the age of 50 compared with that in men of the same age (**Fig. 7.3**).

Syndrome X

The presence of multiple cardiac risk factors in many patients with type 2 diabetes has led to the concept of syndrome X. It has been hypothesized that insulin resistance and hyperinsulinaemia, resulting from environmental and genetic factors, are central to the development of:

- Glucose intolerance
- Hypertension
- Dyslipidaemia
- Coagulopathy

These factors promote accelerated atherosclerosis, explaining the increased risk of macrovascular disease (**Fig. 7.4**).

The DCCT and UKPDS suggest that improving glycaemic control alone appears to have only a marginally beneficial effect in reducing the risk of macrovascular complications in patients with diabetes and controlling these other factors is thus important to substantially reduce the risk.

HYPERTENSION

EPIDEMIOLOGY

Hypertension is up to three times more prevalent in patients with diabetes.

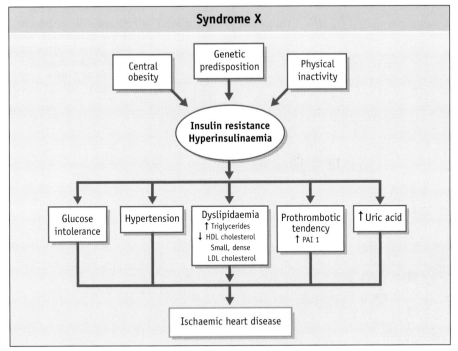

Fig. 7.4 *Pathophysiology and consequences of syndrome X.*

Type 1 diabetes

The excess of affected individuals in type 1 diabetes is almost entirely accounted for by the effect of diabetic nephropathy (see Ch. 9). A sustained rise in BP within the normal range may be one of the first features of nephropathy.

Type 2 diabetes

In patients with type 2 diabetes, obesity is an important contributor to the prevalence of hypertension, but accounts for only about 50% of the excess. Other factors contributing to the development of hypertension include sodium retention and activation of the renin–angiotensin system. Isolated systolic hypertension, which results from a loss of arterial elasticity, is usually seen in elderly people, but occurs about 20 years earlier in diabetic patients.

CLINICAL IMPLICATIONS

Hypertension accelerates the progression of microvascular complications. Even a rising BP within the normal range may be damaging to microvascular endothelium because of the failure of autoregulation (see **Fig. 5.4**, p. 57). There is evidence that patients with diabetes have disturbance of the normal diurnal changes in BP, in particular loss of the nocturnal fall, and this may also contribute to microvascular damage. The importance of hypertension in accelerating microvascular complications can be deduced from the observation that carotid artery stenosis and renal artery stenosis protect against ipsilateral retinopathy and nephropathy respectively.

Hypertension, as an independent risk factor, increases the likelihood of macrovascular complications, especially in those with type 2 diabetes (**Fig. 7.5**).

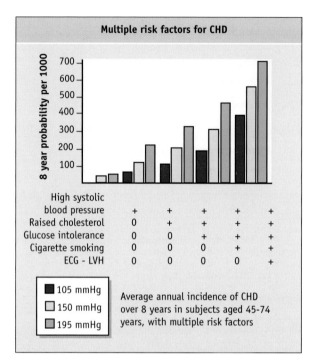

Fig. 7.5   *The impact of additional risk factors on incidence of ischaemic heart disease (from Houston 1989 American Heart Journal 118: 819–829, with permission).*

MANAGEMENT

The threshold for instituting BP-lowering strategies, and the target BP for those on treatment, should be 140/80 in patients with diabetes, because of the vulnerability of their vascular endothelium. This threshold should be lowered by 10 mmHg in those who already have evidence of complications.

Initial management should focus on lifestyle changes to promote BP lowering. These may include:

- Weight reduction
- Limit alcohol intake
- Reduce salt intake
- Increase physical activity
- Smoking cessation

Most patients will subsequently need to commence antihypertensive drug therapy (**Fig. 7.6**). However, there are potential metabolic consequences associated with antihypertensive agents that may need to be taken into consideration when deciding on appropriate therapy (**Fig. 7.7**).

Type 1 diabetes

In patients with type 1 diabetes angiotensin-converting enzyme (ACE) inhibitors are the antihypertensive agent of choice, because of their renoprotective effect (see Ch. 9). If they are

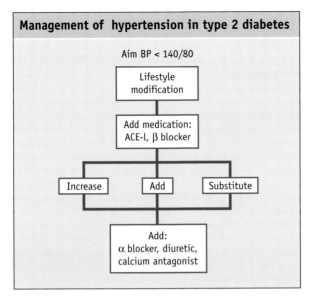

Management of hypertension in type 2 diabetes

Aim BP < 140/80

Lifestyle modification

Add medication: ACE-I, β blocker

Increase Add Substitute

Add: α blocker, diuretic, calcium antagonist

Fig. 7.6 *Algorithm for management of the diabetic patient with hypertension.*

Fig. 7.7 Metabolic effects of antihypertensive therapies

Drug	Total C	TG	HDL-C	Glucose	Insulin sensitivity	Exercise tolerance
Thiazide	↑	↑↑	↓	↑	↓	↔
β blocker	↔	↑↑↑	↓↓	↑	↓	↓
α blocker	↓	↓↓	↑	↔	↑	↔
Calcium antagonist	↔	↔	↔	↔	↔	↔
ACE inhibitor	↔	↔	↔	↔	↔	↔

not tolerated by the patient then the preferred alternatives are A-II receptor antagonists, calcium antagonists or α blockers.

Type 2 diabetes

In patients with type 2 diabetes the same drugs are usually the first-line agents. The ABCD and FACET trials suggested that ACE inhibitors may reduce the risk of morbidity from coronary heart disease in patients with type 2 diabetes. Both studies indicated that calcium antagonists were less effective, although the SYST-EUR study suggested these may be beneficial. In the UKPDS, tight BP control reduced the risk of microvascular and certain macrovascular complications (**Fig. 7.8**), and ACE inhibitors or β blockers were equally effective. The HOT study showed similar benefits of tight BP control (**Fig. 7.9**). Most recently the HOPE study has shown in patients with type 2 diabetes and at least one other cardiovascular risk factor, that the ACE inhibitor ramipril significantly reduced microvascular and macrovascular complications and mortality and, intriguingly, reduced the risk of developing diabetes in non-diabetic individuals with pre-existing heart disease. However, caution is needed when using ACE inhibitors because of the possibility that

Fig. 7.8   The benefits of tight blood pressure control (mean 144/82) in the UKPDS

Events	Risk reduction
Diabetes-related death	32%
Stroke	44%
Heart failure	56%
Progression of retinopathy	34%

Fig. 7.9   The benefits of tight blood pressure control in the HOT study: comparison of diabetic patients with all patients in study

Events	Target BP	Whole study	Diabetic patients
Major CVS	< 80	9.3	11.9
	< 85	10.0	18.6
	< 90	9.9	24.4
Stroke	< 80	3.8	6.4
	< 85	4.7	7.0
	< 90	4.0	9.1
CVS mortality	< 80	4.1	3.7
	< 85	3.8	11.2
	< 90	3.7	11.1

Fig. 7.10   Indications for specific antihypertensive therapy in patients with diabetes

	Choice	Caution
Angina	β blocker	
	Ca antagonist	
Post AMI	β blocker	
	ACE-I	
LVF	ACE-I	β blocker
	Ca antagonist	
PVD	α blocker	β blocker
	Ca antagonist	ACE-I
Impotence	α blocker	β blocker
	ACE-I	Thiazide
Hypoglycaemia		β blocker

LVF = Left ventricular fibrillation; PVD = peripheral vascular disease.

patients may have renal artery stenosis (see below). This is likely when there is evidence of peripheral vascular disease, femoral artery bruits being a particularly useful predictor.

There may be specific indications that favour the use of other agents (**Fig. 7.10**). For example, although β blockers may have adverse metabolic effects and mask hypoglycaemic symptoms they are preferred in patients with ischaemic heart disease. Many patients will require more than one agent – with about 30% needing at least three agents in UKPDS – and diuretics may be of value in this case, as they significantly enhance the effect of ACE inhibitors. It should also be noted that ACE inhibitors and β blockers are often less effective in Afro-Caribbean people, who appear to be at greater risk of developing complications of hypertension.

HYPERLIPIDAEMIA

EPIDEMIOLOGY
In patients with well-controlled type 1 diabetes lipid profiles are no different from the general population. Poor control is associated with elevation in total and low density lipoprotein (LDL) cholesterol, and in triglycerides. Nephropathy, from the onset, is associated with lipoprotein abnormalities, mainly affecting cholesterol levels.

CLINICAL IMPLICATIONS
Type 2 diabetes is associated with a characteristic dyslipidaemia. Inactivation of hormone-sensitive lipase, which is insulin responsive, results in an increase in the concentration of

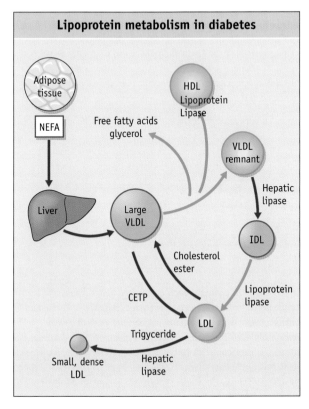

Fig. 7.11 *Lipoprotein metabolism in diabetes: green = decreased activity/concentration, red = increased activity/concentration in type 2 diabetes.*

83

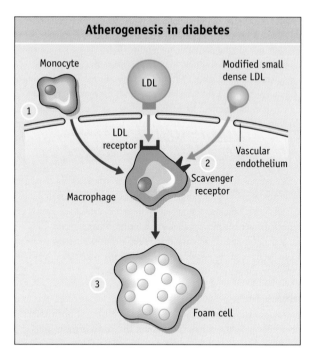

Fig. 7.12   Atherogenesis in diabetes. 1. Endothelium, damaged by protein glycation and hypertension, becomes more permeable to lipoproteins. 2. Small dense LDLs, more readily modified by glycation and oxidation, are taken into macrophages via scavenger pathway, which is not saturable in contrast to conventional LDL-receptor pathway. 3. Lipid-laden macrophages, foam cells, initiate formation fatty streak and generate cascade to sustain atheroma formation.

NEFA delivered to the liver. This leads to excessive very low density lipoprotein (VLDL) production. Also, with inhibition of lipoprotein lipase and activation of hepatic lipase, removal of cholesterol ester from these particles results in the formation of small, dense, triglyceride-rich LDL particles (**Fig. 7.11**). These are highly atherogenic, being more susceptible to oxidation and uncontrolled uptake into macrophages via the scavenger pathway, particularly if they are glycated (**Fig. 7.12**).

MANAGEMENT

Patients with hyperlipidaemia should be given dietary advice initially. The priorities for treatment are, in order:

1. Elevated LDL cholesterol
2. Decreased HDL cholesterol
3. Elevated triglycerides

Statin therapy

The large multicentre trials of statin therapy in patients with ischaemic heart disease demonstrated that the benefit of cholesterol lowering in patients with diabetes is at least as great as in non-diabetics. Thus statins are the first-line agents in diabetic patients with ischaemic heart disease and elevated cholesterol, although there is some evidence that the beneficial effects of statins are diminished in those with hypertriglyceridaemia. The same strategy should be employed in those without heart disease in whom hypercholesterolaemia is the main abnormality. The cholesterol level at which intervention is indicated in patients without ischaemic heart disease may be determined from risk factor tables.

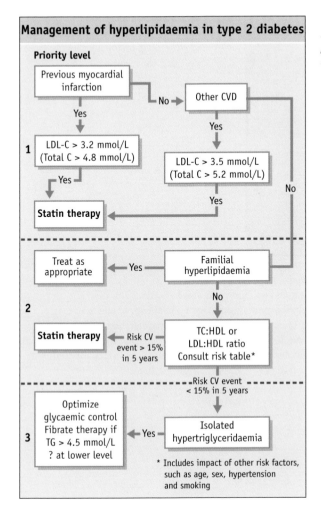

Fig. 7.13 *Algorithm for management of the diabetic patient with hyperlipidaemia.*

Other agents

Fibrates may be indicated in patients with triglyceride levels greater than 5 mmol/L, either alone or in combination with a statin (**Fig. 7.13**). Other lipid-lowering drugs are rarely used. Resins lower cholesterol levels but elevate triglyceride levels. Nicotinic acid aggravates glucose intolerance, but the longer acting derivative, acipimox, may improve glycaemic control by lowering levels of NEFA.

ISCHAEMIC HEART DISEASE

EPIDEMIOLOGY AND CLINICAL IMPLICATIONS

Patients with diabetes usually have more severe and extensive coronary artery atherosclerosis than do non-diabetics (**Fig. 7.14**). Ischaemic heart disease also presents at an earlier age in those with diabetes. However, autonomic neuropathy may diminish visceral pain perception. If so, then cardiac ischaemia is not associated with characteristic pain and may go

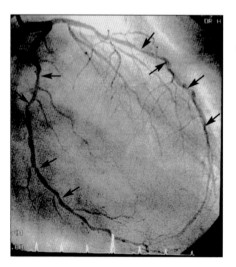

Fig. 7.14   *Coronary angiogram in patient with type 2 diabetes showing extensive coronary atheroma (arrows).*

unrecognized. Microvascular damage may affect the coronary circulation, exacerbating the effect of coronary artery narrowing and resulting in diabetic cardiomyopathy.

The relative risk of myocardial infarction is increased up to threefold and acute myocardial infarction is the cause of death in 30% of patients with diabetes. There is a 25–40% risk of death during hospitalization following myocardial infarction, which is up to three times that for non-diabetic individuals. A number of factors may contribute to this poor prognosis:

- More extensive atherosclerosis
- Diabetic cardiomyopathy
- Larger infarct size
- Dysrhythmia*
- Impaired pain perception*
- Impaired coronary artery vasodilatation*
- Coagulopathy
- Metabolic milieu

*Probably a reflection of autonomic neuropathy

Fig. 7.15   Benefits of acute and secondary prevention therapy in patients with diabetes

Therapy	Number treated to save one life
Insulin/glucose infusion	9
β blocker	11
Thrombolysis	27
Statin therapy	10
ACE inhibitor	36

MANAGEMENT

The DIGAMI (Diabetes Insulin Glucose infusion in Acute Myocardial Infarction) study has shown the benefit of insulin therapy in patients suffering an acute myocardial infarction

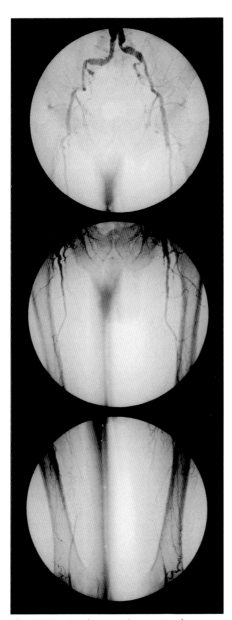

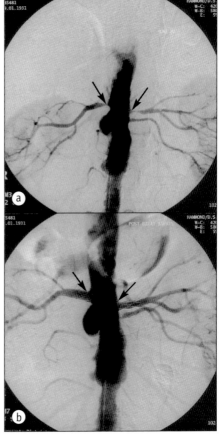

Fig. 7.16 *Angiogram demonstrating arterial irregularity with multiple narrowings in the lower limb arterial tree in a patient with type 2 diabetes.*

Fig. 7.17 *(a) Bilateral proximal renal artery stenosis (arrowed) in a patient with type 2 diabetes: before and (b) after stenting (arrowed).*

87

(AMI). There was almost a 30% reduction in mortality one year after AMI, with the greatest benefit seen in patients not previously taking insulin who were at low cardiac risk. Patients presenting with AMI and blood glucose levels of more than 11 mmol/L, regardless of whether they have a prior diagnosis of diabetes, should be treated with intravenous insulin and glucose to control blood glucose levels tightly and acutely. They should preferably be maintained on subcutaneous insulin for 3 months thereafter.

Diabetic patients should also be given standard therapies for treatment and prevention of myocardial infarction, such as thrombolysis, aspirin, β blockers, ACE inhibitors and statins, all of which are at least as beneficial in patients with diabetes as in non-diabetics (**Fig. 7.15**). Many patients are denied thrombolysis because of concerns about haemorrhage from proliferative retinopathy, but this should not be regarded as a contra-indication.

Coronary artery bypass surgery should be considered in patients with diabetes in the same way as in those without diabetes, but the diffuse disease extending into smaller vessels often makes it difficult to find a suitable site on which to graft. Angioplasty is usually less beneficial because of the multiple narrowings.

PERIPHERAL VASCULAR DISEASE

CLINICAL IMPLICATIONS
Macrovascular disease affecting the arteries to the lower limbs is an important factor in the pathogenesis of the diabetic foot (see Ch. 11). Atheromatous disease is usually extensive (**Fig. 7.16**) and extends more distally than in non-diabetic patients, which makes reconstructive surgery more difficult.

EPIDEMIOLOGY
Patients with peripheral vascular disease frequently have renal artery stenosis (**Fig. 7.17**), which may affect as many as 20% of patients with type 2 diabetes. The diagnosis should be considered in patients with the following symptoms:

Symptoms of renal artery stenosis

- Resistant hypertension
- Renal impairment, in the absence of increased urinary protein excretion
- Deteriorating renal function on ACE inhibitor therapy
- Flash pulmonary oedema

MANAGEMENT
The investigation of choice in such patients is renal angiography. Stenting may be effective in relieving the stenosis, although often there is little improvement in renal function or amelioration of hypertension.

chapter 8

Diabetic Eye Disease

EPIDEMIOLOGY

Diabetic retinopathy is the commonest cause of blindness in people aged 16 to 64. Diabetic eye disease accounts for 12% of all new registrations for blindness and 8% of those for partial sightedness.

Five years after diagnosis about 20% of patients with type 1 diabetes have detectable retinopathy, and by 20 years over 90% will be affected, of which 50% will have proliferative retinopathy (PDR) (**Fig. 8.1**). In 20% of cases this PDR will eventually be sight threatening and approximately 2% of patients with type 1 diabetes will become blind.

Twenty per cent of patients with type 2 diabetes have retinopathy detectable at diagnosis, and up to 80% 10 years later. Maculopathy is the commoner threat to sight in these patients, with 15% of older patients at risk.

PATHOPHYSIOLOGY

Retinal arteries are end-arteries and autoregulation is important in protecting the retinal microcirculation against damage from BP fluctuations. Pericytes, which line the endothelium, control the diameter of the capillaries and proliferation of the endothelium, and constitute a blood–retinal barrier. In patients with diabetes the pericytes are lost. Also, hyperglycaemia results in hyperperfusion and endothelial damage (**Fig. 8.2**).

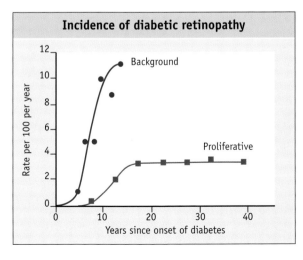

Fig. 8.1 *Incidence of diabetic retinopathy according to the duration of type 1 diabetes (from Mogensen and Standl (eds) 1989 Prevention and Treatment of Diabetic Late Complications. Walter de Gruyter, with permission).*

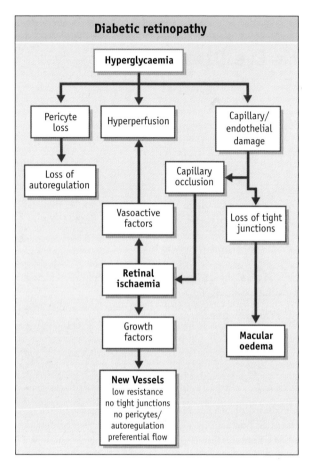

Fig. 8.2 *Pathophysiology of diabetic retinopathy.*

Initial capillary damage is associated with extravasation of blood and protein. Later there is capillary occlusion, which is associated with retinal ischaemia and new vessel formation. These new vessels are particularly prone to damage because of the following features:

- Low resistance
- Failure of autoregulation due to lack of pericytes, so they receive blood flow preferentially
- Lack of tight junctions

These factors predispose to vitreous and preretinal haemorrhage. Fibrous tissue that is formed as the haemorrhage resolves can cause traction retinal detachment. If widespread, it can even impair vision, as can unresolved vitreous haemorrhage (**Fig. 8.3**).

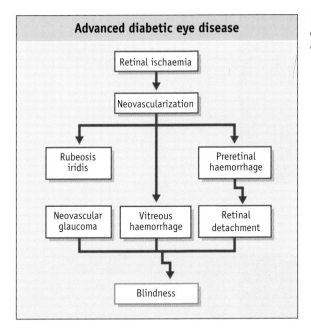

Fig. 8.3 *The progression of advanced diabetic eye disease.*

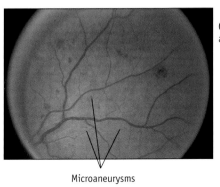

Other patches are haemorrhages

Fig. 8.4 *Microaneurysms and haemorrhages in early background diabetic retinopathy.*

Microaneurysms

CLINICAL FEATURES

Patients rarely experience symptoms related to retinopathy. Vitreous haemorrhage may cause an acute loss of vision, or give the impression of floaters in the field of vision. Severe ischaemic retinopathy and maculopathy may cause deterioration in visual acuity. However, screening identifies most lesions.

The earliest lesions are microaneurysms, which are evidence of endothelial dysfunction; as their numbers increase, they are usually associated with small retinal haemorrhages (**Fig. 8.4**). Other, later, manifestations of background retinopathy are hard exudates, which result from leakage of lipid into the outer layer of the retina, and cotton-wool spots (soft exudates), which indicate infarction in the nerve layer (**Fig. 8.5**). The presence of five or more cotton-wool spots implies significant ischaemia, and other features of preproliferative

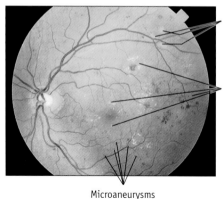

Pale milky blotches
cotton wool spots

White patches
hard exudates
Haemorrhages
as before

Microaneurysms

Fig. 8.5   *Hard exudates and cotton-wool spots in background diabetic retinopathy.*

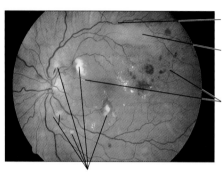

Venous abnormalities
looping + beeding

Particularly
pale area of
retina

IRMAs
abnormal thin
irregular blood
vessels (red)

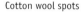

Cotton wool spots

Fig. 8.6   *Retinal pallor and IRMAs in preproliferative diabetic retinopathy.*

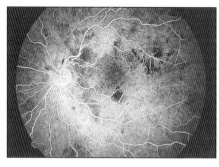

Dark patches
ischaemic
regions

Dots
Microaneurysms

Venous looping and
IRMAs visible

Fig. 8.7   *Fluorescein angiogram showing areas of retinal ischaemia (same patient as in Fig. 8.6).*

retinopathy may also be seen. These intraretinal microvascular abnormalities (IRMAs) and venous changes reflect the response of the retinal circulation to ischaemia (**Fig. 8.6**).

Retinal ischaemia (**Fig. 8.7**) stimulates the formation of new blood vessels (**Fig. 8.8**), and rupture of these vessels results in preretinal or vitreous haemorrhage.

Visual loss is associated with a number of clinical features:

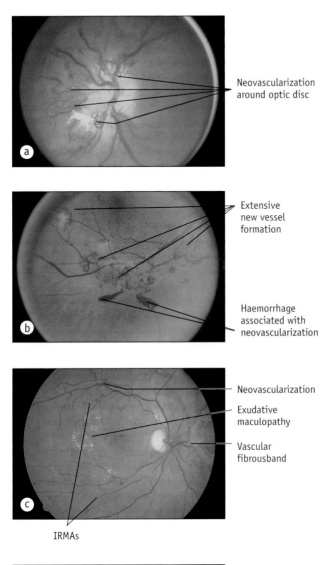

Neovascularization around optic disc

Extensive new vessel formation

Haemorrhage associated with neovascularization

Neovascularization

Exudative maculopathy

Vascular fibrousband

IRMAs

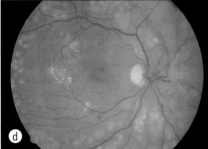

Fig. 8.8 *Proliferative diabetic retinopathy: neovascularization: (a) neovascularization affecting the disc (NVD); (b) neovascularization affecting the peripheral retina (NVE); (c) neovascularization with fibrosis and exudative maculopathy; (d) same patient as (c) immediately after laser therapy.*

Clinical features associated with loss of vision

- **Advanced eye disease**   Fibrous proliferation (**Fig. 8.9**) following resorption of haemorrhage, which may result in retinal detachment
  Rubeosis iridis (**Fig. 8.10**) and neovascular glaucoma, which results from extensive retinal ischaemia or detachment
- **Maculopathy**   Macular oedema
  Extensive macular hard exudate (**Fig. 8.11**)
  Macular ischaemia

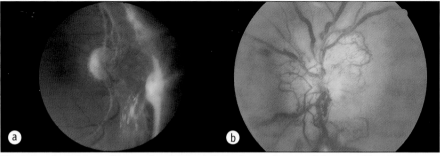

Fig. 8.9   *Retinitis proliferans in advanced diabetic eye disease: (a) severe fibrosis associated with neovascularization to one side of the optic disc; (b) vitreous haemorrhage causing greenish hue and obscuring the retina, although neovascularization can be seen.*

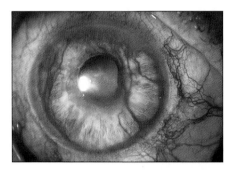

Fig. 8.10   *Rubeosis iridis in advanced diabetic eye disease (from Mr J Hillman, with permission).*

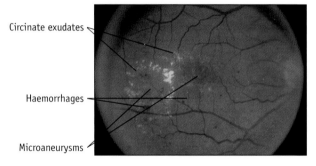

Circinate exudates

Haemorrhages

Microaneurysms

Fig. 8.11   *Background diabetic retinopathy affecting the macula in maculopathy.*

The only evidence of maculopathy, particularly that due to oedema, may be an unexplained loss of visual acuity, and patients who experience this should be referred for ophthalmological assessment.

MANAGEMENT

PREVENTIVE TREATMENT

Prevention or delaying of retinopathy can be achieved by good glycaemic control and lowering of BP. In the DCCT the development of retinopathy was delayed in the intensively treated patients without retinopathy at randomization (**Fig. 8.12**). There was an almost 30% reduction in new cases, and progression was delayed by up to 75% in those patients with retinopathy initially (**Fig. 8.13**). The UKPDS showed similar benefits of intensive glycaemic control in patients with type 2 diabetes. However, tightening of glycaemic control can at first worsen the retinopathy (**Figs 8.12, 8.13**). Possible mechanisms for this phenomenon are a decrease in blood flow worsening the ischaemia, or the effect of increased IGF-I levels. The latter are stimulated by insulin but also increase in puberty and pregnancy, so this may explain the worsening of retinopathy seen in these situations.

Lowering of BP in hypertensive patients leads to a slowing of the rate of progression of retinopathy. Recent data from the EUCLID study suggest that ACE inhibitor therapy may also prevent the development and progression of retinopathy in patients with type 1 diabetes, irrespective of BP. In type 2 diabetes the UKPDS showed that tight BP control delayed the progression of retinopathy and reduced the need for photocoagulation, and that ACE inhibitors and β blockers were equally effective.

Smoking and hyperlipidaemia accelerate the progression of retinopathy and should be tackled. Aspirin therapy has not proved to be of benefit.

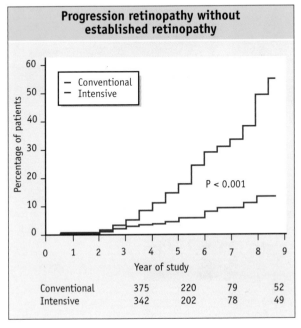

Fig. 8.12 *Effect of intensive insulin therapy in patients without retinopathy – progression of retinopathy in conventional and intensive treatment groups in the DCCT (from the Diabetes Control and Complications Trial Research Group 1993. New England Journal of Medicine 329: 977–986, with permission).*

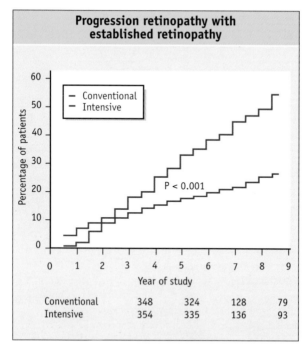

Fig. 8.13 *Effect of intensive insulin therapy in patients with retinopathy – progression of retinopathy in conventional and intensive treatment groups in the DCCT (from the Diabetes Control and Complications Trial Research Group 1993. New England Journal of Medicine 329: 977–986, with permission).*

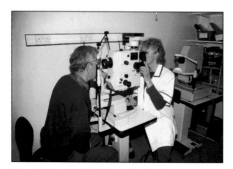
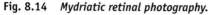

Fig. 8.14 *Mydriatic retinal photography.*

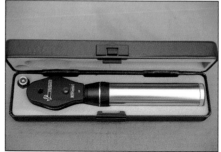

Fig. 8.15 *Ophthalmoscope for indirect fundoscopy.*

Screening programmes

The lack of symptoms associated with significant retinopathy means that screening programmes need to be in place to identify affected individuals before sight is threatened. Screening may be performed by one of two methods:

- Retinal photography (**Fig. 8.14**), preferably through a dilated pupil, since non-mydriatic photography has not, as yet, been fully validated
- Indirect ophthalmoscopy (**Fig. 8.15**) by
  — a diabetologist
  — an optometrist

Whichever method is employed, the criteria for a screening investigation must be satisfied. These include:

- Sensitivity and specificity > 80%
- Efficient patient call-up and recall system
- Annual screening interval
- Access to an ophthalmologist if an abnormality is identified
- Low technical failure rate
- Audit and quality control programmes

Patients must also be made aware that other assessments are needed to ensure good eye health (**Fig. 8.16**). These are most readily accessible through optometry services.

If significant retinopathy is identified then urgent or early ophthalmological assessment, depending on the nature of the lesion, is mandatory (**Fig. 8.17**). Fluorescein angiography (see **Fig. 8.7**, p. 92) may be helpful in assessing the extent of ischaemia and identifying lesions before focal laser therapy.

PHOTOCOAGULATION AND SURGERY

Pan-retinal photocoagulation (**Fig. 8.18**) ablates all regions of the retina except those essential for central vision, the macula and its nerve efferents. This concentrates the blood supply on the untreated retina, therefore reducing ischaemia and thus removing the stimulus to neovascularization and causing new vessels to regress. If used as soon as high risk PDR develops, this technique can reduce the risk of severe visual loss by over 90%. However, there is a risk of a decrease in visual acuity and visual field loss associated with full pan-retinal photocoagulation.

Focal laser photocoagulation is an effective treatment for maculopathy, with burns being delivered in a grid pattern aimed at leaking microaneurysms.

Photocoagulation is performed using an argon laser. An anaesthetic, such as proxymetacaine hydrochloride, is applied topically to the cornea. A contact lens is applied and burns are delivered using direct visualization (**Fig. 8.19**).

Vitreoretinal surgery has improved the prognosis for sight in patients with advanced diabetic eye disease. Surgical vitrectomy, in particular, may be beneficial in certain patients suffering vitreous haemorrhage or retinal detachment.

VISUAL AIDS

Unfortunately, visual impairment still affects a minority of patients and can be very disabling. Routine management of diabetes can become difficult, particularly for those

Fig. 8.16   Recommended annual eye assessment for the patient with diabetes

- Visual acuity; refraction if indicated
- Measurement of intraocular pressure
- Slit-lamp examination:
  - anterior segment, particularly for cataract
  - macular thickening
- Retinal examination with dilated pupil:
  - either ophthalmoscopy
  - or retinal photography

Fig. 8.17   Criteria for referral for specialist ophthalmological opinion

Immediate assessment	• Vitreous haemorrhage
	• Retinal detachment
	• Neovascular glaucoma
Urgent referral	• Rubeosis iridis
(see within 1 week)	• Fibrous proliferation
	• Preretinal haemorrhage
	• New vessels (disc or elsewhere)
	• Decreased visual acuity ($\geq$ two lines)
	• Non-proliferative retinopathy with macular involvement
Semiurgent referral	• Preproliferative retinopathy
(see within 6 weeks)	— venous changes
	— IRMAs
	— multiple haemorrhages or cotton-wool spots
	• Large exudates within major temporal vascular arcades
Non-urgent referral	• Cataract

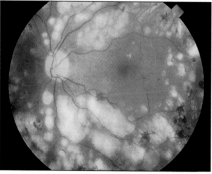

Fig. 8.18   *Extensive laser burns following panretinal photocoagulation.*

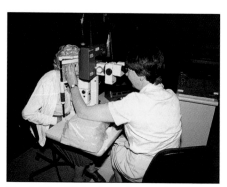

Fig. 8.19   *Diabetic patient undergoing panretinal photocoagulation.*

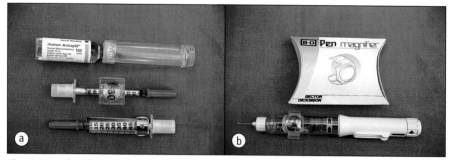

Fig. 8.20   *(a, b) Magnifying aids for insulin syringes and pens to assist the visually impaired diabetic patient.*

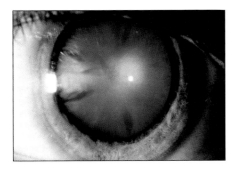

Fig. 8.21 *Cataract in a diabetic patient.*

patients treated with insulin, although there are various visual aids (**Fig. 8.20**) to assist such patients, including speaking blood glucose meters. Patients with visual impairment should be aware of potential benefits (see Ch. 3) and should be informed of local and national patient support groups.

OTHER EYE COMPLICATIONS

NEOVASCULAR GLAUCOMA

Widespread retinal ischaemia may stimulate neovascularization of the iris – causing rubeosis iridis (see **Fig. 8.10**, p.94). Obstruction of aqueous humour drainage by these new vessels leads to increased intraocular pressure, which is termed neovascular glaucoma. This carries a poor prognosis for vision.

There is some evidence to suggest that, even in the absence of iris neovascularization, diabetic patients have higher than average intraocular pressures.

CATARACT

Cataract is a common problem in diabetic patients (**Fig. 8.21**), with a higher prevalence at any given age than in the general population. Cataract extraction may expose unrecognized retinopathy and may result in deterioration of pre-existing retinopathy.

chapter 9

Diabetic Nephropathy

EPIDEMIOLOGY

Diabetic nephropathy is the commonest cause of end-stage renal failure worldwide. The earliest clinical feature of diabetic nephropathy is microalbuminuria, which has a prevalence of about 60% in patients with type 1 diabetes of 30 years' duration. However, less than 50% of these patients will progress to end-stage renal failure, and this number appears to be decreasing over time as the effects of tighter glycaemic control become apparent. The peak incidence of nephropathy occurs after about 20 years' disease duration, and declines sharply with duration over 30 years. The prevalence of diabetic nephropathy is much lower in type 2 diabetes, with less than 10% of individuals affected. Patients of Afro-Caribbean and Asian origin have much higher prevalence rates than Caucasians.

There is familial clustering of diabetic nephropathy, implying a genetic predisposition. Over 95% of patients with diabetic nephropathy also have retinopathy; therefore the absence of the latter complication may be evidence of an alternative cause for renal impairment (**Fig. 9.1**).

Other factors are associated with the development of nephropathy including:

- Poor glycaemic control
- Hypertension
- Cigarette smoking
- Elevated LDL cholesterol

Fig. 9.1   Renal impairment in the diabetic patient independent of diabetic nephropathy

Consider if:
- No retinopathy, particularly in type 1 diabetes
- No proteinuria
- Rapid decline in renal function
- Acute nephritic syndrome
- Red cell casts or marked haematuria

Commoner in patients with diabetes:
- Hypertensive nephropathy
- Renovascular disease
- Renal papillary necrosis
- Chronic pyelonephritis

PATHOPHYSIOLOGY

The stages of diabetic nephropathy are:

1. Hyperfiltration
2. Microalbuminuria
3. Overt proteinuria
4. Declining glomerular filtration rate
5. End-stage renal failure

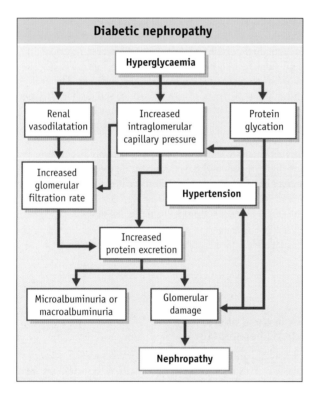

Fig. 9.2   *Pathophysiology of diabetic nephropathy.*

Hyperfiltration and increased renal size can be demonstrated in all patients at diagnosis of type 1 diabetes, and are a result of increased renal blood flow. They resolve once glycaemic control is established, but subsequently recur in some patients. This results from the interplay of endothelial dysfunction, haemodynamic factors and changes in the extracellular matrix (**Fig. 9.2**). Widespread endothelial dysfunction in these patients may explain the coexistence of macrovascular disease and nephropathy.

In the characteristic lesion of diabetic nephropathy, the Kimmelstiel–Wilson, there is nodular glomerulosclerosis, with glomerular basement membrane thickening and mesangial expansion. Increasing pore size in the glomerular basement membrane, loss of negative charge and increased glomerular capillary pressure underlie the transition through microalbuminuria to macroalbuminuria. Hypertension, which is aggravated by salt and water retention in patients with nephropathy, in turn increases capillary pressure so accelerating the glomerular damage.

CLINICAL FEATURES

MICROALBUMINARIA

The earliest feature of diabetic nephropathy is microalbuminuria. This is defined as follows:

Definition of microalbuminaria

- 30–300 mg/24 hours in a 24 hour collection
- 20–200 µg/min in an overnight collection
- Urine albumin:creatinine ratio 3.0–30 mg/mmol on a spot early morning urine

Up to 80% of patients with type 1 diabetes will develop nephropathy over the next 10 years, compared with about 20% of patients with type 2 diabetes. However, microalbuminuria is a strong predictor of macrovascular disease risk in type 2 diabetes, probably because it reflects widespread endothelial dysfunction. It is correlated with the following factors:

- Poor glycaemic control
- Age
- Hypertension
- Smoking

The incidence of macrovascular complications is increased two- to fivefold in patients with microalbuminuria, with an even more marked increase in cardiovascular mortality.

Therefore it is recommended that all patients with diabetes are screened annually for microalbuminuria (**Fig. 9.3**).

Hypertension usually accompanies microalbuminuria. Indeed, the earliest change may be a rise in BP within the normal range. On average the BP will be about 135/85 at onset of microalbuminuria, increasing to 145/95 with proteinuria and again to 160/100 once creatinine starts to rise.

PROTEINURIA

Overt proteinuria, which is Dipstix positive, represents established nephropathy. These patients will almost certainly progress to end-stage renal failure. The rate of progression can be determined by serial reciprocal creatinine plots (**Fig. 9.4**).

MACROVASCULAR COMPLICATIONS

Macrovascular complications are a common problem once established proteinuria occurs. About 40% of patients will develop ischaemic heart disease over the first 6 years, and there is an almost 40-fold increase in cardiovascular mortality compared with the normal population. The median survival time for patients developing proteinuria is 10 years.

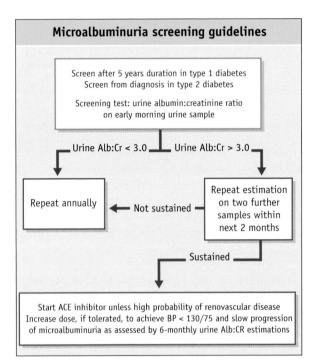

Fig. 9.3 *Guidelines for microalbuminuria screening.*

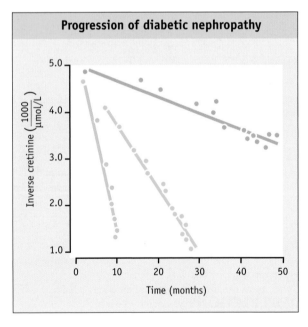

Fig. 9.4 *The reciprocal creatinine plot as a guide to progression of nephropathy.*

An important consideration is the need for vascular imaging. Myocardial infarction is a common cause of death after renal transplantation, but this could be reduced by coronary artery bypass surgery. However, use of contrast media may acutely worsen renal function;

therefore contrast investigations should be done, where possible, before the creatinine exceeds 250 μmol/L.

OTHER RENAL DISEASES

Renal impairment in diabetes is not necessarily due to nephropathy. Hypertension and renovascular disease are important causes in patients with type 2 diabetes, and other renal diseases may occur irrespective of diabetes. Presence of the following clinical features suggests an alternative cause:

Clinical features suggesting other renal disease

- Absence of retinopathy
- Absence of micro/macroalbuminuria
- Persistent haematuria or red cell casts
- Rapid deterioration in previously normal renal function or rapid onset of overt proteinuria

Where these are found, patients should be evaluated for other forms of renal disease by renal imaging (usually ultrasound initially), an immunological screen and often renal biopsy.

MANAGEMENT

The onset and progression of nephropathy can be prevented or delayed by good glycaemic control. In the DCCT the risk of progressing from normoalbuminuria to microalbuminuria in type 1 diabetes was reduced by almost 40%, and from microalbuminuria to proteinuria by almost 55% (**Fig. 9.5**). A similar benefit in type 2 diabetes was seen with intensive glycaemic control in the UKPDS.

BP control, aiming for a target of less than 130/80, delays the progression of nephropathy, by decreasing albuminuria and slowing the decline in glomerular filtration rate.

DRUG THERAPY

ACE inhibitors appear to have a renoprotective effect that is additional to their antihypertensive action. This is probably because they preferentially dilate the efferent glomerular arteriole, thus reducing intraglomerular pressure. This action also accounts for the worsening renal function seen in patients with renal artery stenosis treated with ACE inhibitors. The use of captopril has been shown to reduce the risk of dialysis, transplantation or death in patients with type 1 diabetes and overt proteinuria by 50%. It appears to be an effect of this class of drugs generally, as other ACE inhibitors have also been shown to slow the rate of progression of microalbuminuria in patients with type 1 and type 2 diabetes.

In patients with type 1 diabetes, ACE inhibitor therapy should be introduced in all patients with microalbuminuria, whether they are normotensive or hypertensive, and the dose increased to control the BP and retard progression of microalbuminuria.

Reduction of dietary protein intake to less than 0.6 g/kg per day may slow the rate of progression of established nephropathy, but such a diet is poorly tolerated.

Total and LDL cholesterol levels rise and HDL cholesterol levels fall with worsening renal impairment. Statin therapy may slow the rate of progression of nephropathy. More importantly, patients with nephropathy need diligent surveillance for and aggressive management of macrovascular complications (**Fig. 9.6**).

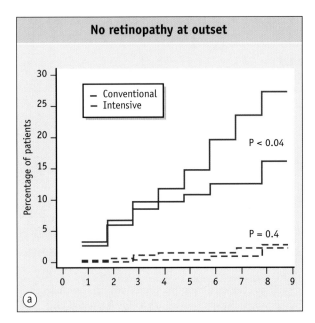

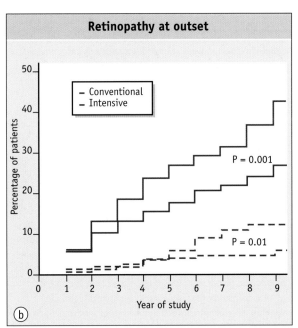

Fig. 9.5   *Effect of intensive insulin therapy on progression of nephropathy (a) in patients without retinopathy at outset and (b) in patients with retinopathy at outset (solid line = microalbuminuria; dashed line = albuminuria) (from The Diabetes Control and Complications Trial Research Group 1993 New England Journal of Medicine 329: 977–986, with permission).*

Patients should be referred for further management to a specialist renal unit once serum creatinine exceeds 200 μmol/L. Oral hypoglycaemic agents, with the exception of second-generation sulfonylureas such as gliclazide, are excreted renally and so should be avoided. It is probably preferable to convert all patients to insulin.

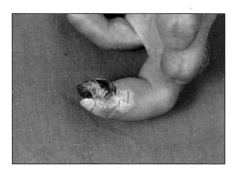

Fig. 9.6 *Diabetic patient with chronic renal impairment complicated by digital gangrene.*

RENAL REPLACEMENT THERAPY

Renal replacement therapy with dialysis or renal transplantation is effective for patients with diabetic nephropathy. In the UK, continuous ambulatory peritoneal dialysis (CAPD) is favoured for diabetic patients. It is inexpensive, allows patients to remain independent and does not require vascular access. Haemodialysis is preferred in the USA.

Transplantation is usually considered when serum creatinine reaches 500 μmol/L, in patients less than 65 years of age and without severe vascular disease. The 5-year survival is over 60% for cadaver and 80% for live-related grafts. After transplantation, frequent problems include the sequelae of other complications such as myocardial infarction, foot ulceration and amputation. Cardiovascular disease is the usual cause of death, although sepsis is not uncommon.

chapter 10

Skin and Soft Tissue Problems in Diabetes

SKIN DISEASES ASSOCIATED WITH DIABETES

Skin diseases associated with diabetes can be classified as:

> **Classification of skin diseases associated with diabetes**
>
> - Collagen disorders
> - Diabetic dermopathy
> - Diabetic bullous disease
> - Skin infections
> - Other associated conditions

COLLAGEN DISORDERS

The commonest collagen disorder affecting the skin is necrobiosis lipoidica (**Fig. 10.1**), which is characterized by atrophic, yellow plaques associated with prominent telangiectasiae, usually on the shin. Over 75% of those affected have glucose intolerance, whilst at least 1% of patients with diabetes experience this condition, usually young Caucasian women. However, there is no relationship between the natural history of the necrobiosis and glycaemic control. It is the result of hyaline degeneration of collagen and the histological appearance is similar to that of granuloma annulare (**Fig. 10.2**). There is controversy as to whether this condition is also associated with diabetes. Necrobiosis may respond to topical or locally injected steroids, but treatment is usually ineffective. Camouflage creams may be used to mask the lesions.

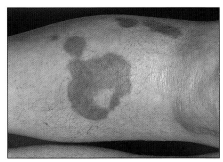

Fig. 10.1 *Necrobiosis lipoidica.*

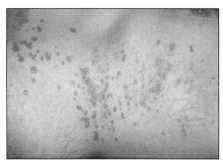

Fig. 10.2 *Granuloma annulare.*

109

Glycation of the collagen in skin and soft tissues, with thickening and loss of elasticity, results in a variety of different conditions including Dupuytren's contracture, scleroedema and carpal tunnel syndrome. Cheiroarthropathy may affect as many as 35% of patients, and is characterized by limitation of movement of the small joints of the hands, the overlying skin having a waxy appearance. When the patient is asked to hold their hands together, as if in prayer, there is a characteristic failure of occlusion (**Fig. 10.3**).

DIABETIC DERMOPATHY
This condition may affect as many as 50% of diabetic patients, and is commoner in men. The initial lesions are small red papules, which scale over to leave brown atrophic scars (**Fig. 10.4**). The usual site for the lesions is the shin, although bony prominences may be affected. Microvascular changes may be observed in histological specimens, but the cause of this condition remains obscure.

DIABETIC BULLOUS DISEASE
Diabetic bullae are a rare complication of diabetes, usually affecting young males with long-standing diabetes (**Fig. 10.5**). The bullae are intraepidermal, and present as tense blisters most commonly on the limbs, and especially the feet. The autoimmune blistering disease, bullous pemphigoid (**Fig. 10.6**), may also be more common in patients with diabetes.

SKIN INFECTIONS
Superficial skin infections, such as folliculitis, abscesses (**Fig. 10.7**) and erysipelas (**Fig. 10.8**), probably occur more frequently in patients with diabetes. *Staphylococcus aureus* is a common pathogen.

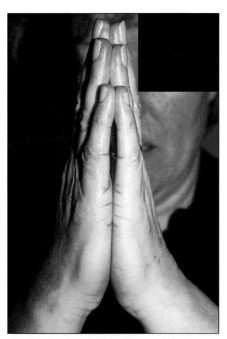

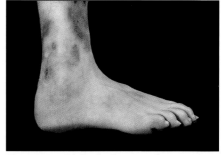

Fig. 10.4   *Diabetic dermopathy.*

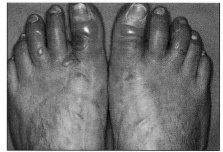

Fig. 10.3   *'The prayer sign' – diabetic cheiroarthropathy.*

Fig. 10.5   *Diabetic bullae.*

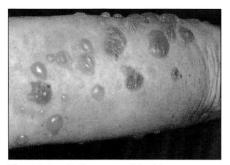

Fig. 10.6 *Bullous pemphigoid.*

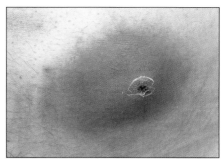

Fig. 10.7 *Skin abscess in a diabetic patient.*

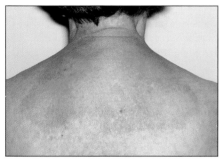

Fig. 10.8 *Erysipelas in a diabetic patient.*

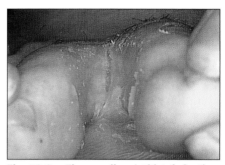

Fig. 10.9 *Tinea pedis – 'athlete's foot'.*

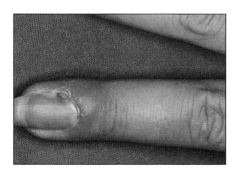

Fig. 10.10 *Chronic paronychia due to C. albicans infection.*

Poor glycaemic control is associated with *Candida albicans* infections, particularly vulvovaginitis and balanitis. Oral fluconazole may be more effective than topical therapy at eradicating these infections.

Dermatophyte infections (or tinea pedis) are common in patients with diabetes. They are often widespread, particularly in the web spaces of the feet (**Fig. 10.9**). Systemic therapy, usually with terbinafine, may be necessary.

A variety of nail infections may occur, including dermatophyte infection, and acute or chronic paronychia. This is usually due to candidal infection (**Fig. 10.10**), but may be caused by staphylococcal infection.

111

OTHER ASSOCIATED CONDITIONS

The following are cutaneous markers of diabetes:

Cutaneous markers of diabetes

- Vitiligo, which is a marker of autoimmune disease*
- Acanthosis nigricans, which is a marker of insulin resistance (see Fig. 2.15, p.14)
- Periungual telangiectasiae, which probably reflects microvascular disease

Lipoatrophy and lipohypertrophy

Insulin injection sites may show evidence of lipoatrophy (**Fig. 10.11**) or lipohypertrophy (**Fig. 10.12**). Lipoatrophy is thought to result from a local immune response against the injected insulin. Lipohypertrophy is due to the local lipogenic action of insulin.

Secondary causes

Secondary causes of diabetes may be associated with skin conditions. These include the bronze pigmentation of haemochromatosis, necrolytic migratory erythema, and the pathognomonic rash of the glucagonoma syndrome (see Ch. 22).

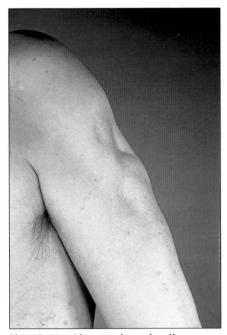

Fig. 10.11 *Lipoatrophy at insulin injection site.*

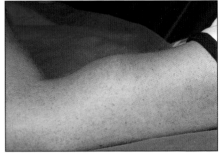

Fig. 10.12 *Lipohypertrophy at insulin injection site.*

OTHER CONNECTIVE TISSUE DISORDERS

Diabetic osteopathy is a patchy osteopenia associated with resorption of the distal metatarsals and proximal phalanges, and appears to be a self-limiting condition. Diabetic osteolysis is a disabling condition characterized by joint pain and effusion that usually affects the hip or knee. It is most commonly seen in women with type 2 diabetes over the age of 50. It may respond to low dose glucocorticoids.

INFECTIOUS DISEASES IN DIABETES

Patients with diabetes are more prone to infection because hyperglycaemia impairs leukocyte function and hence bacterial killing. In addition there are a number of infections that are particularly associated with diabetes, including:

- Gas-forming bacterial infections (**Figs 10.13, 10.14**)
- Papillary necrosis – sloughing of the renal papillae leading to acute renal failure as a consequence of pyelonephritis
- Pneumonia due to *Staphylococcus aureus* or *Klebsiella* infection (**Fig. 10.15**)
- Necrotizing fasciitis due to Group A (β haemolytic) *Streptococcus* infection
- Malignant otitis externa – an aggressive infection with *Pseudomonas aeruginosa*, which can invade intracranially but appears to respond well to quinolones (**Fig. 10.16**)
- Mucormycosis – a saprophytic infection, usually rhinocerebral and presenting with involvement of nasal sinuses. There is a risk of intracranial spread (**Fig. 10.17**), or pulmonary. Treatment is with surgical debridement and amphotericin B, but both methods carry a high mortality

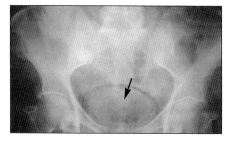

Fig. 10.13 *Emphysematous cystitis due to gas-forming bacterial infection; the bladder is outlined by air (arrowed).*

113

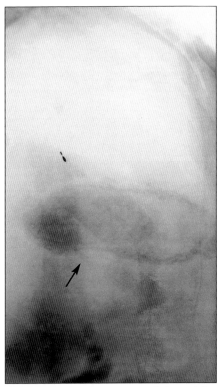

Fig. 10.14 *Emphysematous cholecystitis due to gas-forming bacterial infection; the gall bladder is outlined by air (arrowed).*

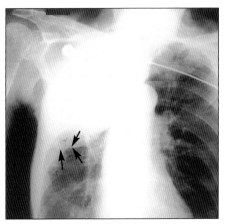

Fig. 10.15 *Klebsiella pneumonia affecting the right upper lobe in a patient with diabetes. Note the downward-sloping of the horizontal fissure due to upper lobe expansion, which is often seen with this infection (arrowed).*

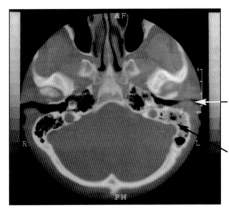

Fig. 10.16 *CT scan showing opacification of the auditory canal (arrowed) due to malignant otitis externa.*

Soft tissue thickening in external auditory canal

Loss of mastoid airspaces due to filling with exudate

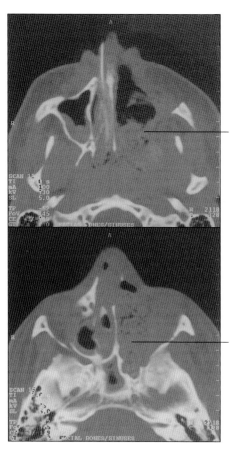

Soft tissue
mass with
extensive bone
destruction

Soft tissue
mass eroding
back into
skull bone

Fig. 10.17 *CT scan
showing destruction of
the paranasal sinuses and
a soft tissue mass
(arrowed) due to
rhinocerebral
mucormycosis.*

chapter 11

Diabetic Neuropathy

INTRODUCTION

The diabetic neuropathies are diverse disorders of nerve function associated with diabetes. The pathophysiology and natural history vary according to the type of neuropathy. The most useful classification is into chronic progressive and acute neuropathies (**Fig. 11.1**).

In the largest epidemiological study of neuropathy Pirart showed a prevalence at diagnosis of 8%, rising to 50% at 25 years' duration of diabetes (**Fig. 11.2**). In those with type 2 diabetes, where hyperglycaemia may have been present for some time, the prevalence of neuropathy seen at diagnosis is about 10%. However, an acute neuropathy is also seen rarely in patients with type 1 diabetes, and resolves over a few months once treatment is instituted.

The most common of the neuropathies is the 'classical' diffuse symmetrical sensorimotor neuropathy. The prevalence of this neuropathy depends on how it is defined. On the basis of electrophysiological abnormalities over 50% of patients will develop nerve dysfunction, although clinically significant neuropathy probably affects only 20%. Even amongst the second group of individuals, only 25–50% will suffer from foot ulceration, the most important consequence of peripheral neuropathy, and crippling chronic pain is a rare feature. Diffuse sensorimotor neuropathy is associated with the following features:

Fig. 11.1 Classification of the diabetic neuropathies

Type of neuropathy	Natural history	Sensory dysfunction	Motor dysfunction
Diffuse sensorimotor-symmetrical	Progressive	+++	+
Small fibre neuropathy – autonomic	Progressive	+++	0
Acute mononeuropathy – cranial neuropathies,	Recovery in 3 to 6 months	+	+++
Truncal radiculopathy Femoral amyotrophy	Recovery in 12 to 18 months	+	+++
Acute painful neuropathy	Recovery in 6 to 12 months	+	0
Pressure palsies	Recovery is site dependent	++	++

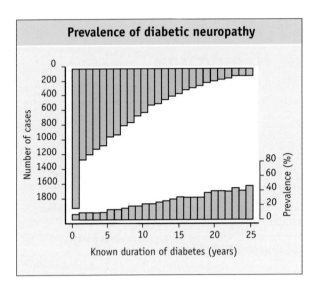

Fig.11.2 *The prevalence of diabetic neuropathy with duration of disease, showing the number of patients evaluated at each point in time. (From Pirart 1978 Diabetes Care 1: 168–188, with permission from* **The American Diabetes Association***).*

- Duration and severity of diabetes. The latter is evidenced by the presence of other complications such as retinopathy or microalbuminuria, rather than the degree of glycaemic control, which correlates only with electrophysiological changes
- Smoking
- Height. This probably reflects the length of the peripheral nerves and hence their vulnerability.
- Male sex

Autonomic neuropathy is often associated with diffuse, symmetrical sensorimotor neuropathy but is usually asymptomatic. However, a small proportion of patients has mostly small fibre neuropathy, which is characterized by loss of temperature sensation and often markedly symptomatic autonomic dysfunction.

The other neuropathies are rare, and probably affect less than 1% of all patients with diabetes. They are unpredictable and usually resolve completely. However, they occur more frequently in older men and are often associated with a period of poor glycaemic control.

DIFFUSE SYMMETRICAL SENSORIMOTOR NEUROPATHY

PATHOPHYSIOLOGY

The main histological features of diabetic peripheral neuropathy are:

Features of diabetic peripheral neuropathy

- Distal axonal loss
- Loss of large and small fibres
- Focal demyelination and regeneration

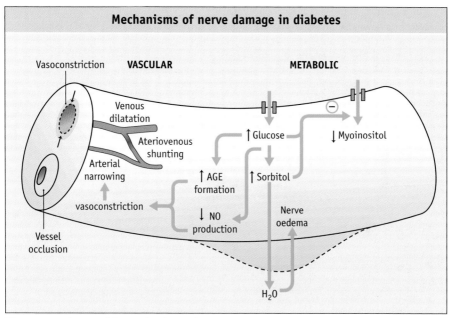

Fig. 11.3 *The possible mechanisms of nerve damage in diabetic peripheral neuropathy.*

Distal axonal loss suggests a metabolic neuropathy, since nerve metabolism is controlled proximally, close to the nerve root. This makes the distal axon more vulnerable. When nerve fibres are lost, the large fibres are particularly affected; small fibre loss is more variable. In focal demyelination and regeneration, the focal nature of the lesions suggests ischaemic damage.

The electrophysiological consequence of these changes is a slowing in nerve conduction velocity, with a rise in the threshold for sensory perception.

There is controversy over the mechanisms by which peripheral nerve damage occurs in diabetes, but, as indicated above, it seems likely to be due to a combination of both metabolic derangement and ischaemia (**Fig. 11.3**).

Glucose uptake by peripheral nerves is an insulin-independent process, and so is determined by circulating blood glucose levels. The following mechanisms have been proposed by which increased glucose uptake causes nerve damage:

- Accumulation of osmotically active sugars from the metabolism of glucose via the polyol pathway (see **Fig. 11.8**, p.123), causing water influx and nerve swelling
- Depletion of myoinositol, causing impaired sodium transport and thus altered membrane potential and slowed nerve conduction
- Depletion of glutathione, reducing defences against free-radical damage
- Depletion of nitric oxide, reducing vasodilatation and promoting ischaemia
- Generation of AGEs and glycosylation of proteins such as tubulin, impairing axonal transport

This is known as the 'metabolic hypothesis'.

Nerve ischaemia results from a combination of three processes. First, there is basement membrane thickening in the vasa nervorum – the blood vessels that supply the peripheral nerves. There is also endothelial dysfunction, which results in impaired vasodilatation, in part as a consequence of the metabolic changes. The third component comprises factors reducing blood flow and increasing blood vessel occlusion, such as increased fibrinogen levels and platelet aggregation.

The resulting nerve hypoxia probably accounts for the failure of nerve conduction to increase in response to exercise as expected in normal individuals.

CLINICAL FEATURES

There is considerable variation between individuals in the manifestations of diffuse symmetrical sensorimotor neuropathy. The main symptoms and signs are:

Clinical features of diffuse, symmetrical sensorimotor neuropathy

Symptoms:
- Loss of sensation:
  — anaesthesia: 'numbness'
  — loss of pain perception
- Altered sensation:
  — paraesthesiae: 'pins and needles'
  — dysaesthesiae: e.g. 'walking on pebbles/broken glass/cotton wool'
- Pain:
  — burning – constant or intermittent
  — hyperaesthesia/allodynia (contact hypersensitivity): e.g. bedclothes causing pain
  — neuralgia – lancinating pain
  — cramps; restless legs

Signs:
- Sensory loss:
  — diminished pain and temperature thresholds initially
  — loss of touch perception – monofilament
  — loss of vibration sensation – tuning fork, biosthesiometer
- Diminished/absent tendon reflexes
- Muscle wasting and weakness is rare but motor dysfunction results in foot deformities
- Autonomic dysfunction is common but usually asymptomatic
- Neuropathic oedema
- Foot ulceration

Signs of neuropathy are commonly found in the absence of symptoms, but, conversely, a small number of patients have genuine symptoms that are seemingly out of proportion to the signs elicited. Sensory symptoms and signs are much more common than motor abnormalities. The pattern of sensory disturbance is symmetrical and distal, the 'glove and stocking' distribution, although involvement of the upper limbs is less common. Sensory loss is an important risk factor for ulceration, whereas pain can be very disabling (see below). Foot deformities that reflect altered motor function, such as loss of plantar arches and toe clawing due to unopposed action of the long extensor tendons, lead to abnormal pressure loading, which predisposes the foot to ulceration. Neuropathic oedema probably reflects increased capillary blood flow due to the effects of autonomic dysfunction on the microcirculation.

A few individuals show more selective patterns of neuropathy including:
- A predominantly motor, diffuse neuropathy of subacute onset, which is not associated with poor glycaemic control, together with the notable clinical finding of fasciculation of the dorsal interossei in the feet

- A small fibre neuropathy causing loss of pain and temperature sensation, which is associated with significant symptomatic autonomic neuropathy

The diagnosis is usually not in doubt, although other possible causes of peripheral neuropathy, both hereditary and acquired, should be considered. Usually the only difficulty is in distinguishing between neuropathic and ischaemic pain, particularly if rest pain occurs at night and is aggravated by contact.

Tests for neuropathy

In the clinic setting testing for neuropathy is part of the overall assessment to identify 'at-risk' feet (see below). This usually includes:

- *Pinprick sensation*. This is a qualitative assessment using, for example, Neurotips (**Fig. 11.4**)
- *Touch sensation*. This is done most accurately using Semmes–Weinstein monofilaments (**Fig. 11.4**); inability to feel a 10 g filament at the point of buckling predicting risk of foot ulceration
- *Vibration sensation*. This is usually performed qualitatively using a 128 Hz tuning fork (**Fig. 11.5**)
- *Tendon reflexes*. Diabetes complicated by neuropathy and cerebrovascular disease is one of the causes of absent ankle jerks with extensor plantar responses

In patients in whom neuropathy is identified, vibration sensation may be assessed quantitatively using a biosthesiometer (**Fig. 11.6**). In this test, an electromagnet activates a spring-loaded stimulator. The threshold for vibration sensation is represented by the voltage required. A threshold that is greater than 25 V confers at least a threefold increase in the risk of foot ulceration.

Other tests for pain and thermal sensory thresholds are largely used as research tools.

TREATMENT

Treatment strategies can be divided into those that prevent the development of neuropathy and those that relieve the symptoms of neuropathy (**Fig. 11.7**).

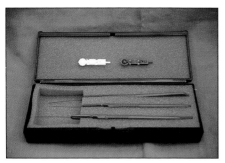

Fig. 11.4 *Three 10 g Semmes–Weinstein monofilaments for testing touch sensation (in box) with two Neurotips (red and white) for testing pinprick sensation.*

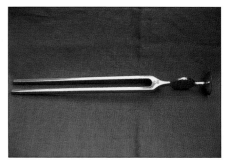

Fig. 11.5 *A 128 Hz tuning fork for testing vibration sensation.*

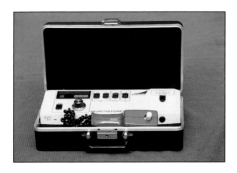

Fig. 11.6   *A biosthesiometer for quantitative analysis of vibration sensation.*

Fig. 11.7   Treatment options in chronic diffuse symmetrical sensorimotor neuropathy

Treatment	Benefit
Prevention:	
• Aldose reductase inhibitors	Possible electrophysiological improvement but little clinical benefit
• γ linolenic acid	Possible improvement in symptoms and electrophysiological parameters
Symptom relief:	
• Adhesive film e.g. Opsite	Contact pain (allodynia)
• Tricyclic antidepressants	Chronic burning pain
• Capsaicin (topical)	Chronic burning pain
• TENS	Chronic burning pain
• Anticonvulsants:	
— gabapentin, lamotrigine	Chronic burning pain
— carbamazepine, phenytoin, valproate	Lancinating pain (neuralgia)
• Local anaesthetic e.g. mexilitine, lignocaine	Lancinating pain
• Clonazepam	Restless legs

Prevention

Improved glycaemic control   Good glycaemic control is important to inhibit the progression of chronic diabetic neuropathy. The DCCT demonstrated a 60% reduction in the progression of clinical neuropathy in those individuals with tight glycaemic control; there was also a reduction in the risk of developing neuropathy in the intensively controlled group. Furthermore, there is also evidence, albeit in a small number of patients, that combined renal–pancreas transplantation improves nerve dysfunction, even in severely affected individuals. In practice, although diabetic neuropathy is not reversible its progression is highly variable and may be delayed by improving glycaemic control.

Other preventative strategies are of more doubtful efficacy.

Aldose reductase inhibitors   Aldose reductase is the rate-limiting enzyme in the polyol pathway, and its inhibitors reduce the metabolism of glucose to sorbitol (**Fig. 11.8**). Such agents effectively prevent diabetic neuropathy in animal models. However, in humans minor electrophysiological improvements seen with their use do not appear to translate into clinically significant changes. This may be because use of these drugs has to date been limited to patients with established neuropathy, where damage is irreversible. However, at present there is no indication for their routine use.

Gamma linolenic acid   A possible mechanism for the development of ischaemia in diabetic neuropathy is the inhibition of prostacyclin synthesis, which favours vasoconstriction. Gamma linolenic acid bypasses the first step in its synthetic pathway (**Fig. 11.9**), so promoting prostacyclin production. It has been shown in small clinical studies that when administered alone, or as a constituent of evening primrose oil, gamma linolenic acid improves both nerve conduction velocities and symptoms in patients with diabetic neuropathy.

Other treatments   Other treatments that are presently experimental include the use of:
- Aminoguanidine, which prevents formation of AGEs
- Antioxidants, such as probucol, which limit free radical damage to nerves
- Vasodilators, such as ACE inhibitors, which may reduce nerve ischaemia
- Nerve growth factors, which may promote nerve regeneration
- L-carnitine, which may improve energy generation within the nerve

Symptom relief

The mainstay of management for patients with significant neuropathy is education to reduce the risk of foot ulceration (see below) and symptom relief. The conventional treatments for neuropathic pain are:
- *Tricyclic antidepressants, usually imipramine or amitriptyline.* These prevent reuptake of both noradrenaline (norepinephrine) and serotonin, and their dual action appears to be important for pain inhibition. A low dose is used initially, and is usually given at night to provide additional sedation, since sleep disturbance is common

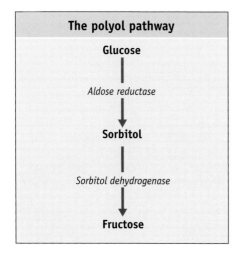

Fig. 11.8 *The polyol pathway: aldose reductase inhibitors block the conversion of glucose to sorbitol.*

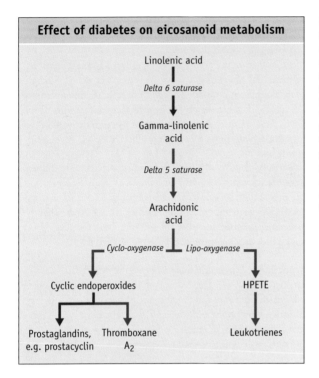

Effect of diabetes on eicosanoid metabolism

Linolenic acid

↓ *Delta 6 saturase*

Gamma-linolenic acid

↓ *Delta 5 saturase*

Arachidonic acid

Cyclo-oxygenase   *Lipo-oxygenase*

Cyclic endoperoxides   HPETE

Prostaglandins, Thromboxane   Leukotrienes
e.g. prostacyclin A_2

Fig. 11.9   *The effect of diabetes on eicosanoid metabolism. The reactions indicated by red lines are those inhibited in diabetes – the production of the vasoconstrictor thromboxane A2 over the vasodilator prostacyclin is favoured; g linolenic acid bypasses the initial metabolic block. HPETE = hydroxyperoxyeicosatetra traenoic acid.*

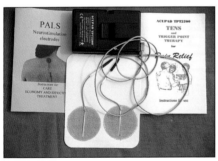

Fig. 11.10   *A TENS device, showing control box, leads and electrodes, which are placed proximal to the affected area.*

- *Carbamazepine*. This acts as a membrane stabilizer and prevents lancinating pains–comparable to its action in trigeminal neuralgia. Doses up to 1g daily may be needed
Newer alternatives include:
- *Capsaicin*. This is an alkaloid found in capsicum peppers that depletes nerve endings of substance P, a nociceptive neurotransmitter. It is applied topically twice daily. However, it may aggravate pain when first applied owing to the initial release of substance P from nerve endings
- *Adhesive plastic films, for example Opsite*. These are particularly effective in stopping contact pain. They probably act, in part, by providing an alternative sensory stimulus, the 'gating' theory of pain relief
- *Transcutaneous electrical nerve stimulation (TENS)* (**Fig. 11.10**). This similarly works on the 'gating' principle. Controversy exists over its efficacy in diabetic neuropathy but some patients appear to benefit

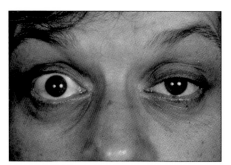

Fig. 11.11   *Oculomotor palsy in a patient with diabetes: unusually there is partial ptosis.*

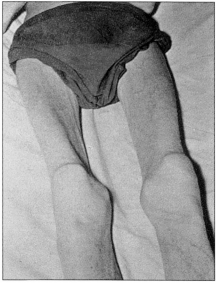

Fig. 11.12   *Bilateral femoral amyotrophy with neuropathic cachexia; the profound muscle wasting was associated with marked weight loss.*

In practice, amitriptyline is usually the first-line therapy. Other strategies are then either substituted or added as appropriate. About 75% of patients will experience adequate symptom relief using these measures. However, in a small proportion all attempts to alleviate symptoms prove futile.

ACUTE NEUROPATHIES

PATHOPHYSIOLOGY

The characteristic feature of the acute neuropathies is that they almost always resolve over time, as they probably result from acute ischaemia of a nerve trunk or its roots. They are possibly more common in association with type 2 diabetes.

Acute mononeuropathies include cranial neuropathies and truncal radiculopathies. The commonest cranial neuropathy is an oculomotor (IIIrd nerve) palsy, although VIth nerve palsies may occur. In a diabetic oculomotor palsy (**Fig. 11.11**) the outer nerve fibres are least affected. In consequence, the pupil is usually spared and ptosis is very rarely seen. Truncal radiculopathy is rare and usually causes neuropathic pain, but occasionally it results in muscle weakness and focal bulging of the thoracic or abdominal wall.

Femoral amyotrophy (amyotrophy of Garland) is probably due to femoral nerve root ischaemia. There is marked pain, weakness and wasting of the thigh (**Fig. 11.12**), with loss of the knee jerk on the affected side. In 50% of cases the problem becomes bilateral, and recurrence has been reported after an apparently complete recovery. Other causes of femoral radiculopathy should be excluded, and imaging of the lumbar spine should be performed – with a plain radiograph at least and possibly magnetic resonance imaging (MRI).

Acute painful neuropathy is often precipitated by improved glycaemic control. The term 'insulin neuritis' has been used in those patients developing this syndrome after insulin therapy has been started. Usually the lower limbs are affected in a symmetrical, distal distribution. It has been postulated that a decrease in nerve blood flow accompanying the fall in blood glucose concentrations may precipitate the disorder. This situation is similar to the transient worsening of retinopathy that is seen on commencing intensive glycaemic control.

MANAGEMENT

All the acute neuropathies usually resolve over a period of 6 to 18 months. Therefore, once any alternative diagnoses have been excluded, patients should be reassured about the prognosis. Glycaemic control should be optimized, because poor glycaemic control may play a part in the pathogenesis of these complications. There is also evidence that improved control, possibly with the introduction of insulin, may accelerate recovery of nerve function. Treatment is otherwise symptomatic, and includes measures for pain control similar to those described above for chronic neuropathy.

PRESSURE PALSIES

Patients with diabetes have an increased risk of developing pressure palsies. This is possibly because less pressure than normal is required to compromise an already ischaemic nerve. Or it may be that limited joint mobility as a result of glycosylation of connective tissue proteins predisposes nerves to entrapment. The commonest type is median nerve palsy due to carpal tunnel syndrome (**Fig. 11.13**). This is amenable to surgical decompression, although there is some evidence that diabetic patients do not recover their nerve function so readily as other individuals. Ulnar nerve entrapment at the elbow is also surgically remediable. Lateral popliteal nerve palsy is less easily treated, and often the resultant foot drop is permanent. If so, an orthotic appliance is required to correct the deformity.

NEUROPATHIC PAIN

Pain may occur with either acute or chronic neuropathy. It results from small fibre damage, although the exact cause for pain syndromes remains unclear. Lancinating, neuralgia-type pain is thought to follow ectopic generation of nerve impulses, whereas chronic, burning

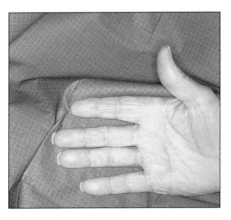

Fig. 11.13 *Wasting of the thenar eminence in a patient with carpal tunnel syndrome; this patient also had a significant peripheral neuropathy complicated by foot ulceration (see Fig. 11.26).*

pain may be due to nerve ischaemia. Painful neuropathy is often associated with insomnia and depression, both of which may be helped by the use of tricylic antidepressants. Severe painful neuropathy may rarely be associated with marked wasting, weakness and loss of up to 60% of body weight – a condition termed 'neuropathic cachexia' (**Fig. 11.12**).

AUTONOMIC NEUROPATHY

EPIDEMIOLOGY

Autonomic neuropathy (**Fig. 11.14**) is much more common in type 1 diabetes than in type 2. Symptomatic disease is most common in females aged between 20 and 40 years. Signs of autonomic nerve dysfunction may be identified in as many as 4% of those with type 1 diabetes of 1 year's duration, and as many as 30% show such signs after 5 years. However, symptomatic autonomic neuropathy is much less common, with a prevalence of only 0.5–1%.

PATHOPHYSIOLOGY

The pathophysiology of autonomic neuropathy appears to be the same as in diffuse sensorimotor neuropathy, with which it is closely associated. In a few cases, antibodies against sympathetic ganglia have been found. In a subset of patients, usually young females, autonomic dysfunction is associated with iritis. This suggests that there may be an

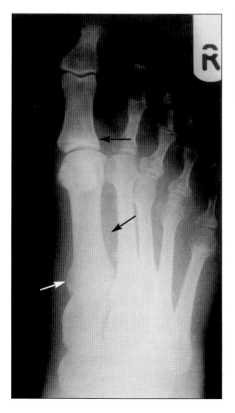

Fig. 11.14 *Calcification of the media in the small arteries of the foot (arrowed) in patient with autonomic neuropathy: note the metal object (arrowed) impaled under the right metatarsophalangeal joint, which became embedded there unnoticed by the patient.*

autoimmune aetiology. Parasympathetic involvement usually precedes clinically evident sympathetic nerve dysfunction. Symptoms are often intermittent, however, and the natural history is highly variable; many patients show little evidence of progression.

CLINICAL FEATURES AND MANAGEMENT

A wide spectrum of visceral functions may be deranged in autonomic neuropathy, for which different treatment options are appropriate (**Fig. 11.15**).

Cardiovascular involvement

Cardiovascular involvement usually presents as postural hypotension. Most patients experience at most mild dizziness on standing; however, occasionally symptoms may be very debilitating including loss of consciousness on standing. Such patients should be advised to stand up slowly and exercise their leg muscles before standing to increase the venous return.

Glycaemic control should also be optimized to prevent polyuria and dehydration; hypotensive agents such as diuretics and tricylic antidepressants should be avoided.

If these measures are ineffective, in most cases the symptoms will respond to fludrocortisone, given in a dosage of up to 1 mg daily. Other treatment options include midodrine, an α_1-adrenoreceptor agonist (vasoconstrictor), given in doses up to 10 mg t.d.s., or the subcutaneous somatostatin analogue octreotide, which causes splanchnic vasoconstriction.

Other cardiovascular problems include neuropathic oedema, a result of increased capillary blood flow, and cardiac arrhythmia, which may account for rare cases of

Fig. 11.15   Clinical features of autonomic neuropathy and treatment options

Clinical features	Treatment options
• Cardiovascular	
— postural hypotension	Fludrocortisone, Midodrine,
— cardiac arrhythmias	Octreotide
— neuropathic oedema	
• Gastrointestinal	
— gastroparesis	Prokinetics: metoclopramide, erythromycin
— diarrhoea	Codeine, loperamide, antibiotics
• Sweating abnormalities	Anticholinergics
• Erectile dysfunction	Intracavernosal prostaglandin E_1, papaverine, oral sildenafil, sublingual apomorphine
• Osteopenia/ neuroarthropathy	? Bisphosphonates
• Neuropathic bladder	
• Respiratory arrest	
• Loss of visceral pain	
• Blunting of response to hypoglycaemia	

unexplained sudden death in type 1 diabetes. Small vessel calcification is a frequent radiological finding in patients with diabetes (**Fig. 11.14**); it is thought to result from the increased blood flow resulting from autonomic dysfunction.

Gastrointestinal involvement

The whole of the gastrointestinal tract may be affected by autonomic dysfunction, usually as a result of disordered motility. Gastroparesis can cause abdominal bloating and rarely vomiting, which is occasionally intractable. It is often difficult to demonstrate, however. The commonest radiological abnormality is delayed emptying of radiolabelled liquids. Prokinetic agents may improve gastric emptying, but in severe cases patients may have to be admitted to hospital for intravenous rehydration and enteral feeding.

Diabetic diarrhoea is probably due to a combination of dysmotility and bacterial overgrowth. It is usually intermittent and watery in nature, with nocturnal exacerbations and frequent incontinence. Codeine, loperamide or antibiotics, particularly oxytetracycline and erythromycin, directed at the bacterial overgrowth, may ease symptoms.

Sweating

Sweating abnormalities are common, but frequently overlooked. Gustatory sweating usually occurs after the person has eaten spicy food or cheese. There is profuse sweating, in a distribution following the superior cervical ganglion – over the face, neck and upper thorax. The problem is thought to be due to aberrant nerve regeneration. Symptoms may be very distressing, and although relieved by anticholinergic agents such as poldine, the side-effects of these agents, particularly dry mouth and also urinary retention and tachycardia, limit their usefulness. Clonidine has reportedly been helpful in some cases.

Other sweating abnormalities include drenching night sweats that are unrelated to hypoglycaemia. Conversely, there may be loss of sweating in the feet, skin dryness and cracking predisposing to ulceration.

Other features

Neuropathic osteopenia (**Fig. 11.16**) is probably due to increased bone blood flow. It contributes to neuroarthropathy (see below).

Erectile dysfunction affects up to 40% of diabetic men. Although multifactorial in aetiology, is most often due to neuropathy (see Ch. 3).

Neuropathic bladder is uncommon, usually occurring only at an advanced stage. Bladder emptying is impaired, and intermittent self-catheterization or long-term indwelling catheterization may be necessary, along with antibiotic therapy for the frequent infections.

Respiratory arrest is a rare occurrence and of uncertain clinical significance.

Loss of visceral pain sensation is particularly well recognized in the phenomenon of silent myocardial infarction, a frequent problem in patients with diabetes. It may result in delays in diagnosis and thrombolytic therapy, and therefore a worsened prognosis. This loss of sensation may also mask acute intra-abdominal pathology, such as a perforated viscus.

Autonomic neuropathy also blunts the counter-regulatory hormone response to hypoglycaemia (see Ch. 5). This slows recovery from hypoglycaemia, but is unlikely to contribute significantly to hypoglycaemia unawareness.

Tests

There are a number of readily performed autonomic function tests (**Fig. 11.17**). These look for evidence of:

- *Loss of cardiac reflexes*. These reflect parasympathetic function
- *Postural hypotension*. These reflect sympathetic function

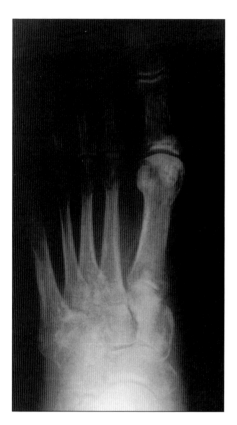

Fig. 11.16   *Patchy porosis of the foot bones, more marked distally, in patient with autonomic neuropathy.*

Fig. 11.17   Simple bedside tests of autonomic function

Test	Normal response	Abnormal response
Heart rate variation on deep breathing: maximum – minimum (b.p.m.)	> 15	< 10
Heart rate increase on standing (b.p.m.):		
15 seconds after	> 15	< 12
30:15 second ratio	> 1.04	< 1.00
Heart rate response to Valsalva manoeuvre: maximum:minimum	> 1.21	< 1.00
BP response to standing: fall in systolic pressure after 2 minutes (mmHg)	< 10	> 30
BP response to sustained handgrip: increase in diastolic pressure (mmHg)	> 16	< 10

More sophisticated testing may be used to look for:

- *Pupillary abnormalities.* Abnormalities include a decrease in pupil diameter and sluggish dilatation, which requires a high resolution infrared camera. These abnormalities are often the first sign of autonomic dysfunction
- *Sweating abnormalities.* These use warming or cholinergic agents and a dye such as chinizarin, which changes colour in the presence of sweat

The prognosis for patients with significant autonomic dysfunction is poor, 10 year mortality being as high as 50%. Death is usually a result of renal failure, but a small number of cases due to sudden death are presumed to be secondary to cardiac arrhythmia or respiratory arrest.

CHARCOT NEUROARTHROPATHY

EPIDEMIOLOGY

Charcot arthropathy affects 0.1–0.5% of patients with diabetes. It usually presents in patients aged 40–60 years, and is more common in those with type 1 diabetes. It is bilateral in up to 40% of cases. The joints affected are usually those of the forefoot, the tarsometarsal or the midfoot (intertarsal) regions. The calcaneal or ankle joints are rarely involved. It may present acutely with a swollen red foot mimicking a septic arthritis, or as a chronically unstable deformed foot (**Figs 11.18 and 11.19**).

PATHOPHYSIOLOGY

A number of factors are thought to contribute to the development of neuroarthropathy:

- Microfractures of the weakened bone due to abnormal stresses followed by abnormal bone formation – this is thought to be the initiating lesion
- Autonomic neuropathy causing increased blood flow, which results in thinning and weakening of bone (see **Fig. 11.16**)
- Glycosylation of connective tissue proteins, which limits joint mobility and causes abnormal load bearing
- Peripheral neuropathy causing loss of sensation, so that the patient is unaware of the trauma

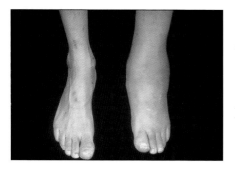

Fig. 11.18 *Charcot neuroarthropathy of the midfoot: the normal right foot is shown for comparison.*

131

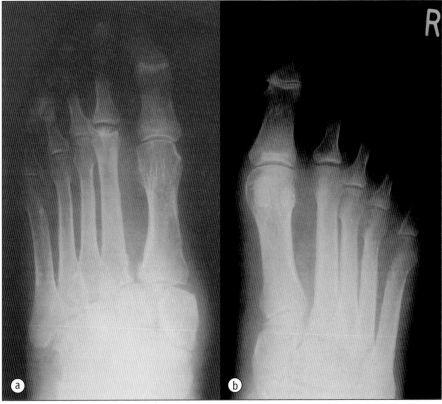

Fig. 11.19   *Plain radiograph of the foot, showing Charcot neuroarthropathy affecting the intertarsal joints (the normal right foot is shown for comparison).*

MANAGEMENT

Strategies directed at preventing the diabetic foot (see below) will reduce the risk of neuroarthropathy. Bisphosphonates have been used in an attempt to prevent deterioration of Charcot neuroarthropathy because they inhibit bone turnover, so may stop progression when microfractures occur. In a small study pamidronate appeared to have had a beneficial effect in five patients. If patients present acutely the process may be halted by strict avoidance of weight bearing for at least 12 weeks.

The chronic Charcot foot must be protected against ulceration by use of appropriate footwear and other measures to reduce abnormal pressure on prominent areas. In severe disease arthrodesis may be considered. Amputation may rarely be necessary as a last resort.

THE DIABETIC FOOT

EPIDEMIOLOGY

The major complication of diabetic neuropathy is foot ulceration. It is the commonest cause for admission of patients with diabetes, accounting for 25% of the in-patient care for these patients. Between 5 and 10% of patients will suffer from a foot ulcer, and 1% will undergo an amputation, which is 15 times the risk for the non-diabetic population. Once a diabetic

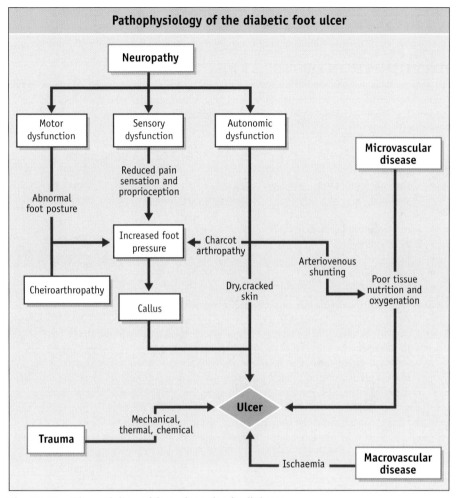

Fig. 11.20 *The aetiology of foot ulceration in diabetes.*

patient has had an amputation there is a 50% chance of losing the other limb or dying within the following 3 years. The cost of foot ulcer care in the last decade has been estimated to be £13 million in the UK and $500 million in the USA. Prevention of diabetic foot disease is therefore both a clinical and an economic imperative – a fact that has been recognized in both Europe and the USA with initiatives to reduce amputations due to diabetic foot disease by 50–75% over 5 years.

PATHOPHYSIOLOGY

A number of factors contribute to diabetic foot disease (**Fig. 11.20**). The most important of these is neuropathy, which is present in the majority of patients with foot ulcers, only 11% being purely ischaemic. A lack of pain perception, which makes the patient unaware of trauma, is in turn more likely to occur as a result of the abnormal posture of the foot, and puts the patient at risk of ulceration. Callus, which forms at sites of abnormal pressure loading, is prone to breakdown in response to trauma, forming an ulcer. Ischaemia due to large or small vessel disease contributes to poor wound healing and progression of ulceration, hypoxia and impaired nutrition; all of these predispose to ulcer infection.

IDENTIFICATION OF THE 'AT RISK FOOT'

All patients with diabetes should have their feet inspected annually to identify those at risk of ulceration. Furthermore, certain patients are at greater risk and should have more frequent inspections. These include elderly patients, particularly if they are isolated or confused, and also patients with:

- Previous foot ulcer
- Peripheral neuropathy:
  — somatic, or
  — autonomic
- Peripheral vascular disease
- Foot deformity
- Callus
- Visual impairment
- Nephropathy

It is the onus of the clinic doctor to remove the shoes, and inspect both the shoes – for foreign objects and suitability – and the feet (**Fig. 11.21**).

Assessment of neuropathy is as described above. The association of neuropathy with callus is a good predictor of ulcer risk. The neuropathic foot is usually a warm, red foot and appears deceptively healthy, but is as much at risk as the cold, ischaemic foot. If vascular insufficiency is suspected then doppler examination of the pulse pressure in the feet is helpful in identifying those patients who require further investigation, which is usually done by means of arteriography (see Ch. 6). It is also important to identify coexisting conditions that, although not specific to diabetes, may contribute to diabetic foot problems. These include:

Fig. 11.21   Identification of the 'at-risk foot' – clinical pointers to risk factors

Features	Examination
Foot deformity	Clawing/overriding toes
	Loss of plantar arches
	Charcot deformity
	Diminished joint mobility
	Callus
Neuropathy	Sensory loss
	Warm, dry skin
	Distended foot veins
	Muscle weakness/wasting
Ischaemia	Pedal pulses
	Doppler examination
	Cold feet

- Dermatophyte (fungal) infection of the nails or skin
- Paronychia
- Ingrowing toenail
- Onychogryphosis
- Eczema
- Psoriasis
- Varicose ulceration

MANAGEMENT OF THE 'AT RISK FOOT'

If the foot is not at risk then education about nail care, foot hygiene and footwear should be provided and an annual review performed. Those patients with feet at high risk require more intensive education, targeted to the needs and abilities of the individual patient. Advice should be personalized as much as possible, although the following key points need reinforcing with all patients:

- Inspect the feet daily using a mirror for the plantar aspect; pay particular attention to areas between the toes and to pressure areas
- Bathe feet in tepid water daily; always check the water temperature before getting into a bath, preferably with a thermometer, or alternatively with the elbow
- Keep the feet away from other sources of heat such as hot water bottles, fires and radiators
- Keep the skin moist by applying lotion after drying
- Always wear protective footwear; do not go barefoot indoors or on the beach
- Check shoes before wearing, change shoes regularly, have the feet measured when buying shoes and buy lace-up shoes with plenty of room; training shoes are often an acceptable way of providing support with style. Choice of hosiery is also important, sports socks providing good protection by evening-out pressures over the foot
- Attend a chiropodist/podiatrist for regular skin and nail care

There are no specific therapeutic measures to prevent diabetic foot disease and prevention is largely dependent on at-risk individuals following this advice. It has been shown, however, that effective education can have a dramatic effect in reducing amputation rates. It is also important to educate other healthcare professionals, particularly over the care of vulnerable feet in acutely unwell patients. Judicious use of foam leg-troughs, for example, can reduce the risk of pressure necrosis of the heel (**Fig. 11.22**).

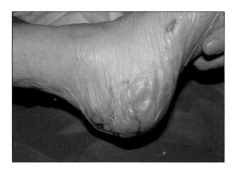

Fig. 11.22   *Early pressure damage to the heel in a patient with diabetic neuropathy.*

Fig. 11.23   Wagner classification of foot ulcers

Grade	Ulcer characteristics
0	High risk foot, no ulcer
1	Superficial ulcer without clinical evidence of infection
2	Deeper ulcer, often with cellulitis, but no abscess or bone involvement
3	Deep ulcer with bone involvement or abscess formation
4	Localized gangrene: toe, forefoot, or heel
5	Gangrene of the whole foot

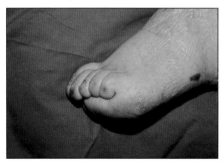

Fig. 11.24   *The at-risk foot (Wagner 0): clawed toes; loss of plantar arches; dry and flaking skin; and bleeding at pressure points, i.e. the tips of digits and on the lateral aspect.*

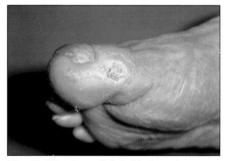

Fig. 11.25   *Superficial skin breach on medial aspect great toe (Wagner 1).*

FOOT ULCERS

Foot ulceration may be graded according to the Wagner classification (**Figs 11.23–11.28**).

When assessing a foot ulcer it is important to consider these factors:

- *The site.* Ischaemic ulcers usually occur on the great toe, the medial and lateral surfaces of the forefoot or the heel, whereas neuropathic ulcers usually occur under the metatarsal heads, at the tips of the toes or between the toes

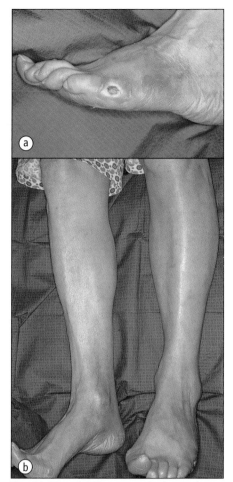

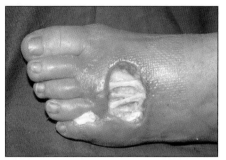

Fig. 11.27 *Deep, wide ulcer with extensive cellulitis, exposure of tendons and almost certain bone involvement (Wagner 3).*

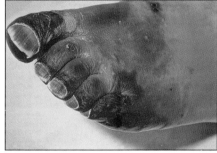

Fig. 11.26 *(a) Deep, punched-out ulcer on the lateral aspect of the foot, with surrounding cellulitis (Wagner 2); (b) lower limbs in the same patient showing clawed, overriding toes and dilated foot veins indicating autonomic dysfunction.*

Fig. 11.28 *Localized forefoot gangrene (Wagner 4).*

- *The depth of the ulcer.* Cursory examination may suggest an ulcer is superficial but it is important to probe the ulcer to determine the depth accurately; if the probe detects bone then osteomyelitis can be assumed to be present
- *The presence of exudate.* If trapped *under* callus this can cause extensive tissue destruction
- *The presence of infection.* The commonest sign is erythema, but there may be purulent discharge, or crepitation indicating the presence of gas-forming organisms
- *The presence of ischaemia.* Ischaemic ulcers are usually painful, in contrast to neuropathic ulcers; signs include cold feet, trophic changes such as hair loss and nail atrophy, in addition to weak or absent pulses; doppler examination should be performed to quantify foot pulse pressures

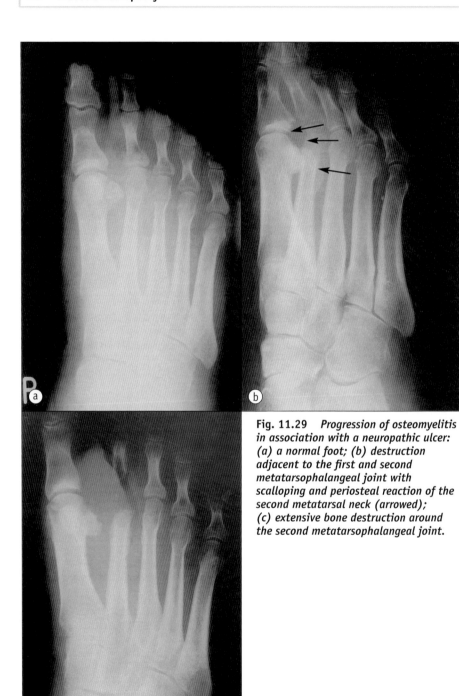

Fig. 11.29   Progression of osteomyelitis in association with a neuropathic ulcer: (a) a normal foot; (b) destruction adjacent to the first and second metatarsophalangeal joint with scalloping and periosteal reaction of the second metatarsal neck (arrowed); (c) extensive bone destruction around the second metatarsophalangeal joint.

Management of foot ulceration involves:

- *Debridement of callus.* This is preferably done with a scalpel, rather than chemical or other methods
- *Relief of pressure.* This may be achieved by padding or shoe inserts, but if healing is slow to occur then either casting or strict non weight-bearing is necessary; suitable casts include light plaster-of-Paris casts to the knee, or removable fibreglass Scotchcasts; casting is not appropriate in the presence of significant infection or ischaemia
- *Treatment of the infection.* Effective antibiotic combinations include co-amoxiclav (Augmentin) and metronidazole, or clindamycin and ciprofloxacin
- *Evaluation of peripheral vascular disease.* Vascular reconstruction should be performed where appropriate
- *Good glycaemic control*
- *Treatment of pedal oedema.*

Patients with grade 3, 4 or 5 lesions should be admitted to hospital. Although in grade 1 or 2 lesions the value of plain radiographs is questionable, it is mandatory in more severe lesions so as to identify bone involvement (**Fig. 11.29**) or the presence of gas-forming organisms.

Abscesses require incision and drainage, and extensive soft tissue infection or osteomyelitis, or both, requires prolonged administration of intravenous antibiotics. The organisms most commonly cultured vary from mainly gram-positive cocci in grade 2 lesions to mainly anaerobes and gram-negative rods in grade 3, 4 and 5 lesions.

Patients with localized gangrene require arteriography. If vascular reconstruction is possible it should be performed. The gangrenous tissue can either be removed surgically or left to autoamputate. If there is diffuse vascular disease, which is inoperable, then major amputation, preferably below the knee, should be undertaken. This should be the primary procedure in patients with grade 5 lesions. There is little benefit in performing a limited amputation on a patient if it fails to heal and more radical amputation is subsequently required, since rehabilitation is then much more difficult.

The use of dressings for ulcers is controversial. There is no evidence that newer, more expensive dressings confer any advantage, and indeed occlusive dressings may cause wound deterioration. After debridement packing of the ulcer crater with a saline-soaked gauze will promote formation of granulation tissue. Otherwise covering of the ulcer with a dry, sterile, non-adherent gauze dressing, of sufficient depth to absorb ulcer exudate, is probably the best option. Newer treatments to promote ulcer healing, such as growth factor preparations and engineered skin dressings, are currently under evaluation. In cases of failed ulcer healing or chronic osteomyelitis, hyperbaric oxygen may improve tissue healing, and both are recognized indications for this therapeutic modality in the USA.

A specialist team comprising a physician, chiropodist or podiatrist, specialist nurse and orthotist, with involvement of surgeons where appropriate, provides the best ulcer management. Once an ulcer is successfully healed it should be remembered that recurrence will occur in two-thirds of patients; therefore careful monitoring is required and appropriate footwear should be provided. It is also important to recognize the psychological effects of foot ulceration. Patients are often anxious about the possibility of amputation and distressed by the unattractive footwear that may be offered to them. Patients may also rarely inflict trauma on their own feet – the Munchausen diabetic foot. A holistic approach to the diabetic foot is therefore required, involving a number of different healthcare professionals as appropriate, and reinforcing footcare advice so that the patient is able to play an active role in ulcer prevention.

chapter 12

Diabetes in Special Groups

CHILDREN AND ADOLESCENTS

Although the onset of type 1 diabetes can occur at any age, the majority of patients are diagnosed in childhood or adolescence, with the peak incidence at the age of 12 years. Children usually present with classical symptoms, although they occasionally have non-specific symptoms, such as abdominal pain or growth failure. Most children do not need to be admitted at the time of diagnosis, as ketoacidosis at presentation is becoming increasingly rare. Initial out-patient care needs intensive support and education.

PREPUBERTY

The insulin requirements of the prepubertal child are usually between 0.2 and 0.5 U/kg per day, although this is highly variable, and many will go through a 'honeymoon phase' where insulin requirements become negligible. Children should be encouraged to manage their diabetes independently; self-administration of insulin is usually possible from the age of 6 years. Most children are managed with a twice-daily (bd) regimen (see Ch. 4, p. 45). Hypoglycaemia can be a cause for concern, especially in young children, who may not recognize the symptoms:

Symptoms of hypoglycaemia in children

- Feels faint
- Nausea
- Irritability
- Tearfulness
- Abdominal pain
- Blurred vision
- Pallor
- Sweating
- Feels cold
- Hunger
- Destructive behaviour
- Drowsiness
- Headache
- Slurred speech
- Tremor
- Tachycardia

Frequent mild to moderate hypoglycaemia may cause intellectual impairment (see Ch. 6).

Wherever possible exercise should be planned and insulin doses adjusted accordingly. In holidays, when energy expenditure is likely to be increased, the total insulin dose often needs to be lowered.

Diet can be a problem. The dietary recommendations are the same as for adults (see Ch. 3). It is important to provide sufficient energy for exercise and growth, and it is therefore preferable to regulate the intake of 'children's foods' and sweets, rather than to ban them.

Poor glycaemic control will stunt growth, and growth charts are a useful way of analysing the efficacy of control. Subtle autonomic changes such as abnormal heart rate variability and pupillary dilatation may be observed prepubertally, but not retinopathy and nephropathy.

Social interaction becomes increasingly important with age, and the impact of diabetes care must be minimized. Rigid guidelines should be avoided to limit harming independence and self-esteem. Schools need to be educated if a pupil has diabetes, with an identified person having responsibility, where necessary, for insulin administration, diet and management of hypoglycaemia.

PUBERTY

During puberty children become insulin resistant because of increasing levels of growth hormone (GH) and sex steroids, and insulin requirements usually rise to about 1.5 U/kg per day, falling to about 1 U/kg per day thereafter. These physiological changes, coupled with the psychological changes associated with adolescence, often lead to a period of poor glycaemic control. This should be avoided as much as possible since significant microvascular complications start to appear with the onset of puberty. In a few cases with a long duration of diabetes, rapid progression of retinopathy may occur peripubertally.

A separate adolescent diabetic clinic, with the support of a psychologist, may be valuable in helping teenagers through this difficult transition period. Brittle diabetes (**Fig. 12.1**) is most common in teenagers. Its clinical features are:

Clinical features of brittle diabetes

- Adolescent, young adult
- Female preponderance
- Poor glycaemic control
- Overweight/obese
- Psychological disturbance
- Eating disorders
- Menstrual irregularity
- Poor pregnancy outcome
- Increased prevalence of diabetic complications
- Probable increased mortality

A number of factors contribute to poor glycaemic control at this age:

- Behavioural problems
- Psychological disturbance
- Eating disorders
- Dietary non-compliance
- Erratic mealtimes
- Insulin errors/omissions
- Exercise
- Pubertal hormone flux
- Growth spurts
- Menstruation
- Pregnancy
- Seasonal variation

Fig. 12.1   Classification of brittle diabetes

A Incapacitated	B Regular lifestyle interruptions at least thrice weekly
1	Hyperglycaemia
2	Hypoglycaemia
3	Mixed pattern

Fig. 12.2   Consequences of eating disorders in adolescent diabetes

- Non-compliance with therapy
  — omission of insulin
  — underdosing with insulin
- Non-compliance with diet
  — binge eating
  — anorexia
  — excess intake to avoid hypoglycaemia
- Laxative abuse
- Poor glycaemic control
- Excessive risk of complications

Eating disorders are a particular concern. They are particularly common amongst teenage girls, and probably occur more frequently in those with diabetes. This may reflect the emphasis on diet in the management of diabetes, and the diabetic patient has an additional means of weight control in their insulin dosage. Such behaviour can have serious consequences (**Fig. 12.2**).

PREGNANCY

PREGNANCY IN ESTABLISHED DIABETES

Pregnancy in the patient with diabetes is associated with increased risks for both mother and fetus. These risks can be minimized by maintaining good glycaemic control both preconceptually and during pregnancy. Thus diabetic pregnancy needs to be planned and patients should be counselled before conception about the risks and requirements. Issues that should be addressed include:

- *Congenital malformations.* These affect 2 to 4% of diabetic fetuses, compared with 1% in non-diabetic pregnancies (**Fig. 12.3**); the risk is closely correlated with glycaemic control in early pregnancy
- *Maternal/perinatal morbidity and mortality.* These rates have fallen rapidly with improvements in diabetic and obstetric care, but are still greater than in the normal population
- *Diabetic complications.* Some women may experience rapid progression of retinopathy and nephropathy

Fig. 12.3   Congenital malformations associated with diabetic pregnancy

Malformation	Frequency in diabetic mothers (approximate %)	Compared with general population (approximate)
• Neural tube defects	2	10 ×
• Caudal regression syndrome — sacral agenesis, phocomelia	0.5	200 ×
• Cardiac anomalies	4	5 ×
• Renal anomalies — renal agenesis, ureteral duplication	3	15 ×
• Gastrointestinal anomalies — duodenal/anorectal atresia	2.5	4 ×

Fig. 12.4   Inheritance of diabetes (Type 1)

	Mother affected	Father affected	Both parents affected
Risk	1–3%	6–9%	20–30%

- *Inheritance of diabetes* (**Fig. 12.4**)
- *Strict glycaemic control.* Women should preferably be on a basal-bolus insulin regimen before conception. Women with type 2 diabetes should stop oral hypoglycaemic agents, which are potentially teratogenic
- *Stopping smoking and avoiding alcohol*
- *Folate supplementation.* The intermediate risk of neural tube defects has led to a recommendation that diabetic women should take 4 mg daily once they are planning conception until the 12th week of gestation
- *Fertility.* This is usually no different in the woman with diabetes unless control is very poor

Management

During pregnancy   During pregnancy the parameters of good glycaemic control are a preprandial glucose level of less than 5 mmol/L and postprandial glucose level of less than 7 mmol/L. During the first trimester in a normal pregnancy, fasting glucose levels fall and postprandial levels rise. Insulin requirements for the diabetic patient may fall initially. However, increasing insulin resistance during subsequent trimesters, which is largely due to the metabolic effects of human placental lactogen (HPL), mean that insulin requirements have usually doubled by the end of pregnancy.

Frequent monitoring of complications, particularly retinopathy (**Fig. 12.5**), is necessary as these may accelerate rapidly in some women. Retinopathy may initially worsen as a consequence of improved glycaemic control (see Ch. 8). Subsequent progression of retinopathy may occur in up to 50% of women, but regression often occurs postpartum. In

Fig. 12.5 Monitoring of retinopathy in diabetic pregnancy

	Preconception	During pregnancy
None or minimal background retinopathy	Ophthalmological assessment	12-weekly review
Significant background retinopathy	Laser treatment for maculopathy	6-weekly review
Preproliferative or proliferative retinopathy	Laser treatment if indicated	1–6-weekly review depending on progression

women with proliferative retinopathy, laser therapy prepregnancy significantly reduces the risk of progression.

Diabetic women may rarely develop a marked nephrotic syndrome during pregnancy. In patients with overt nephropathy, acceleration may occur; this is probably due to the increased demands on the kidney in pregnancy. Women with end-stage renal failure are usually infertile, and should probably be counselled to avoid pregnancy until after renal transplantation.

Hypertension will contribute to the acceleration of complications and should be aggressively treated with non-teratogenic agents, such as methyldopa or β blockers. Pre-eclampsia is more common in diabetic than in women and is often more aggressive.

Fetal monitoring with serial ultrasonography is particularly important during the third trimester. Poor glycaemic control stimulates fetal hyperinsulinaemia, which has a number of consequences. These include:

- Macrosomia
- Organomegaly
- Neonatal hypoglycaemia
- Polycythaemia
- Respiratory distress
- Jaundice

The commonest of these is macrosomia (**Fig. 12.6**). This can result in problems with delivery, such as shoulder dystocia.

Delivery

The timing of delivery is controversial. There are concerns about the increased risk of unexplained fetal death in diabetic pregnancy progressing beyond term. Some centres still induce labour at 38 weeks' gestation, whereas others allow a pregnancy to go to full term. Premature labour is managed with sympathomimetic drugs, such as salbutamol, to delay progression, and glucocorticoids, to stimulate maturation of fetal lungs. Both drugs may stimulate severe hyperglycaemia and possibly ketoacidosis, and large doses of insulin may be required to control blood glucose levels.

Once labour is established the blood glucose levels should be controlled using an intravenous insulin infusion (see below). If blood glucose levels are not well controlled the resulting fetal hyperinsulinaemia may provoke neonatal hypoglycaemia postpartum.

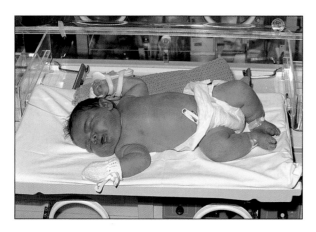

Fig. 12.6 *A macrosomic neonate.*

After delivery

After delivery insulin requirements fall rapidly. Therefore women should be advised to return to their prepregnancy insulin dosage or, if this is not known, to halve their final pregnancy dose. Breast feeding should be encouraged, and insulin requirements may fall by a further 25% if it is established. Women should be advised about restarting contraception.

DIABETES DIAGNOSED DURING PREGNANCY

Gestational diabetes (GDM) is diabetes first diagnosed during pregnancy. About 0.01% of those diagnosed during pregnancy will have type 1 diabetes, and they may present at any stage of the pregnancy. In others the diagnosis is made during the second or third trimester as the insulin resistance increases, unmasking β-cell insufficiency.

Management

Screening for GDM is highly variable. Some centres screen all women with a 50 g glucose tolerance test (GTT) (**Fig. 12.7**); others screen only women at high risk. High risk factors include:

- Obesity
- Family history of type 2 diabetes
- Previous GDM
- Previous macrosomic infant, stillbirth
- Ethnicity (Asian, Afro-Caribbean)
- Persistent glycosuria

Following an abnormal screening test, a number of different criteria exist for the diagnosis of GDM using either a 75 g or a 100 g GTT. (The former is favoured in the UK, the latter in the USA.) Women defined as having GDM or gestational impaired glucose tolerance (IGT) should be given dietary advice and monitor their blood glucose levels. If glucose levels are greater than 5 mmol/L preprandially or greater than 7 mmol/L postprandially then insulin therapy should be started, usually with short-acting insulin before meals initially. Subsequent

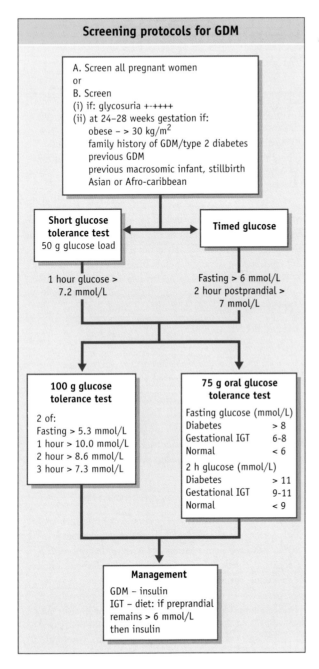

Fig. 12.7 *Screening protocols for gestational diabetes (GDM).*

fetal monitoring and management of labour should be the same as for those women with established diabetes.

Most women with GDM will have normal blood glucose levels postpartum. A GTT at 6 weeks' postpartum will identify those few women who are still diabetic. The remaining women should be advised that they will probably develop GDM in subsequent pregnancies,

147

and have a lifetime risk of developing type 2 diabetes of about 30%. This risk can be minimized by adopting a healthy lifestyle, and in particular avoiding obesity.

SURGERY

Surgery promotes hyperglycaemia, and possibly ketosis, in insulin-deficient patients. This is because of the counter-regulatory hormone response and suppression of insulin secretion. There may also be a risk of hypoglycaemia due to prolonged restriction of calorie intake peri- and postoperatively. Tight control of blood glucose levels is important in promoting recovery and wound healing, and in avoiding infection.

MANAGEMENT

The diabetic patient undergoing an operation will usually need admission at least one day prior to surgery. Patients on longer-acting sulfonylureas should be changed to shorter-acting agents a few days before surgery to reduce the risk of hypoglycaemia. Both those patients with type 2 diabetes who have significant fasting hyperglycaemia preoperatively and those with type 1 diabetes will need to be managed with intravenous insulin in the perioperative period (**Fig. 12.8**). Particular care is needed with patients whose operation requires them to be on cardiopulmonary bypass, since the use of glucose-rich solutions and inotropes will increase insulin requirements.

ELDERLY CARE

There is a gradual increase in blood glucose levels with normal ageing, and so the prevalence of diabetes also rises; 10–20% of people over the age of 65 are affected. The high prevalence of other physical problems and social problems (**Fig. 12.9**) in the elderly makes management of diabetes more difficult for these patients. For example, financial strictures may result in dietary problems, whilst cognitive impairment precludes self-management of diabetes.

MANAGEMENT

Diabetes is a particular problem for the institutionalized elderly. Almost $2 billion is spent on nursing home care for people with diabetes in the USA. The prevalence of diabetes in nursing homes may be as high as 30%, although many patients remain undiagnosed. It is important that these patients have access to chiropodists, optometrists and diabetes nurses, and it is often beneficial to provide protocols for management of hypoglycaemia, hyperglycaemia, diet and footcare.

The aims of management in the elderly will depend on the individual. The healthy 75-year-old person has a life expectancy of at least 10 years, and therefore should be treated as aggressively as younger patients to reduce the risk of complications. However, where life expectancy is much less, the aims are to relieve symptoms, prevent acute complications and prevent foot problems, which are a particular concern in the elderly.

Elderly patients should be treated with short-acting second generation sulfonylureas, such as gliclazide, to minimize the risk of hypoglycaemia (see Ch. 4). Metformin may need to be withdrawn if renal function declines, as is likely with increasing age. Insulin therapy should not be denied to elderly patients. Non-specific symptoms of lethargy and malaise often reflect hyperglycaemia and patients can feel much better when insulin

Protocol for perioperative diabetes management

HARROGATE HEALTH CARE TRUST
THE PERIOPERATIVE MANAGEMENT OF DIABETES:
GUIDLINES AND PRESCRIPTION

GENERAL POINTS
Aim to maintain blood glucose 4–10 mmol/L
Frequently measure blood glucose (BM) e.g. Preop; QID
Postop; 1 hrly for 4 hrs then 2 hrly overnight then 4 hrly if stable
Try to put the patient first on the list
Discuss with Anaesthetist and Surgeon early

		Morning surgery	Afternoon surgery
Diet-controlled diabetic	**Preop**	BM < 10 = treat as normal BM > 10 = treat as INSULIN	BM < = treat as normal BM > = treat as INSULIN
	Postop	May need insulin after major surgery	May need insulin after major surgery
Oral hypoglycaemics		BM < 10 = treat as INSULIN BM > 10 = treat as follows:	BM < 10 = treat as INSULIN BM > = 10 treat as follows:
Able to eat within 24 hrs postop	**Preop**	Starve from midnight Omit am tablets	Starve after breakfast Give breakfast tablets
	Postop	Restart tablets when eating	Restart tablets when eating
Unable to eat within 24 hrs postop	**Preop**	Starve from midnight Omit am tablets Gluc/insulin from 0800	Starve after breakfast Give breakfast tablets Gluc/insulin from 0800
	Postop	Restart tablets when eating	Restart tablets when eating
INSULIN	**Preop**	Starve from midnight Usual insulin until midnight Omit all am subcut insulin Gluc/insulin from 0800	Starve after breakfast Usual insulin until midnight. Omit all am subcut insulin Gluc/insulin from 0800
	Postop	IV Glucose/insulin until patient eats 2nd meal, then usual s/c regime	IV Glucose/insulin until patient eats 2nd meal, then usual s/c regime

Fig. 12.8 *Guidelines for perioperative management of diabetes.*

therapy is commenced. There is a small rise in incidence of type 1 diabetes around the age of 80, particularly in women, and this possibility should not be overlooked (see Ch. 2) as these patients will suffer symptomatically if treated with oral hypoglycaemic agents.

Fig. 12.9   Physical and social problems in the elderly having an impact on diabetes care

Physical:
- Visual impairment
  — reduced acuity: cataract, maculopathy
  — visual field loss: retinopathy, glaucoma
- Communication problems
  — dysphasia
  — dysarthria
- Cognitive impairment
- Loss of coordination or manual dexterity
  — cerebrovascular disease
  — neurodegenerative disease
  — arthritis
  — neuropathy

- Reduced mobility
  — cerebrovascular disease
  — neurodegenerative disease
  — arthritis
  — neuropathy
- Cardiorespiratory disease

Social:
- Bereavement
- Withdrawal
- Social isolation
- Poverty
- Lack of appropriate food
- Loss of autonomy
- Residential or nursing home care

ETHNIC GROUPS

The prevalence of diabetes is much higher in certain ethnic groups, particularly Afro-Caribbeans, Asians and Hispanic Americans. These groups often have a higher prevalence of other problems such as hypertension and ischaemic heart disease.

MANAGEMENT

Management considerations are no different, although response to therapies such as antihypertensive medication may differ. Cultural and dietary differences may cause problems. For example, animal insulins are probably best avoided in Asian patients and special consideration needs to be given to the management of diabetes during periods of religious fasting.

Literature to educate different ethnic groups should take these differences into consideration, and, where necessary, should be translated into different languages.

PRISON

MANAGEMENT

Management of the diabetic prisoner needs particular attention. Following arrest, there are frequent reports of hypoglycaemia being mistaken for inebriation. Once in prison the lack of flexibility in diet, the lack of exercise and prohibition of blood glucose self-monitoring all cause problems with glycaemic control.

chapter 13

Endocrinology – Introduction

Managing patients with endocrine disorders is a fascinating and continuing challenge. The variety of disorders encountered, the range of presentations from the subtle to the gross, and from the stereotyped to the atypical, are excitements met in every clinic. Added to this is the almost unparalleled capacity to transform patients' lives for the better – not only with acute emergencies but also with chronic conditions over the entire range of age and glandular involvement. The clinical skills of diagnosis and management – the art of clinical endocrinology – are the focus of this part of the book.

But this is only half the story, for the accuracy of diagnosis and range of therapy, as well as the intellectual satisfaction of good practice, are based on sound science. Indeed, endocrinology as a clinical discipline is grounded on a clear understanding of physiology. In endocrinology, the research into basic sciences has led the way in revealing principles of cellular control, using cutting-edge technologies that have fed many other specialties. This continues even more strikingly to be the case, necessitating an understanding of areas such as molecular biology that are moving rapidly from the laboratory to the clinic.

Definition of endocrinology

- The study of hormones – the site and control of their synthesis and secretion, their blood-borne effects on distant organs and the disorders of hormone production and response, constitute the basis of endocrinology. Hormones play a central role in regulating growth, reproduction and a wide range of metabolic processes

---

REGULATION OF HORMONES

Classically, hormones are thought to act steadily over a long time course, coordinating measures to ensure constancy of the internal milieu, or homeostasis, in the face of variations in external factors such as temperature, food, demands of physical activity, diurnal and seasonal changes, reproduction and challenges posed by trauma or infection. An important element in the regulation of many hormones is the negative feedback loop. This may be ostensibly simple, such as a stimulatory action on organs elevating compound x, which can in turn directly inhibit the secretion of the hormone. An example is parathyroid hormone (PTH), which stimulates a rise in the extracellular ionized calcium concentration (symbolized as $[Ca^{2+}]$) by enhancing gut absorption, bone resorption and renal tubular reabsorption of Ca^{2+}, which in turn inhibits the PTH secretion (**Fig. 13.1a**). In contrast, an elevation in postprandial glucose stimulates insulin secretion; this drives glucose into many tissues

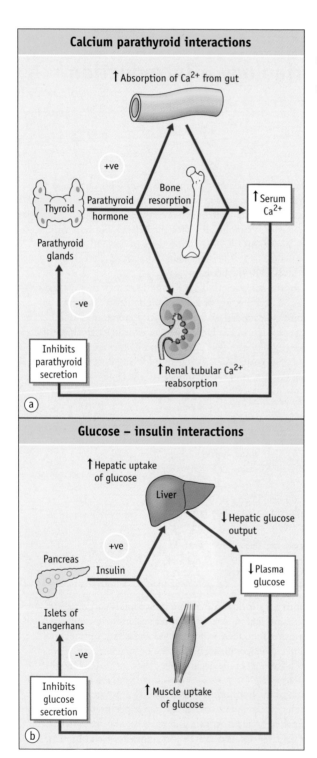

Fig. 13.1
(a) Calcium–PTH interactions;
(b) glucose–insulin interactions.

thereby lowering the plasma glucose concentration, and as this happens the level of insulin secretion falls (**Fig. 13.1b**).

These two examples oversimplify the events occurring in vivo, however, by ignoring other metabolic interactions – for instance in the first example that of PTH and Ca^{2+} with magnesium and vitamin D metabolism (**Fig. 13.2a**). In the second example, the reversal of hypoglycaemia involves not just inhibition of insulin output, but the stimulation of an array of counter-regulatory influences including catecholamines, glucagon, growth hormone (GH, or somatotrophin) and cortisol (**Fig. 13.2b**). This illustrates a further common phenomenon: redundancy of response such that many coordinated secretions occur in defence of a vital physiological parameter, one or more of which may be defective without necessarily compromising safety. Other conditions eliciting plurihormonal responses include acute hypovolaemia, hypotension and physical stress such as trauma and sepsis (**Fig. 13.3**).

Negative feedback relationships may coordinate the secretion of pairs of glands, classically exhibited in the pituitary–target-gland axes, such as the hypothalamo-pituitary–thyroid axis (**Fig. 13.4a**) and the hypothalamo-pituitary–adrenal-cortex axis (**Fig. 13.4b**). Similarly, tonic secretion of estradiol from the ovary tonically inhibits luteinizing hormone (LH) secretion unless the estradiol concentration exceeds a critical level for a critical period, at which point it evokes a transient positive feedback effect, producing the preovulatory LH surge (**Fig. 13.5**). Independent influences on pituitary hormone

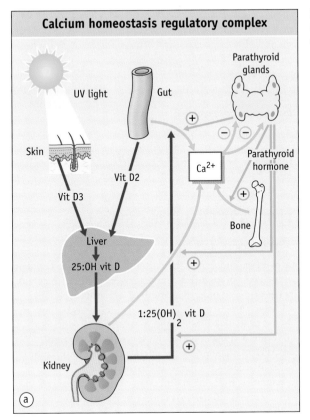

Calcium homeostasis regulatory complex

Fig. 13.2 *(a) Calcium homeostasis regulatory complex.*

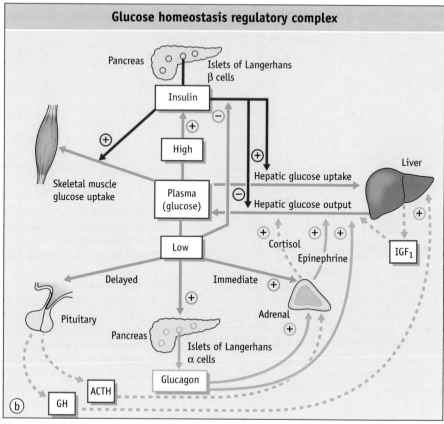

Fig. 13.2 *(b) Glucose homeostasis regulatory complex.*

secretion from the central nervous system are mediated by the neurovascular link between the hypothalamus and the pituitary.

ENDOCRINE AND OTHER SYSTEMS OF CELL REGULATION

The endocrine and nervous systems overlap. Endocrine stimulation can be rapid and brief as well as slow and steady. Many glands consist of modified neurons (e.g. in the hypothalamus and adrenal medulla). Many hormones display a pulsatile pattern of secretion, especially those of the anterior pituitary gland, which are driven by episodic hypothalamic output. Many peptide hormones are distributed in several different locations and act in different fashions; for instance, somatostatin is found in the hypothalamus, cerebral cortex and pancreatic islets of Langerhans. The APUD (amine-precursor uptake and decarboxylation) hypothesis was formulated (by Pearse) to account for the wide distribution of neuroendocrine cells by embryonic migration from the neural crest. Though challenged and modified, this hypothesis has proved a seminal influence on endocrine theory, including an explanation of the source of ectopic hormone secretion from many tumours.

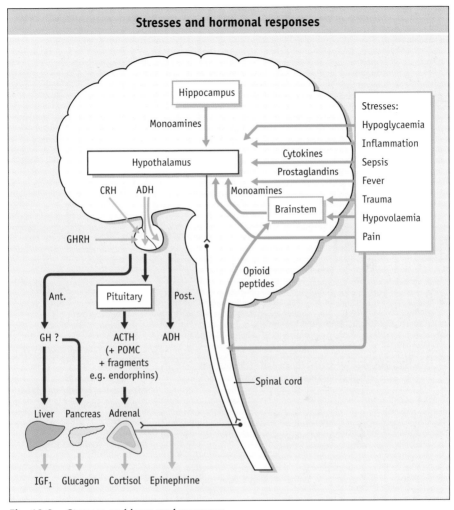

Fig. 13.3 *Stresses and hormonal responses.*

The different tiers of cellular regulation involve similar mechanisms, differing only in the spatial relationships between effector and responder cells (**Fig. 13.6**). These can be grouped into two main areas of action – long distance and local:

Long-distance actions are mediated by:
- Networks of nerves (nervous system), or
- Bloodstream (*endocrine system*)

or locally:
- Affecting the producer cell itself (*autocrine*), or
- Neighbouring cells (*paracrine*)

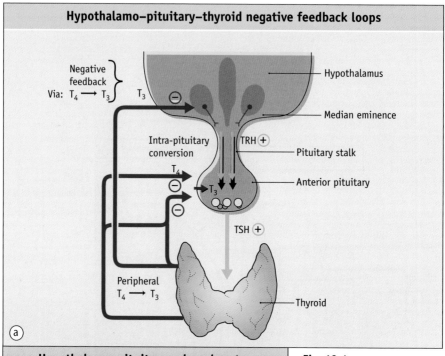

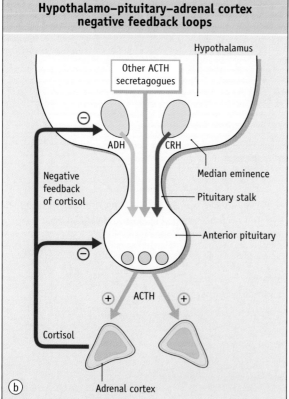

Fig. 13.4
(a) Hypothalamo-pituitary–thyroid negative feedback loops;
(b) hypothalamo-pituitary–adrenal cortex negative feedback loops.

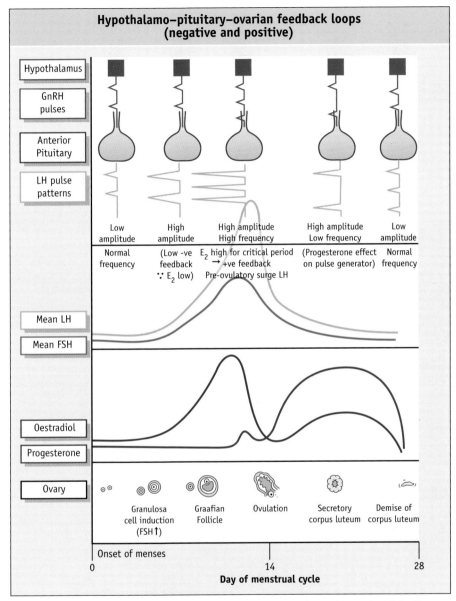

Fig. 13.5 *Hypothalamo-pituitary–ovarian feedback loops (negative and positive).*

This wider pattern encompasses long-distance and local immunoregulation by cytokines and related compounds, which have actions and receptors similar to those of classical hormones. These mechanisms advance our growing understanding of the intimate relationships between the endocrine, nervous and immune responses in health and disease.

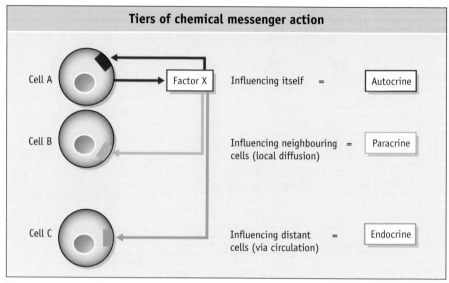

Fig. 13.6   *Tiers of chemical messenger action (endocrine, autocrine and paracrine).*

CELLULAR REGULATION BY HORMONES

Endocrine regulation depends critically upon the specificity of hormone receptors, their sites of distribution, numbers and affinities (which vary, being affected by factors such as current and past hormonal exposure).

Two main types of receptor exist, as determined by the lipid solubility of their cognate hormones:

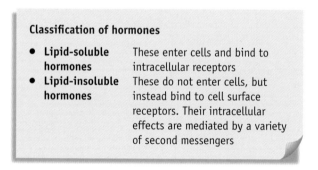

Classification of hormones

- **Lipid-soluble hormones**   These enter cells and bind to intracellular receptors
- **Lipid-insoluble hormones**   These do not enter cells, but instead bind to cell surface receptors. Their intracellular effects are mediated by a variety of second messengers

Examples of lipid-soluble hormones include steroids, thyroid hormones and vitamin D. Despite the chemical diversity of these substances, their intracellular receptors comprise a homologous superfamily with a constant pattern of different regions. Some show a remarkable conservation of amino acid sequence (**Fig. 13.7**).

The lipid-insoluble hormones include many peptide hormones and amines. Their second messengers include cyclic AMP (cAMP), Ca^{2+}, diacylglycerol (DAG) and the more recently described JAK-STAT pathways. Important intermediates between the receptor and the catalytic production of the second message are heterotrimers of G proteins, which are

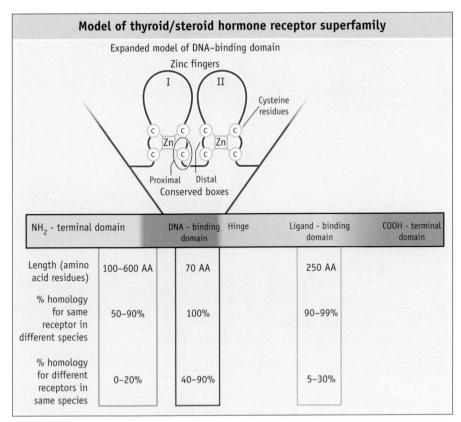

Fig. 13.7 *Model of thyroid/steroid hormone receptor superfamily.*

activated by hormone binding to the receptor. They link by guanine nucleotide binding and metabolism of the receptor and catalytic units. Stimulatory and inhibitory examples of these intermediates exist for the cAMP pathway (**Fig. 13.8**) and the inisitol phosphate–IP$_3$/DAG pathway (**Fig. 13.9**). These second messengers act on specific subcellular organelles, including the nucleus, allowing pleiomorphic responses and interaction between different hormones and their intracellular actions.

NUCLEAR ACTION OF HORMONES

Many important cellular processes are ultimately genetically regulated via synthesis of proteins having enzymatic, structural or contractile functions within cells. Alternatively, they may be exported into the extracellular fluid as hormones, antibodies or carrier proteins.

LIPID-SOLUBLE HORMONES

Hormones acting via intracellular receptors do so mainly at the nucleus. Steroid receptors in the unoccupied state are associated with 'chaperone molecules' including heat-shock proteins, which may prevent activation of the genome in the absence of ligand. Steroid hormone binding to receptor leads to conformational change, shedding of chaperone molecules and translocation to the nucleus. The DNA-binding domain may take the form of zinc fingers. These bind *trans*-acting and *cis*-regulatory elements on the DNA promoter sites

159

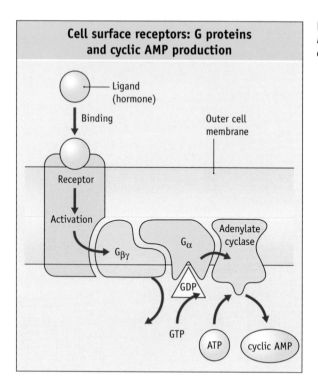

Fig. 13.8   *Cell surface receptors: G proteins and cAMP production.*

upstream from the relevant genes, which are then stimulated by ribonucleic acid (RNA) polymerase II to undergo transcription to messenger RNA (mRNA).

Thyroid hormones bind with other agents such as retinoids to form heterodimers. These in turn bind with hormone receptor response elements in the genome. There are no heat-shock proteins associated with these hormone receptors.

LIPID-INSOLUBLE HORMONES

Cell-surface-acting hormones can also influence the nucleus. In this case it is via their second messengers. For instance, cyclic AMP is thought to act largely through protein kinase A, and thence several compounds including CREB, CREM and AFT-1. IP_3 stimulates the mobilization of Ca^{2+} from intracellular stores. This in turn binds to calmodulin and similar proteins, which when thus activated influence genomic activity. The alternative pathway of DAG acts via protein kinase C and the transforming factor AP-1 (a heterodimer of the cellular oncogenes *c-fos* and *c-jun*) on the phorbol ester (or TPA) response elements.

A PRACTICAL APPROACH TO CLINICAL INVESTIGATION

Most clinical disorders in endocrinology involve either hyper- or hyposecretion. Therefore hormonal measurements, usually in blood, are needed for assessment.

SINGLE BLOOD TESTS

These may provide reliable information in many circumstances. For example, thyroid hormones are relatively stable and measurement of plasma thyroxine (T_4) and thyroid-

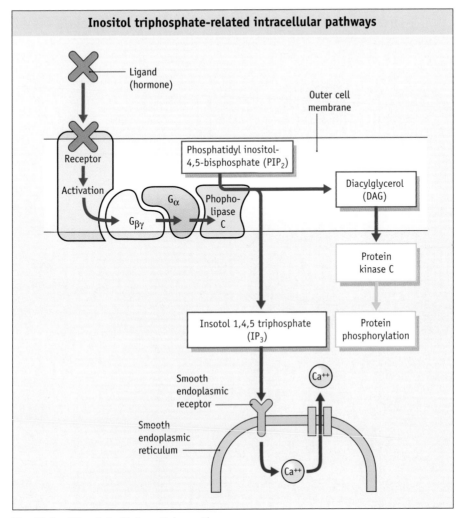

Inositol triphosphate-related intracellular pathways

Fig. 13.9 *IP₃-related intracellular pathways.*

stimulating hormone (TSH) often suffice. However, population-derived reference ranges usually reflect the mean plus or minus two standard deviations (σ) – hence 5% of normal people have results outside this range. Furthermore, healthy individuals regulate plasma thyroxine concentration within a much narrower band. It is debatable whether any mild disorder that shifts hormone values outside this personal band, but within the population-based reference range, represents a disease state requiring treatment. As blood tests become increasingly sensitive and accurate, there is an increasing trend towards early intervention, but a sense of proportion must be retained. It is sensible therefore to repeat the test and seek corroborative evidence.

Likewise, the existence of primary hyperparathyroidism is strongly suggested by the simultaneous measurement of plasma calcium and PTH, though one should always consider the possibility of hypocalciuric hypercalcaemia. It may also be misleading to rely on total calcium/albumin measurements to give a 'corrected calcium' figure. For instance, a

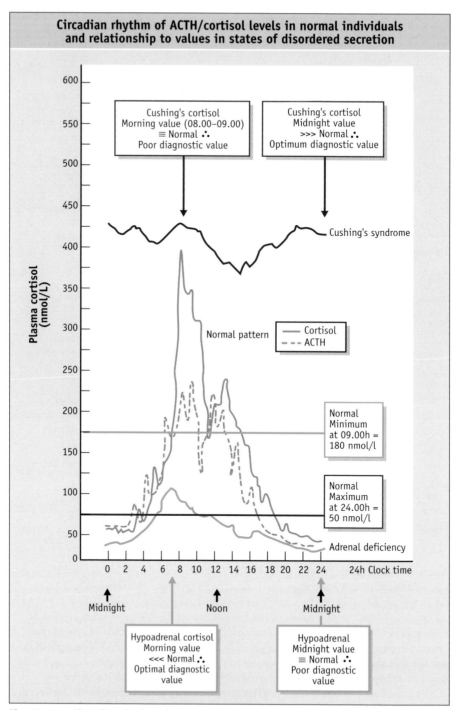

Fig. 13.10 *Circadian rhythm of ACTH/cortisol levels in normal individuals and relationship to values found in states of disordered secretion.*

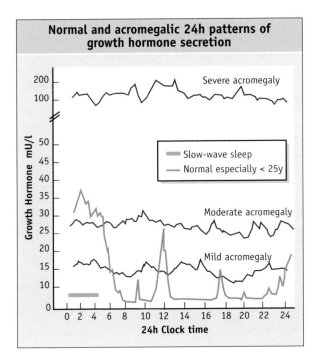

Fig. 13.11 *Normal pattern of GH secretion and use of single blood samples in the diagnosis of acromegaly ($a_1, a_2, a_3 < 2mU/L$ = not acromegaly; b mid spontaneous peak 8 mU/L = could be mild acromegaly; c mid big spontaneous peak 22 mU/L = could be moderate acromegaly; NB avoid sleep sampling, can be high in slow-wave sleep).*

significant γ-globulin paraprotein may produce the rare finding of high total calcium but normal albumin, and thus raised 'corrected calcium' but normal ionized calcium.

Many hormones show considerable variation in plasma levels, including pulsatile secretion and rhythmic or stress-induced changes. Sampling should therefore take account of such variability. If the clinical question is one of possible hypersecretion, diagnosis is optimized by sampling when the value would normally be at its lowest, and conversely with hypersecretion. The test for cortisol secretion exemplifies this: check at the normal circadian nadir (midnight) for suspected hypersecretion, and at 8 to 9 a.m., the normal maximum, for hypoadrenalism (**Fig. 13.10**).

Single blood samples may aid screening especially if the likelihood is low; for instance, a single undetectable GH value eliminates the possibility of acromegaly. High values can be normal, however – for instance, if sampling has by chance captured the peak of one of the few, brief daytime pulses of GH. In this event, further investigations are required (**Fig. 13.11**).

DYNAMIC TESTS

When single samples prove inconclusive, the next step is often to use dynamic tests (e.g. **Fig. 15.10**, p.185), often with serial, carefully timed blood samples after a pharmacological stimulus.

If hypersecretion is suspected, suppressive manoeuvres are employed. For example, in acromegaly administration of oral glucose will not suppress GH as it does in normal people. In contrast, where hyposecretion is suspected a stimulation test is needed. For instance, induction of hypoglycaemia with insulin normally allows assessment of the reserve for secretion of adrenocorticotrophin (ACTH)/cortisol and GH in response to stress. Stimulation tests may also, paradoxically, be useful in some hypersecretory states – especially where these are intermittent (e.g. insulinoma or phaeochromocytoma). However, these interventions may be hazardous and so should be avoided wherever possible.

ANATOMICAL LOCALIZATION OF SITES OF ABNORMAL SECRETION

It is frequently important to know the location of such sites. For instance, many hypersecretory states are due to neoplasms, albeit often benign, and are thus potentially curable by surgery. Tumours may also, conversely, impair hormone secretion. The exact size and position of some tumours (e.g. pituitary tumours) are particularly important to assess because of the threat to local structures such as the optic chiasm. Localization is therefore a necessity for planning surgery and judging prognosis.

The source of abnormal hormone secretion is commonly uncertain, however. For example, hyperparathyroidism may be due to a single adenoma, two adenomas, four-gland hyperplasia, supernumerary or ectopic glands (e.g. mediastinal). Virilization may be due to abnormalities in secretion of either one or both ovaries, or one or both adrenals. In ectopic ACTH production, a number of organs may be the cause. Common sites are the lung, thymus, pancreas and thyroid (medullary cell carcinoma).

IMAGING MODALITIES

These include:

- **Ultrasound** — Ovaries (especially transvaginal), scrotum, thyroid, parathyroids
  Endoscopic/operative: pancreas, duodenum
- **CT scanning** — Thorax, especially volume acquisition (spiral), adrenals, pituitary, pancreas
- **MRI scanning** — Pituitary (modality of choice), adrenals
- **Isotope scanning** — Thyroid (rarely used: Plummer's disease, thyroiditis, with amiodarone)
  Parathyroids (with sestamibi)
  Many neuroendocrine tumours, carcinoids (with octreotide)
  Phaeochromocytomas and related tumours (with meta-iodo benzyl guanidine, or MIBG)
  Adrenals (with selenocholesterol)

chapter 14

Endocrine Emergencies

INTRODUCTION

Prompt recognition and proper management of endocrine emergencies are usually gratifyingly well rewarded, whereas failure to do so may have serious, and even lethal, consequences. This dictates consideration of the possible aetiological involvement of endocrine emergencies in various acute medical situations, even those that are rare. The therapeutic dividend of course continues from the acute situation, as therapy is often lifelong – for instance when endocrine replacement is introduced.

Often the most severe emergencies occur either de novo or in patients with unrecognized prior disease. This requires medical staff to be aware of such possibilities, selection of appropriate tests and formulate effective management plans. Management may require the use of non-specific resuscitation measures and then correction of pathophysiological abnormalities before a definitive diagnosis is made. Diagnosis should, however, be delayed as little as possible in case the management strategy needs modifying. It is vital to check the differential diagnosis in order to consider the nuances of different management plans, which may be important in acute situations, and to prepare for the next stage of treatment – for example the possibility of tumour resection and on-going hormone replacement.

PATHOPHYSIOLOGICAL MECHANISMS

Since endocrine regulation is paramount in maintaining homeostasis, failure of the regulatory mechanisms may underlie many acute metabolic emergencies, though intercurrent illness often provokes the final breakdown. The following is a summary of the essential points relating to pathophysiological mechanisms and factors underlying the failure of salt and water, calcium, glucose and immune regulation. Mechanical effects may also be important.

Salt and water metabolism

In the pathology of salt and water metabolism, the extracellular and intracellular compartments may be affected separately. The most common abnormalities affect plasma volume; depletion is especially common. Losses may occur from the renal and gastrointestinal tracts, and also from the skin.

Relative water: solute losses determine plasma electrolytic concentrations. The following ions and hormones play a role in regulation:

- Sodium concentration is *not* a direct measure of content. Renal sodium loss is mainly controlled by aldosterone, although natriuretic peptides have a minor role
- The plasma ionic potassium concentration is influenced by corticosteroids and acutely also by insulin

- Water metabolism is mainly regulated by vasopressin. Also, free water generation requires cortisol and thyroid hormones
- Excess cortisol levels have a mineralocorticoid effect (see Ch. 18)

Calcium metabolism

In the maintenance of calcium balance, the major physiological regulators are PTH, vitamin D metabolites and calcitonin. An emergency situation can arise from either excess or deficiency of calcium, or from magnesium deficiency:

- Hypercalcaemia may be caused by excess of PTH or vitamin D, cortisol deficiency, or hyperthyroidism. In the malignant form an imbalance of PTH-related peptide, cytokines, $1\propto$-25(OH)$_2$ vitamin D, or osteolytic secondaries may be seen. Hypercalcaemia can provoke vomiting and a vicious exacerbatory cycle
- Hypocalcaemia causes electrophysiological and neuromuscular changes, such as seen in tetany
- Hypomagnesaemia can also cause tetany, as well as refractory hypocalcaemia

Glucose metabolism

Neuronal activity is largely determined by the extracellular concentration of glucose. For most cell types, the entry of glucose into the cell interior is insulin dependent. Either an excess or a deficiency of glucose can lead to an acute situation:

- Hypoglycaemia is usually caused by an excess of insulin, but rarely by that of IGF-II. Childhood hypoglycaemia is common with GH and cortisol deficiency, and glycogen storage disease
- Hyperglycaemic syndromes include diabetic ketoacidosis, hyperosmolar non-ketotic coma and lactic acidosis. Hyperglycaemic crises cause dehydration from osmotic diuresis. In the metabolic derangement of acidosis, deficits in sodium, potassium, phosphate and bicarbonate need to be corrected

Immune mechanisms and stress

Cortisol is the main influence on the role of stress in immune system dysfunction:

- Cortisol rises in stress to curtail inappropriate cytokine overproduction. Cortisol excess causes neutrophil leukocytosis, lymphopenia and eosinopenia. Extreme hypercortisolism compromises the immune response, so there may be opportunistic infection
- Cortisol deficiency is also associated with stress, particularly in shock, adult respiratory distress syndrome and organ failure. Fever may accompany cortisol deficiency per se

Other hormones are produced in stressful conditions including: catecholamines, glucagon, GH, prolactin (PRL) and vasopressin.

Mechanical effects

Mechanical effects occur, for instance, from acute expansion of an organ, which may result in critical damage. This often occurs in already pathologically enlarged glands. Examples include the pituitary, thyroid, adrenals and ovaries:

- In pituitary apoplexy, haemorrhagic expansion of a pituitary tumour can cause subarachnoid haemorrhage, visual loss, ophthalmoplegia and acute adrenal insufficiency
- In thyroid surgery, asphyxia due to haematoma is a rare early complication, and recurrent laryngeal nerve palsy increases the risk of respiratory arrest. Anaplastic invasive thyroid cancer can also compromise the airways. In multinodular goitre, a bleed into a cyst may cause stridor
- Large adrenal tumours (usually carcinomas) can bleed and expand suddenly. Adrenal apoplexy is a rare cause of sudden addisonian crisis

- In ovarian hyperstimulation syndrome there is increased ovarian size. This may also cause ascites, pleural effusion, vascular collapse or organ failure

ACUTE CLINICAL EMERGENCIES

Emergencies may be categorized according to presentation, which should act as an aide-mémoire to consider relevant possible diagnoses (**Fig. 14.1**).

However, many endocrine conditions can present in a variety of ways, and so the following section describes in turn each of the endocrine disorders and their management.

ORGAN/SYSTEM-RELATED DISORDERS AND THEIR MANAGEMENT

PITUITARY

Pituitary apoplexy

Pituitary apoplexy may cause instant death. Severe consequences include subarachnoid haemorrhage, ophthalmoplegia and hypoadrenalism.

Management   In the immediate management of pituitary apoplexy, the following procedure is suggested:

- Check the levels of urea, electrolytes and cortisol, and the thyroid function urgently
- Arrange for a CT or MRI scan

Fig. 14.1   Endocrine causes of acute clinical emergencies, according to presentation

Coma	Hypoglycaemia, hyperglycaemia, hyponatraemia, hypothyroidism, hypoadrenalism, hypercalcaemia
Fits	Hypoglycaemia, hypocalcaemia, hyponatraemia, pituitary or parapituitary disease, adrenoleukodystrophy
Psychosis/toxic confusional state	Cushing's syndrome, thyrotoxicosis, hypothyroidism, hypercalcaemia, hypocalcaemia, hypoglycaemia, adrenal insufficiency, hyponatraemia
Hypovolaemic decompensation	Hyperglycaemic crises such as ketoacidosis, hyperosmolar non-ketotic coma and lactic acidosis, addisonian crisis, hypercalcaemic crisis, phaeochromocytoma, ovarian hyperstimulation syndrome, gut tumours including carcinoids, gastrinoma, VIP-oma
Arrhythmias/ heart failure	Thyrotoxicosis, phaeochromocytoma, hypercalcaemia, carcinoid syndrome
Vomiting/ diarrhoea/ acute abdomen	Addison's disease, hypercalcaemia, diabetic ketoacidosis, thyrotoxicosis, hypothyroidism, pituitary apoplexy, gut tumours including carcinoids, gastrinoma, VIP-oma
Respiratory obstruction/ arrest	Thyroidectomy, thyroid neoplasms such as anaplastic carcinoma or lymphoma, hypocalcaemia, acromegaly

- Give hydrocortisone 100 mg i.v.
- Perform an urgent neurosurgical assessment

- If there is stress, for instance as a result of infection, surgery or myocardial infarction, then increased hydrocortisone is required. Give two to three times the normal requirements, either by mouth or intravenously/intramuscularly if the patient is collapsed, vomiting, or unable to swallow. However, return to replacement levels as soon as possible (within 48–72 hours)

Hyponatraemia

Hyponatraemia often accompanies hypopituitary decompensation.

Symptoms

Early hyponatraemia [Na⁺] < 120 mmol/L:
- Headache
- Nausea
- Irritability and personality change
- Cramps

Severe hyponatraemia [Na⁺] < 110 mmol/L:
- Confusion
- Seizure
- Coma
- Death

Management
- First assess the plasma volume clinically; measure the CVP if necessary
- Measure the fluid input and output strictly; weigh the patient daily
- Closely monitor the plasma and urine biochemistry, and treat as follows

- For water intoxication with normovolaemia (e.g. in syndrome of inappropriate antidiuretic hormone secretion, or SIADH): restrict fluids
- If the salt loss is greater than the water loss leading to hypovolaemia: replenish with intravenous saline
- If the water loss is greater than the salt loss leading to hypervolaemia: as found with congestive cardiac failure, liver failure and often complicating the use of diuretics
- Also check the cortisol production and thyroid function, and treat any deficiencies

The speed of development as well as the degree of dilution is critical. Note, however, that chronic stable hyponatraemia may be asymptomatic. Rapidly falling osmolality can occur with inappropriately large postoperative dextrose infusions, with untreated hypoadrenalism in stressful illness, or may accompany overdosage of drugs such as desmopressin or carbamazepine.

Management of acute, severe hyponatraemia (normovolaemic)

- Give a cautious infusion of hypertonic saline to increase the plasma ionic sodium concentration by not greater than 10 mmol/L over 24 hours; overrapid correction leads to central pontine myelinolysis, which is often fatal
- When the situation is stable (*not* normal) then restrict fluid to 500–750 ml/day
- Correct any underlying cortisol or thyroid deficiency
- If the condition is ongoing then consider giving demeclocycline, up to 1200 mg/day, which leads to mild nephrogenic diabetes insipidus (DI)

Cerebral salt wasting is uncommon but especially follows surgery of the anterior hypothalamus such as clipping of anterior communicating aneurysms, and more rarely resection of craniopharyngiomas. Massive sodium excretion accompanied by water loss leads to hyponatraemia and polyuria (up to 10 litres per day), in contrast to SIADH (see above). Saline and water replacement rather than fluid restriction is required.

Pituitary tumours

Fits may be caused by neoplasms invading brain tissue (e.g. the temporal lobe) with massive pituitary tumours, and following neurosurgery or radiotherapy.

Management   Carbamazepine is an anticonvulsant that can help, and also treats mild cases of diabetes insipidus.

Pregnancy-induced expansion of prolactinomas is mostly clinically significant only with macroadenomas. Prophylactic surgical debulking of pituitary tumours before pregnancy reduces the risk but does not abolish complications, which include headaches, vomiting and rapid bitemporal visual field loss. Hydrocortisone supplementation should be given, together with rapidly escalating doses of bromocriptine starting at 2.5 mg t.d.s. and increasing to 10 mg t.d.s. (which is surprisingly well tolerated) to shrink the tumour (**Fig. 14.2**). Patients with large prolactinomas may be safely maintained on bromocriptine throughout pregnancy to avoid such problems (there is no evidence of it causing teratogenesis).

Somatotrophic tumours may be particularly susceptible to apoplexy. Acromegaly may cause upper-airway obstruction from macroglossia (**Fig. 14.3**) and mucosal hypertrophy that diminishes laryngeal lumen despite cartilagenous growth, leading to sleep apnoea that is usually obstructive. Because of this, intubation for anaesthesia may be both difficult and hazardous.

THYROID

Thyroid crisis is precipitated by intercurrent illness in a thyrotoxic patient. It has become less common since widespread recognition that it may be precipitated by surgery performed in an untreated thyrotoxic patient.

Clinical features of thyroid crisis

- Pyrexia, often > 41°C
- Cardiovascular decompensation: arrhythmias and heart failure
- Psychological disturbance or even frank psychosis

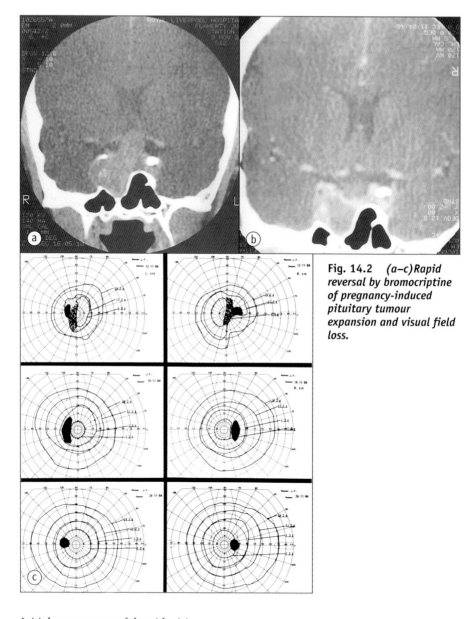

Fig. 14.2 *(a–c)Rapid reversal by bromocriptine of pregnancy-induced pituitary tumour expansion and visual field loss.*

Initial management of thyroid crisis
- First give an oral or nasogastric loading dose of propylthiouracil 300 mg, or carbimazole/methimazole 40 mg
- An hour later give either sodium iodide 1 g i.v., or sodium ipodate
- Propranolol may be added if there is arrhythmia; beware of heart failure
- Sedate with chlorpromazine, which also helps to reduce pyrexia
- Also cool the patient by fanning, or applying icebags
- Rehydrate intravenously, and monitor blood sugar
- Give hydrocortisone 150–200 mg i.v. every 24 hours in three to four divided doses

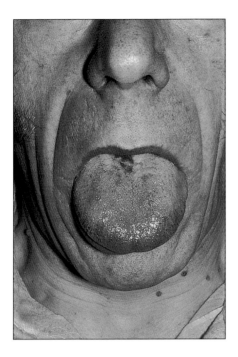

Fig. 14.3 *Macroglossia in acromegaly.*

- Treat underlying causes such as myocardial infarction, pulmonary embolism, or infection

- Amiodarone-induced thyrotoxicosis may progress to crisis; iodine cannot be used
- Lithium carbonate may help, as it blocks thyroid hormone release and improves the mental state
- Use high dose corticosteroids for amiodarone thyroiditis, blocking the conversion of T_4 to T_3

Myxoedema coma

This coma is seen especially in old, undiagnosed or non-compliant hypothyroid patients. There may be environmental cold exposure. Coexisting illness such as pneumonia and other infections, or myocardial infarction, is also common. The condition may be exacerbated by use of sedative drugs.

Most hypothermic patients *look* hypothyroid. Even so, urgently measure the level of TSH. Note, however, that thyroid hormone measurements may be disturbed by artefact.

Management

- First rewarm actively if the core temperature is below 31°C; use a 'space blanket'
- Monitor fluid requirements and electrolytes, and watch out for hyponatraemia
- Monitor the blood glucose level; this may be low or high, and may be associated with pancreatitis
- Retention of carbon dioxide may occur; note that intubation may lead to a risk of ventricular arrhythmia
- Administer T_3 orally or via a nasogastric tube (or intravenously), at a dosage of 2.5 µg 8 hourly for 24 hours, then a double dose daily on the next 2 days up to 10 µg 8 hourly

- Also give hydrocortisone, 50 mg i.v. 8 hourly, in the initial stages of treatment
- Maintain T_3 administration at 10 µg 8 hourly for several days
- Then add 50 µg of T_4 whilst maintaining T_3 at 10 µg 8 hourly for 5 days
- Treat any concomitant illness or complications

Treatment with T_3 is preferable as this is the active thyroid hormone and there may be delayed deiodination of T_4 to T_3, especially in hypothermia and hypothyroidism. Very small doses of T_3 are beneficial and have minimal toxicity but if complications do occur then clearance is rapid. Large doses of T_4 have been recommended when T_3 is unavailable, but this is theoretically inferior.

Myxoedematous madness/psychosis

This occurs typically, but not exclusively, in the elderly. There is commonly a hypersensitivity to psychotropic agents (so these are cleared more slowly than usual).

Management Long-term treatment with thyroxine is beneficial. If the patient is non-compliant then manage this by once-weekly supervised dosing.

Respiratory embarrassment

Clinical features

- Postoperative haematoma (i.e. within 12 hours)
- Bleeding into multinodular goitre
- Recurrent laryngeal nerve palsy (often postsurgery)
- Stridor leading to respiratory arrest
- Malignant invasion (anaplastic carcinoma or lymphoma) with or without recurrent laryngeal nerve involvement

Management
- If there is postoperative haematoma then open the wound and clear the clot
- If there is bleeding into multinodular goitre then use aspiration to remove the altered blood or 'anchovy sauce'-like material
- If stridor occurs then insert a cannula or serum needle through the cricoid membrane prior to formal tracheostomy

ADRENAL CORTEX

Addisonian crisis

With this condition there is usually intercurrent illness supervening on prior weight loss, anorexia, dizziness, lethargy and pigmentation.

Clinical features

- Sudden hypovolaemic shock: adrenal apoplexy and septicaemia (Waterhouse–Friedrichsen syndrome)
- Hyperkalaemia (i.e. a concentration of ionized potassium greater than 8 mmol/L)
- Gastrointestinal features: e.g. vomiting, acute abdomen or diarrhoea
- Profound postural hypotension
- Coma, which is prognostically grave

Management
- Treat on suspicion; a definitive diagnosis can be confirmed later
- Random cortisol levels may be 'normal', and inappropriately low for the level of stress involved
- Administer hydrocortisone 100 mg i.v., followed by 50–100 mg i.v. 6 hourly or by infusion
- Give an infusion of saline: first 1 litre rapidly, then 1 litre 4–6 hourly over the next 24 hours
- Hyperkalaemia usually responds, but fluctuating insulin/glucose levels can lead to dangerous hypoglycaemia
- If there is postictal coma in a male then consider the possibility of adrenoleukodystrophy
- Transfer to the intensive treatment unit for close monitoring of BP, CVP, fluid balance and biochemistry
- Treat precipitating causes such as septicaemia

Cushing's syndrome

This can have a number of acute complications. Malignant hypertension is a rare presentation.

There may be severe hypokalaemic alkalosis, which is suggestive of ectopic ACTH but is not diagnostic. There may also be profound proximal myopathy, which is often exacerbated by hypokalaemia.

IDDM may be seen, but may then disappear with correction of the excess cortisol. Pseudofits may also occur with severe hypercortisolism.

There may be rapid profound osteoporosis, with vertebral collapse leading to paraparesis (**Fig. 14.4**).

Immunocompromise can lead to the occurrence of opportunistic infections such as that by *Pneumocystis carinii*.

Psychiatric problems are prominent in more than 50% of patients with Cushing's syndrome. Frank steroid psychosis may require the administration of metyrapone before any further investigation.

ADRENAL MEDULLA

Phaeochromocytoma

In this condition an acute hypertensive crisis may arise from a preceding normal or elevated BP. Death may occur from cerebral haemorrhage or cardiac tachyarrhythmia.

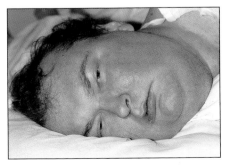

Fig. 14.4 *Severe Cushing's disease causing paralysis from osteoporotic spinal collapse and myopathy.*

Clinical features

- Sudden headache, sweating, sense of impending doom (angor animi)
- Pallor, flushing (and sweating)
- Acute abdomen, mesenteric infarction, ileus, constipation
- Myocardial infarction, myocarditis, heart failure
- Renal impairment
- Hypermetabolism: pyrexia, diabetes mellitus, lactic acidosis
- Exacerbation by bending, abdominal pressure (including pregnancy), micturition (e.g. in bladder tumour)
- Hypotension, especially postcrisis

Acute management

- On suspicion, treat with α-adrenergic blockade
- Administer phenoxybenzamine, a non-competitive antagonist, preferably at least 5–10 mg
- β blockade is often also needed; it must follow α blockade
- Labetalol is inappropriate, as it is far more a β blocker than an α blocker at low dosage, and interferes with assays
- α blockade may reveal hypovolaemia, necessitating blood transfusion
- Transfer to an experienced care centre for further management, especially surgery

DISORDERS OF CALCIUM METABOLISM

Hypercalcaemic crisis

There are a number of causes of this situation including hyperparathyroidism, malignancy, sarcoidosis and vitamin D intoxication. The hypercalcaemia is only loosely related to the ionic calcium concentration; usually the total calcium is greater than 3 mmol/L (12 mg/dl). A vicious spiral may be seen, in which dehydration increases calcium levels, which exacerbates vomiting.

Clinical features

- Hypovolaemic decompensation: vomiting and osmotic diuresis
- Prerenal, renal and postrenal impairment (nephrocalcinosis, renal calculi)
- Thirst, neuromuscular weakness, mental obtundation (common)

Management

- Take a baseline blood count, erythrocyte sedimentation rate (ESR), also check urea and electrolytes, creatinine, calcium, magnesium, phosphate, alkaline phosphatase, albumin, PTH, cortisol, and thyroid function; screen for myeloma

- Infuse 1 litre 0.9% saline as soon as possible, then 1 litre 4–6 hourly
- Monitor calcium and electrolytes; particularly watch the ionic potassium level and replace as needed.
- After rehydration administer pamidronate, 60 mg in 250 ml over 4 hours
- Repeat after 2–3 days
- Treat any underlying precipitating causes such as infection

- If the patient is unresponsive then consider salmon calcitonin 100–200 units or plicamycin 0.15–0.25 mg/kg i.v. (but beware of thrombocytopenia)
- If there is accompanying myeloma, sarcoidosis, or Addison's disease then add corticosteroids

Hypocalcaemia

The major consequence of hypocalcaemia is increased neuromuscular excitability. This infrequently is the cause of refractory epilepsy – which may worsen if treatment is with anticonvulsants inducing hepatic enzymes. Drug-induced osteomalacia may ensue, further lowering calcium concentration. Surgically induced hypoparathyroidism often produces mild tetany, but if this becomes severe and there is concomitant laryngeal nerve damage then there is danger of stridor and even respiratory arrest.

Management of severe hypocalcaemia
- First attend to the airways if there is stridor; prepare for a possible respiratory arrest
- Check the renal function; measures of electrolytes should include calcium, phosphate and magnesium
- Inject 10–20 ml calcium gluconate in a 10% solution over 10 minutes
- Begin oral calcium supplementation, 1 gram or more daily
- Add alfacalcidol 0.5 to 3 µg, or calcitriol 0.25 to 2 µg, as needed

- Replenish magnesium if this is low and the hypocalcaemia remains refractory to treatment

Other endocrine emergencies (e.g. hypoglycaemic and hyperglycaemic comas and gut hormone-induced diarrhoea) are dealt with in the relevant sections of this book.

chapter 15

Hypothalamo-Pituitary Disorders

INTRODUCTION

The hypothalamus and pituitary form a functionally integrated complex. The pituitary gland is suspended by the pituitary stalk from the lowermost part of the hypothalamus. There are two parts to this gland: an anterior lobe that is derived embryologically from an evagination of the stomodeum (foregut), known as Rathke's pouch, and a posterior lobe formed by downward evagination of the brain. The anterior lobe is regulated by chemical factors produced by specialized neurons that terminate in the median eminence of the medial basal hypothalamus. These neurons abut fenestrated capillaries, derived from the arterial system in the anterior circle of Willis, that join to form the hypothalamo-pituitary portal vessels. The portal vessels run down the pituitary stalk to connect with the sinusoidal vessels of the anterior pituitary. In consequence, this system allows the hypothalamic regulatory neurohormones to bathe the pituitary cells (**Fig. 15.1**).

The chemical nature of the hypothalamic regulatory factors has now been elucidated. Most are peptide releasing factors, but hypothalamic inhibition of PRL secretion is mediated largely by dopamine (**Fig. 15.2**). Gonadotrophin-releasing hormone (GnRH) is released in a pulsatile manner; indeed, unremitting sustained exposure to GnRH abolishes pituitary LH secretion (**Fig. 15.3**).

- The posterior pituitary lobe is a storage depot for vasopressin (antidiuretic hormone, or ADH) and oxytocin

The hormones of the posterior lobe are synthesized in the magnocellular neurons of the supraoptic and paraventricular hypothalamic nuclei. They are produced as large precursor molecules that include specific carrier moieties called neurophysins. During axonal passage to the posterior lobe the precursors are cleaved to yield equimolar quantities of the hormones and their carrier neurophysins. Their release is regulated at the hypothalamic level, so hormonal disturbances usually reflect hypothalamic disorder rather than primary pituitary disease.

- The anterior pituitary secretes six major hormones: growth hormone (GH, or somatotrophin), the two gonadotrophins follicle-stimulating hormone (FSH) and luteinizing hormone (LH), thyroid-stimulating hormone (TSH), adrenocorticotrophin (ACTH, or corticotrophin) and prolactin (PRL)

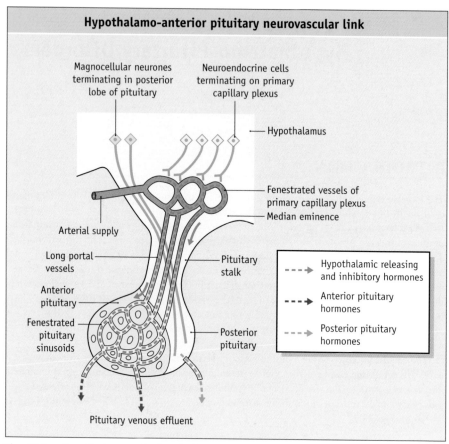

Hypothalamo-anterior pituitary neurovascular link

Magnocellular neurones terminating in posterior lobe of pituitary

Neuroendocrine cells terminating on primary capillary plexus

Hypothalamus

Fenestrated vessels of primary capillary plexus

Median eminence

Arterial supply

Long portal vessels

Pituitary stalk

Anterior pituitary

Fenestrated pituitary sinusoids

Posterior pituitary

- - - → Hypothalamic releasing and inhibitory hormones

- - - → Anterior pituitary hormones

- - - → Posterior pituitary hormones

Pituitary venous effluent

Fig. 15.1   *Hypothalamo-anterior pituitary neurovascular link.*

All the hormones of the anterior lobe except PRL act largely through target glands – including the thyroid, adrenal cortex, gonads and, in the case of GH, the liver, which produces IGF-I (**Fig. 15.4**). GH also stimulates other organs to produce IGF-I, which acts in a local paracrine fashion.

According to the archaeological records, the diseases of GH excess (gigantism and acromegaly) and deficiency (**Fig. 15.5**) were known in antiquity. The identification of pituitary tumours preceded the recognition of the endocrine effects. Acromegaly was first clearly described by Pierre Marie a century ago. Harvey Cushing, besides describing the disease named after him, largely developed a safe technique for neurosurgery of the pituitary, including transsphenoidal and transfrontal approaches, and contributed to the physiological understanding of pituitary function in parallel to others performing animal studies on this gland.

Epidemiological studies of the pituitary are incomplete. Small tumours are commonly found here in autopsy studies of people dying suddenly from accidental causes; most are presumably clinically silent though some stain for PRL. The incidence of clinically significant tumours in the developed world is 20–30 per million per year. Their presentation depends on geography and economics. In Africa the commonest presentation is blindness from a large

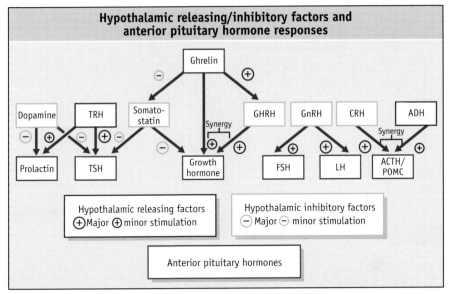

Fig. 15.2 *Hypothalamic releasing/inhibitory factors and anterior pituitary hormone responses.*

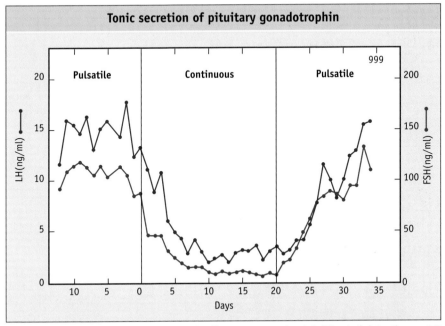

Fig. 15.3 *Differential influence of pulsatile versus sustained GnRH administration on LH release (modified from Belchetz et al. 1978 Science 202: 631–633, with permission).*

179

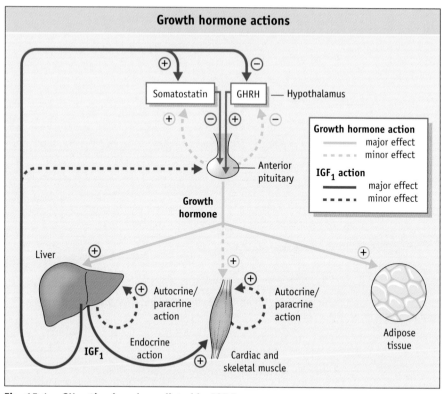

Fig. 15.4   *GH action largely mediated by IGF-I.*

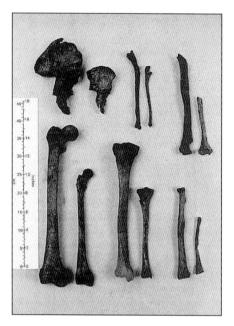

Fig. 15.5   *Skeleton of GH-deficient adult compared with normal-sized skeleton; both were excavated from the same Roman graveyard.*

tumour compressing the optic pathways. However, most tumours are functionless and present with features of a space-occupying lesion with various degrees of hypopituitarism. The recognition of hypersecreting lesions, especially GH and PRL and less frequently ACTH, gonadotrophins and TSH, follows from extra features that are detailed below. The impact of these disorders on mortality and morbidity is increasingly being recognized and defined.

- Acromegaly is estimated to have an incidence of 4–6 new cases per million per year with a prevalence of approximately 40 per million. Overall mortality is twice normal but is reduced to near normal in patients treated so that their mean GH averages less than 5 mU/L (2.5 ng/ml). The major causes of death are cardiovascular, respiratory and cerebrovascular. There is an increased incidence and mortality from colonic cancer

PATHOGENESIS AND PATHOLOGY

PITUITARY TUMOURS

Pituitary tumours are rarely part of multiple endocrine neoplasia, type 1 (MEN-1) syndrome, which may be familial (see Ch. 23). The tumour suppressor gene for this syndrome located on chromosome 11 has been cloned and its common mutations resulting in MEN-1 have been identified. A constitutively active mutation of the stimulatory G protein (*gsp*) has been postulated as the cause of GH-secreting adenomas in up to 40% of cases. Rare familial cases of acromegaly have been recorded but so far the genetic abnormality has not been identified in non-MEN-1 cases. Aggressive tumours of the pituitary have been associated with abnormalities in a number of oncogenes and tumour suppressor genes (**Fig. 15.6**). It has long been noted that in many cases of Cushing's disease either no discrete lesion can be found at surgery or diffuse hyperplastic changes are noted. The blunted rather than fully resistant suppression of cortisol production following dexamethasone administration, the exuberant ACTH response to exogenous corticotrophin-releasing hormone (CRH, also called ACTH-releasing factor) and desmopressin together with the pathological features prompted early ideas that hypothalamic secretion might be responsible. There are alternative explanations, however, such as constitutive activation in the pituitary receptors for releasing factors. Transgenic mice overexpressing the *GHRH* (GH-releasing hormone) gene display initial hyperplasia before developing tumours of somatroph cells. Also, most pituitary tumours studied are monoclonal, which suggests there is true neoplastic transformation.

The pathological characterization of pituitary tumours is based on classical haematoxylin and eosin staining and subsequent trichrome variants. There are three major categories:

Classification of pituitary tumours

- Chromophobe, often functionless tumours (**Fig. 15.7a**)
- Eosinophilic, often producing GH or PRL (**Fig. 15.7b**)
- Basophilic, particularly associated with Cushing's disease (**Fig. 15.76c**)

Fig. 15.6   Oncogenes and tumour suppressor genes possibly related to pituitary tumorigenesis

Oncogenes

G_sP Mutations in G_s protein: 201 Arg → Cys/His or 227Gln → Arg/Leu ? 40% GH secreting adenomas in Caucasian patients, fewer in Japanese

CREB ? facilitating role in somatotroph transformation and GH gene transcription

RAS Found in metastases from pituitary carcinomas and aggressive prolactinoma

PTTG Increased expression in many types, greater expression with more invasive tumours

Tumour suppressor genes

9p Early change in non-functional tumours, rare in somatotrophinomas

9p21 Early change as above, via protein p16, interfering with cell cycle

13q ? via RBI? close situated gene product. Somatotrophinomas, rare: non-functional tumours

10q23 Transition to invasive/metastatic phenotype, in all subtypes or pituitary tumour

11q13 As above? via menin? closely situated gene product

12p13 As above via p27? post-translational action on cell cycle regulation

13q As above: all subtypes

17p Via p53 as above, all subtypes

17p21 Via m23 as above, all subtypes

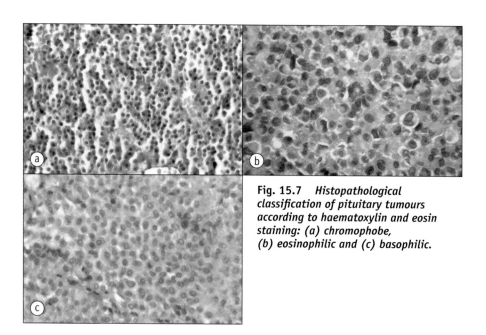

Fig. 15.7   Histopathological classification of pituitary tumours according to haematoxylin and eosin staining: (a) chromophobe, (b) eosinophilic and (c) basophilic.

Sensitive and specific immunostaining techniques reveal the existence of gonadotrophin- and TSH-secreting tumours, oncocytic tumours and functionless tumours staining for synaptophysin and chromogranin. Immunostaining features do not invariably correlate with secretory activity, however.

The invasiveness of pituitary tumours varies greatly, but as with many endocrine tumours this characteristic correlates only poorly with observed features such as mitotic figures or nuclear pleomorphism. Dural invasion is often difficult to recognize at surgery but is commonly the cause of recurrence. Pituitary carcinomas are extremely rare but examples are documented both for PRL-, GH-, ACTH- or TSH-secreting and for endocrinologically functionless tumours. They are defined by the presence of distant metastases within, or much more rarely outside, the CNS.

OTHER HYPOTHALAMO–PITUITARY DISORDERS

For other pathologies in the hypothalamus-pituitary region a number of tests are appropriate:

- **Craniopharyngioma**   The presence of calcified cysts containing β-hCG (beta human chorionic gonadotrophin)
- **Lymphocytic hypophysitis**   Lymphocytes for cd4 (cluster of differentiation 4)
- **Pituitary abscess**   Pus with evidence of bacterial infection
- **Cranial irradiation**   May be associated with cerebral vasculitis
- **Haemochromatosis**   Often marked iron deposition in the pituitary
- **Infarction from apoplexy or Sheehan's syndrome**   Yields pathological features which change with the passage of time from the vascular catastrophe

The application of electron microscopy can sometimes help define pathology while cosecretion of more than one hormone by a single cell, suggested by immunostaining, can be confirmed by demonstration of specific mRNA products.

INVESTIGATION AND DIAGNOSIS

Investigation of hypothalamo-pituitary disorders involves the assessment of endocrine function – whether deficient, excessive or mixed – and delineation of the anatomy, size and topographical relations of any pituitary or parapituitary masses. Assessment of the effects of a mass conventionally focuses on the visual pathways. Quality of life (QOL) evaluation and psychometric testing are increasingly performed, especially in view of the long-term consequences of surgery or other therapeutic interventions (**Fig. 15.8**). Recognition of adult GH deficiency syndrome prompts serial assessment of bone density and body composition as well as cardiovascular risk factors such as lipid profile.

HORMONAL EVALUATION OF PITUITARY FUNCTION

Basal measurements adequately define most aspects of hormonal secretion, including pituitary–thyroid and –gonadal axes, PRL secretion and water metabolism (**Fig. 15.9**). The large variations in GH and ACTH/cortisol levels, which are determined by ultradian, circadian and stress-related mechanisms as well as classical negative feedback loops, often require dynamic testing (**Fig. 15.10**). Nevertheless a single 9 a.m. plasma cortisol measurement can provide adequate evidence of adrenal insufficiency if less than 180 nmol/L (6 µg/dl). Random GH measurements are useful only to exclude the diagnosis of acromegaly – this is unlikely if the value is less than 2 mU/L (1 ng/ml) – or for rough assessment of the degree of GH hypersecretion in known acromegaly since there is a strong correlation between the fasting GH measurement and the mean of serial samples taken over periods up to 24 hours, notwithstanding the frequently observed pulsatility of GH release in acromegaly. Measurement of IGF-I provides an integrated perspective of overall GH secretion. The level of IGF-I tends to be low in hypopituitarism even though it may lie within the age-related normal range in patients in whom stimulatory tests of GH reserve indicate

Fig. 15.8   Psychometric consequences of pituitary disease and treatment by transsphenoidal/transfrontal surgery and radiotherapy*

Treatment	Transsphenoidal surgery	Transfrontal surgery	Medical treatment	Control
Number	23	23	23	23
Mean age (years)	42.7	41.6	38.7	38.9
Years of education	10.9	11.3	11.5	11.6
Estimated duration of illness (years)	8.6	14.9	8.5	–
Estimated premorbid IQ	107.9	109.8	111.0	112.1

Measures	
Premorbid ability	National Adult Reading Test
Attention	Digit subtest of Wechsler Adult Intelligence Scale (Revised)
Memory	Auditory – verbal learning test
	Story recall – from Wechsler Memory Scale
	Recognition – memory test for faces
Executive functions	Controlled oral word association test
	Block design subtest of Wechsler Adult Intelligence Scale (Revised)
	Trail-making test

Results	
	Three or more tests below tenth percentile
	Transsphenoidal = 30.4%, Transfrontal = 43.5%, Medical = 21.7%, Control = 4.3%

Radiotherapy had NO adverse effect on cognitive function

*From Peace et al. Clinical Endocrinology 1998; 49(3): 391–396

Fig. 15.9   Basal blood tests for assessment of pituitary function

Chemistry	Hormones
Electrolytes (Na^+/K^+)	Total/free T_4 (and T_3)
Urea/creatinine	TSH
Osmolality	Prolactin
Calcium profile	FSH/LH
Fasting glucose	α-subunit (if glycoprotein-producing tumour)
Fasting triglycerides	IGF-1
Cholesterol	Growth hormone (acromegaly)
HDL-C	9am cortisol
LDL-C	ACTH (Cushing's disease)
	Midnight cortisol (Cushing's disease)
	Men: testosterone, SHBG
	Women < 50 years: 17β oestradiol

Fig. 15.10 Dynamic tests of hypothalamo-pituitary-adrenal function

Test	Contraindication	Precaution	Protocol	Interpretation
Insulin tolerance test (ITT)	Frank hypoadrenalism Epilepsy Cardiac ischaemia including patients > 70 years old – in whom IHD is likely	Check 9 a.m. cortisol ≥ 180 nmol/L (6 µg/dl) Check history Check history and 12 lead ECG	Fast patient overnight and weigh. Insert venous cannula. Obtain blood for plasma glucose and cortisol (and GH – see below) at 0, 30, 45, 60, 120 min. Inject 0.15 U soluble insulin/kg If patient insulin resistant e.g. obese, acromegalic, Cushings: double dose. If *not* hypoglycaemic by 45 min readminister initial dose and regard this as time zero. If severe response to hypoglycaemia viz coma, fits, chest pain: correct hypoglycaemia with i.v. glucose immediately but continue sampling for stress evoked responses	Normal response: peak cortisol ≥ 550 nmol/L (18 µg/dl) if adequate hypoglycaemia achieved (≤ 2.2 mmol/L) (40 mg/dl) + appropriate symptoms. **NB** Only test validated clinically – ability to withstand surgical stress
Glucagon test	Diabetes mellitus	Prepare for nausea (30%) or vomiting (15%)	Fast patient overnight and weigh. Insert venous cannula. Obtain blood for plasma glucose, cortisol (and GH). Inject glucagon 1 mg i.m. (if weight < 90 kg) 1.5 mg (if weight ≥ 90 kg). Repeat blood samples at 150 and 180 min after glucagon i.m. injection. **NB** Classical subcutaneous test: (same doses but samples at 0, 90, 120, 150, 180, 210 and 240 min)	Non-peak cortisol response ≥ 500 nmol/L (17 µg/dl) Post-glucagon subcutaneous injection peak time more variable, hence need for multiple samples

Fig. 15.10   *(Cont'd)*

Test	Contraindication	Precaution	Protocol	Interpretation
Short Synacthen test	Hypersensitivity to Synacthen (very rare)	Not valid within 2 weeks of pituitary surgery –? longer	Blood sample before and 30 min after tetracosactrin (Synacthen) 250 µg i.m.	Peak cortisol ≥ 600 nmol/L (20 µg/dl) **NB** False positive results common, discouraging use by many investigators
Low dose Synacthen test	Hypersensitivity to Synacthen	Not valid within 2 weeks of surgery	Blood taken before and ? 20, 40, 60 min post-tetracosactrin (Synacthen) 1 µg i.v.	New – few and slightly conflicting date re usefulness. Need own laboratory normal values
Metyrapone (Metopirone)	Frank hypoadrenalism	Prepare for adrenal insufficiency.	Very variable protocols used – poorly standardized using cortisol and 11-desoxycortisol/ ACTH or urine steroids (obsolete)	Does not test stress response. Needs own laboratory normal values

GH deficiency. Conversely levels tend to be raised in acromegaly, and this can be useful for monitoring the level of GH secretion following treatment. The level of IGF-binding protein 3 (IGF-BP3) is also related to mean level of GH secretion, but this measure is less sensitive though more specific than that of IGF-I.

Assessment of cortisol response to stress is essential in patients with pituitary disorders. Various tests are used.

Assessment of GH reserve

- **Insulin tolerance test (ITT)** This is the most powerful stimulus. Peak GH values usually exceed 20 mU/L (10 ng/ml). Lower values are found in old age. Adult onset GH deficiency is defined as ≤ 9 mU/L. (For details and precautions see **Fig. 15.10**)
- **Glucagon test** Peak values are as for ITT (see above)
- **Arginine test** This is used in some centres but responses do not correlate closely with ITT or glucagon in some patients (e.g. after irradiation)
- **Clonidine test** This is of minor value in children but ineffective, so useless, in adults
- **GHRH test** This directly tests pituitary reserve, bypassing vital hypothalamic mechanisms; hence it may give discordant and misleading results
- **Sex hormone priming** Peripubertal individuals should receive testosterone (boys) or ethinyl oestradiol (girls) prior to testing to establish maximum GH secretory capacity (see Ch. 16)

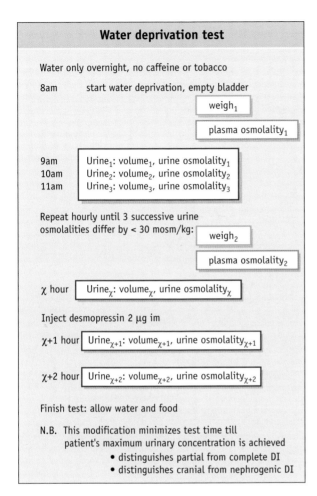

Water deprivation test

Water only overnight, no caffeine or tobacco

8am   start water deprivation, empty bladder

weigh$_1$

plasma osmolality$_1$

9am   Urine$_1$: volume$_1$, urine osmolality$_1$
10am   Urine$_2$: volume$_2$, urine osmolality$_2$
11am   Urine$_3$: volume$_3$, urine osmolality$_3$

Repeat hourly until 3 successive urine
osmolalities differ by < 30 mosm/kg:

weigh$_2$

plasma osmolality$_2$

χ hour   Urine$_\chi$: volume$_\chi$, urine osmolality$_\chi$

Inject desmopressin 2 μg im

χ+1 hour   Urine$_{\chi+1}$: volume$_{\chi+1}$, urine osmolality$_{\chi+1}$

χ+2 hour   Urine$_{\chi+2}$: volume$_{\chi+2}$, urine osmolality$_{\chi+2}$

Finish test: allow water and food

N.B. This modification minimizes test time till
patient's maximum urinary concentration is achieved
- distinguishes partial from complete DI
- distinguishes cranial from nephrogenic DI

Fig. 15.11 *Water deprivation test for assessment of DI.*

Assessment of vasopressin secretion

Frank DI presents with thirst, polyuria including nocturia with the urinary volume exceeding 3 litres over 24 hours, and with a serum sodium level of more than 145 mmol/L. Milder degrees require evaluation with a water deprivation test including documenting response to desmopressin (DDAVP) (**Fig. 15.11**). On occasion, measuring plasma (arginine vasopressin, or AVP) responses to 5% saline infused at 0.04 ml/kg per minute for 2 hours will clarify issues (**Fig. 15.12**).

IMAGING OF THE HYPOTHALAMO-PITUITARY REGION

MRI is the modality of choice in most cases. However, the presence of ferromagnetic material (e.g. some ocular prostheses) is an absolute contraindication. MRI is safe but may prove claustrophobic, noisy and prolonged for some patients. Enhancement with gadolinium very rarely causes adverse reactions. Pituitary adenomas as small as 3 mm can be detected (**Fig. 15.13**). T_1 and T_2 signal characteristics inform about tumour qualities such as water content, haemorrhage and fibrosis. The optic chiasm is visualized well and its relationships to the pituitary well defined (**Fig. 15.14**). The posterior lobe normally appears as a

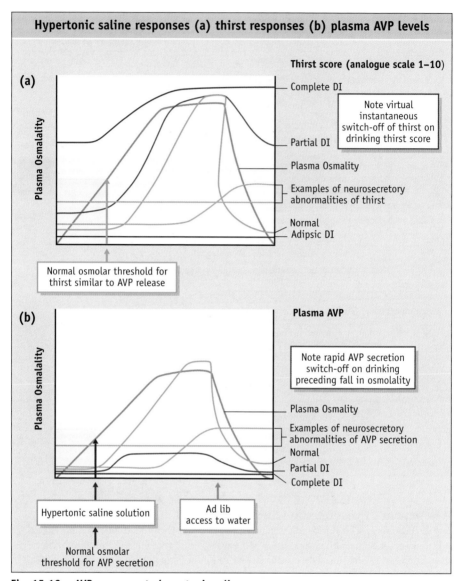

Fig. 15.12   *AVP responses to hypertonic saline.*

hyperintense signal (**Fig. 15.15**). The lateral relations of the pituitary show up well and give evidence of abutment upon or invasion of cavernous sinuses (**Fig. 15.16**).

CT scanning is still useful – especially when access to MRI is limited or delayed. Pituitary tumours are almost as well imaged but chiasmal and cavernosal relations are less so. Bony relations including erosion are particularly well delineated (**Fig. 15.17**). The irradiation load is high so efforts are made to avoid the eye lenses; this may involve the uncomfortable 'hanging head' position to obtain coronal images. Dental fillings may cause streak artefacts. Contrast media give useful information but may be associated with severe reactions.

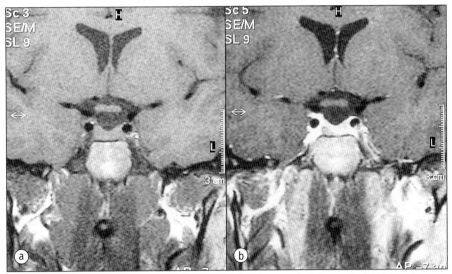

Fig. 15.13 *MRI of pituitary microadenoma (a) before gadolinium – invisible, and (b) after – seen as hypointense area.*

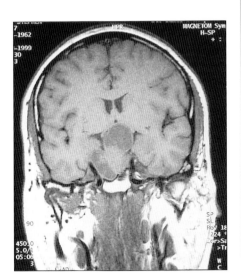

Fig. 15.14 *MRI imaging of a pituitary tumour compressing the optic chiasm.*

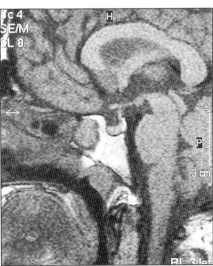

Fig. 15.15 *MRI showing a high intensity signal from the posterior lobe of the pituitary.*

Calcified lesions such as craniopharyngiomas are well demonstrated, but MRI may also be required to show the full extent of tumour (**Fig. 15.18**).

Angiography may be needed to display arterial anatomy – for instance if aneurysms are suspected (**Fig. 15.19**). Ectatic loops of carotid arteries are often seen in acromegaly. Magnetic resonance angiography (MR-A) is of use, though has a lower exclusion value for small aneurysms than conventional angiography.

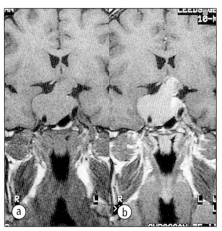

Fig. 15.16   *MRI illustrating a pituitary tumour invading the cavernous sinus (enwrapping the intracavernosal carotid artery), (a) before and (b) after gadolinium.*

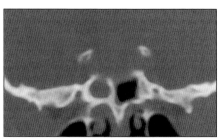

Fig. 15.17   *CT scan demonstrating bony erosion by a pituitary tumour.*

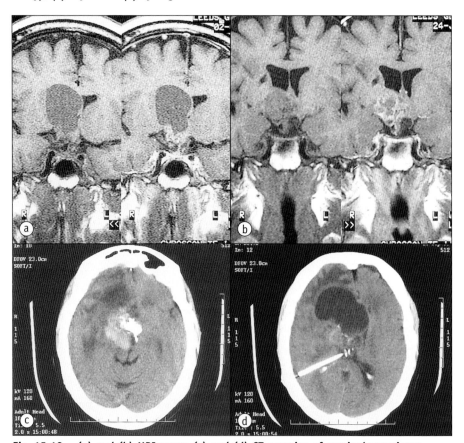

Fig. 15.18   *(a) and (b) MRI versus (c) and (d) CT scanning of craniopharyngioma.*

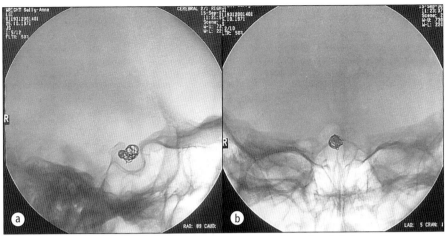

Fig. 15.19 *Cerebral aneurysms in proximity to the pituitary (containing coils introduced to thrombose them).*

INVESTIGATION OF ACROMEGALY

A number of tests may be appropriate:

● Random GH	Values less than 2 mU/L (1ng/dl) exclude acromegaly
● IGF-I	Above the age-matched normal is suggestive – investigate further
● Oral GTT with GH measurements	The normal response is a fall to less than 2 mU/L (1ng/dl) (**Fig. 15.20**)
● MRI	Add, if necessary, MR-A or angiogram, and skull X-rays (**Fig. 15.21**)
● PRL	
● Thyroid function tests	Plus a thyroid scan if goitre is present
● Gonadotrophins and sex steroid measurements	As clinically indicated
● ECG, chest X-ray	Plus echocardiogram if there is hypertension
● Serum calcium, phosphate, 24 hour urinary calcium	Plus if necessary X-ray of the renal tract
● Full blood count	If there is anaemia, bowel symptoms, or a family history of colon cancer add colonoscopy
● Dorsolumbar spine X-ray, DEXA (dual-energy X-ray absorptiometry)	If there is backache, kyphosis, or loss of height
● Nerve conduction studies	If there is neuropathy, especially carpal tunnel syndrome
● Sleep studies	If there is snoring or daytime somnolence
● Skin thickness measurement	(**Fig. 15.22**)
● Ring size measurement	(**Fig. 15.23**)

INVESTIGATION OF CUSHING'S DISEASE

In patients with established Cushing's syndrome (see Ch. 18) the following tests should be performed:

● Low dose dexamethasone test

191

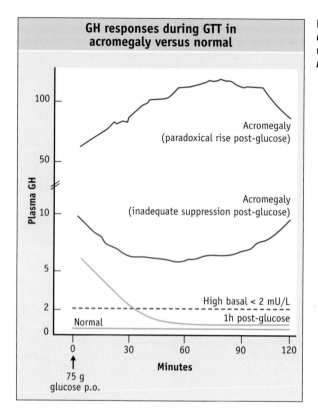

Fig. 15.20 *GTT showing GH responses in a patient with acromegaly and in a normal individual.*

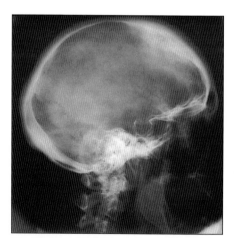

Fig. 15.21 *Skull X-ray of a patient with acromegaly showing an enlarged sella, thickened calvarium, large frontal air sinuses, occipital bossing and prognathism.*

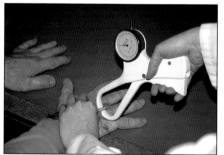

Fig. 15.22 *Skinfold measurements in acromegaly.*

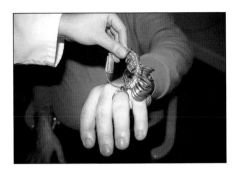

Fig. 15.23 *Ring size measurement in acromegaly.*

- CRH test
- Desmopressin test
- MRI scan
- Inferior petrosal sinus sampling

Petrosal sinus sampling is useful for differentiating pituitary from ectopic sources of ACTH secretion in Cushing's syndrome. Catheters are introduced via the femoral veins and passed under radiological screening up through the heart and jugular veins to the inferior petrosal sinus (IPS). Conventionally, a catheter is inserted each side and a further line established for peripheral venous sampling. After central (right and left) and peripheral blood samples are taken, CRH 100 mg is injected intravenously. Repeat blood samples are taken from both IPSs and the peripheral vein three times over a 15 minute period following the CRH injection for ACTH measurement (in EDTA tubes, sent to the laboratory on ice, rapidly spun and frozen; ensure accurate labelling). Rare but serious complications, including haematoma, thrombosis and brainstem lesions, have led to the development of sequential sampling of each IPS after CRH injection (since the ACTH elevation from pituitary lesions is prolonged), as this has lower morbidity (**Fig. 15.24**). If ACTH values from either IPS exceed twice the simultaneous peripheral value a pituitary source is strongly suggested. Note though that the IPS side with peak ACTH values is not necessarily the side of the pituitary tumour.

CLINICAL FEATURES

PITUITARY TUMOURS

Space-occupying features

- Headache
- Visual disturbance
- Hypopituitarism
- Hydrocephalus, hypothalamic syndrome
- Cerebrospinal fluid (CSF) leak
- Epilepsy

Headache, which is common with pituitary tumours even of modest size, is often attributed to pressure on the dura mater, especially the diaphragma sellae. However, rarely it is due to massive tumours causing raised intracranial pressure.

Pituitary infarction is commonly partial and may be asymptomatic but major episodes cause pituitary apoplexy characterized by the following features:

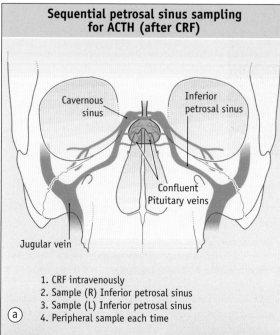

Sequential petrosal sinus sampling for ACTH (after CRF)

Cavernous sinus

Inferior petrosal sinus

Confluent Pituitary veins

Jugular vein

1. CRF intravenously
2. Sample (R) Inferior petrosal sinus
3. Sample (L) Inferior petrosal sinus
4. Peripheral sample each time

(a)

Fig. 15.24   (a–c) Inferior petrosal sinus sampling – sequential technique.

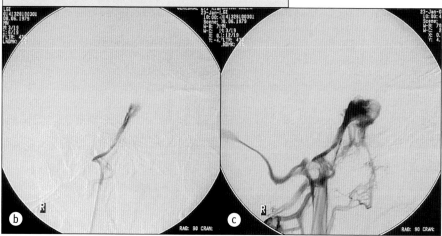

(b) (c)

Features of pituitary apoplexy

- Sudden, severe headache
- Meningism (with evidence of subarachnoid haemorrhage)
- Cavernous sinus involvement – diplopia, ophthalmoplegia, ptosis and facial pain
- Acute anterior pituitary failure – complete or partial including isolated ACTH or TSH deficiency (see Ch. 14)

The most common visual disturbance is chiasmal compression. Classically this begins with upper outer field loss progressing to bitemporal hemianopia or even complete blindness. Clinical testing by confrontation should begin with a red pin (**Fig. 15.25**) as loss of colour vision frequently long predates the inability to see finger movements. Other visual tests include the use of Ishihara colour charts and evidence of relative afferent pupillary defect (**Fig. 15.26**). Assessment of visual acuity should involve the reading of lines of print, as often letters become lost at the beginning and end of lines. Pituitary tumours may be asymmetrical with striking differences in field defects between the right and left eyes. Fundoscopy often reveals optic atrophy with established chiasmal compression (**Fig. 15.27**); papilloedema is rare. Ophthalmoplegia indicates cavernous sinus involvement.

Hypopituitarism due to pituitary tumour characteristically progresses sequentially:

- *GH deficiency.* Is the first detectable feature
- *Gonadotrophin deficiency.* Appears early on, with LH deficiency preceding that of FSH
- *PRL excess.* Is often early but modest; it is due to stalk compression
- *ACTH deficiency.* Is a late feature
- *TSH deficiency.* Is usually last to develop
- *DI.* If present at presentation this strongly suggests a parapituitary disorder

GROWTH HORMONE DEFICIENCY

GH deficiency in childhood is dealt with in Chapter 16. Adult GH deficiency is diagnostically valuable and clinically important (**Fig. 15.28**), since recombinant GH therapy is available. Gonadotrophin deficiency in premenopausal women is generally recognized early on account of primary or secondary amenorrhoea, infertility or loss of libido. Men often delay presentation on developing impotence or loss of libido, though with wider recognition of effective management of erectile dysfunction this pattern is reversing, provided other practitioners check for hormonal causes. Gonadal dysfunction is augmented

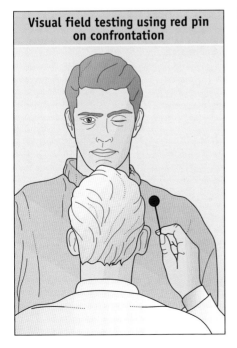

Visual field testing using red pin on confrontation

Fig. 15.25 *Visual field testing by confrontation using a red pin.*

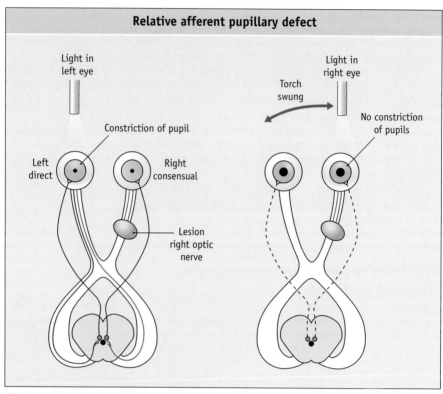

Fig. 15.26   *Relative afferent pupillary defect.*

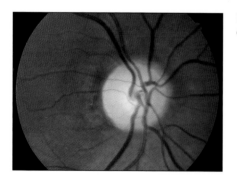

Fig. 15.27   *Optic atrophy after chiasmal compression.*

by hyperprolactinaemia – this is principally due to reduction in the frequency of GnRH release. Galactorrhoea is not common or correlated with level of PRL excess and is rare in men.

HYPERPROLACTINAEMIA

Hyperprolactinaemia may be caused by any of the following:

- Prolactinoma
- Functionless pituitary adenoma (a stalk effect)

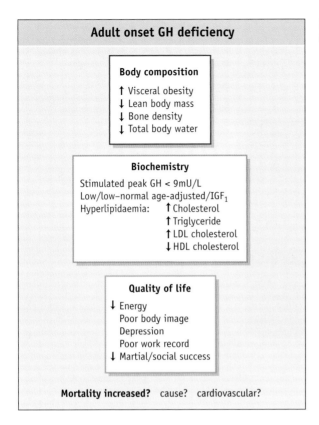

Fig. 15.28 *Features of adult onset GH deficiency.*

- Hypothalamic disease due to tumour, granuloma, or irradiation
- Primary hypothyroidism
- Dopamine antagonists such as phenothiazines, butyrophenones, metoclopramide and domperidone
- Opioid peptides and alkaloids
- Oestrogen – in high dosage, or pregnancy
- H_2 antagonists – such as intravenous (not oral) cimetidine
- Polycystic ovary syndrome (PCOS)
- Acromegaly
- McCune–Albright syndrome (**Fig. 15.29**)
- Chronic renal failure
- Hepatic cirrhosis
- Chest wall disease

Microprolactinomas (less than 10 mm maximum diameter) are common and do not cause space-occupying problems, with the occasional exception of headache; nor are they usually associated with other hormone deficiencies, with the exception of the expected hypogonadism and less often GH deficiency. Macroadenomas secreting PRL contrast with large functionless tumours causing hyperprolactinaemia by stalk compression that interferes with delivery of hypothalamic dopamine, thus disinhibiting normal pituitary lactotrophs. Clinical distinction between the two tumours usually depends on the level of PRL secretion: values over 8000 mU/L (400 ng/ml) strongly suggest macroprolactinoma, whereas those less

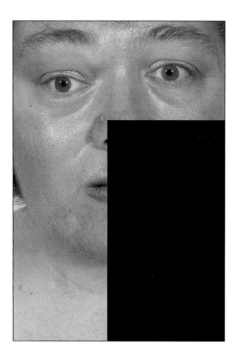

Fig. 15.29 *McCune–Albright syndrome with café au lait pigment, facial asymmetry, hyperprolactinaemia and acromegaly.*

than 2000 mU/L (100 ng/ml) suggest a stalk effect. Macroprolactinomas may shrink markedly with dopamine agonist therapy (see below).

Hypothalamic lesions such as craniopharyngiomas, or those caused by surgical damage or irradiation, may cause modest hyperprolactinaemia by diminishing dopaminergic tone.

HYPOPITUITARISM

ACTH deficiency may present either chronically or acutely, precipitated by intercurrent illness.

Clinical features

Chronic:
- Fatigue
- Disproportionate pallor of skin compared with the mucous membranes (i.e. not due to anaemia)
- Orthostatic hypotension
- Hyponatraemia
- Low grade pyrexia of unknown origin (sepsis excluded)

Acute:
- Haemodynamic collapse
- Nausea and vomiting
- Obtunded consciousness associated with severe hyponatraemia
- Prerenal uraemia (less commonly than in primary adrenal failure)
- Hypoglycaemia

TSH deficiency presents with the usual features of hypothyroidism but is often milder than primary hypothyroidism. Myxoedema is not usually seen in secondary hypothyroidism although the skin is often dramatically cold and dry to the touch.

TUMOURS WITH EXTRASELLAR EXTENSION

Large tumours can extend upward compressing the hypothalamus and third ventricle. Hydrocephalus may result in dementia, loss of balance and abnormalities of micturition. Invasion of the temporal lobes can cause epilepsy. Many neural problems develop, often years later, after surgery or radiotherapy. Tumours eroding through the pituitary fossa and sphenoid bone can lead to the subarachnoid space communicating with the nasopharynx, resulting in CSF rhinorrhoea and the potential for meningitis.

HYPERSECRETING PITUITARY TUMOURS

Cushing's disease – see Ch. 18.

ACROMEGALY

GH excess causing gigantism (**Fig. 15.30**) prepubertally occurs rarely. Apart from the increased growth of long bones leading to an ultimate height often in excess of 2 metres, this is associated with kyphoscoliosis and distortions of the rib cage. The pituitary tumours are frequently large.

Adult onset acromegaly is most frequently diagnosed in patients in the middle years of life, but retrospective analysis of photographs often discloses developing features becoming apparent 10 or more years before diagnosis (**Fig. 15.31**).

Clinical features

- Enlargement of hands (becoming fleshy, so rings need enlarging) (**Fig. 15.32**) and of feet (becoming broader)
- Thick skin with deep creases, increased sweating and sebum production (**Fig. 15.33**)
- Hypertension, left ventricular hypertrophy and congestive cardiac failure
- Soft tissue enlargement – such as in the nose, tongue (**Fig. 15.34**), larynx, or viscera
- Prognathism and increased interdental spacing (**Fig. 15.35**)
- Visual field defects
- Obstructive sleep apnoea
- Goitre, which is multinodular, and sometimes toxic
- Hyperprolactinaemia, hypogonadism and galactorrhoea
- Osteoporosis
- Osteoarthritis
- Colonic polyps and carcinoma
- Impaired glucose tolerance and diabetes mellitus
- Carpal tunnel syndrome
- Hirsutism (**Fig. 15.36**)
- Hypopituitarism
- Myopathy

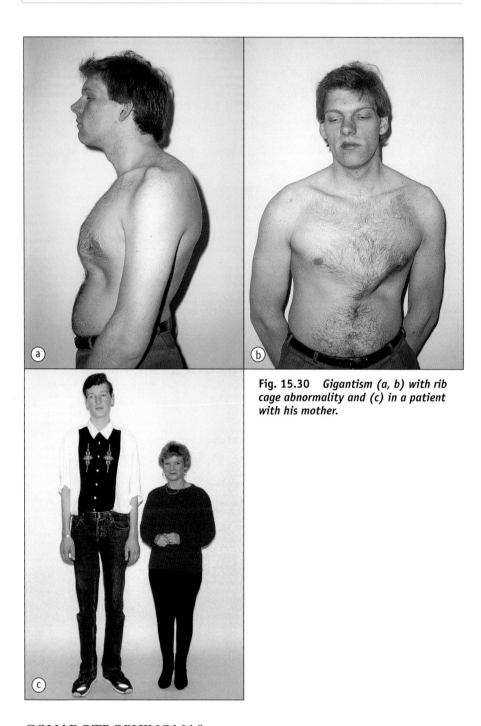

Fig. 15.30   *Gigantism (a, b) with rib cage abnormality and (c) in a patient with his mother.*

GONADOTROPHINOMAS

These have only relatively recently been recognized as a distinct entity. Some claim they constitute the majority of 'functionless' pituitary tumours as judged by immunostaining and

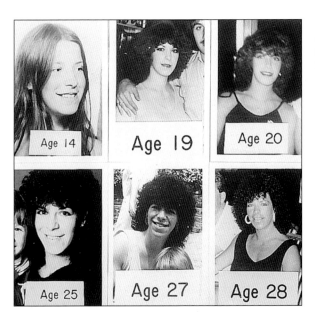

Fig. 15.31 *Chronological sequence of photographs showing slow development of acromegaly.*

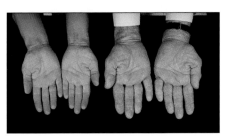

Fig. 15.32 *Large spade-like fleshy hands in acromegaly (compared with normal hands).*

secretion in cell culture after removal at surgery. However, the serum gonadotrophin levels are normal and in addition this claim does not account for the well-recognized inclusion of normal pituitary tissue in many pituitary tumours. Even raised gonadotrophin levels cannot help diagnosis in postmenopausal women – hence the readier recognition of tumours hypersecreting gonadotrophins in men. They usually dominantly secrete FSH with or without excess glycoprotein α-subunit production, LH, LHβ or indeed any other combination. They have been characterized as benign tumours with low rates of dural invasion which eventually present having grown large and causing primarily visual symptoms as well as hypopituitarism. Against this concept of indolent growth is the capacity of documented gonadotrophinomas to recur rapidly postoperatively accompanied by deteriorating vision, which is only partially abrogated by radiotherapy. Men with these tumours often have extremely large testicles caused by an increase in seminiferous tubules.

TSH-OMAS

These are rare, causing thyrotoxicosis with goitre but no eye signs of Graves' disease. Levels of T4 and T_3 are raised, accompanied by normal or raised TSH levels and often excess glycoprotein α-subunit production. Less frequently TSH-omas also secrete PRL, GH or

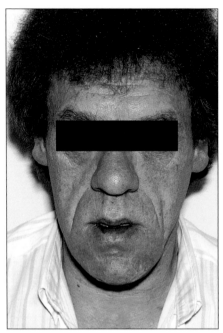

Fig. 15.33   *Thick skin with deep creases in acromegaly.*

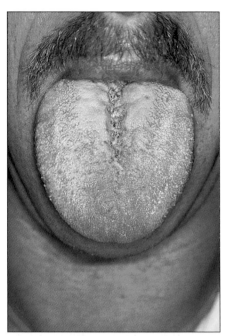

Fig. 15.34   *Macroglossia in acromegaly.*

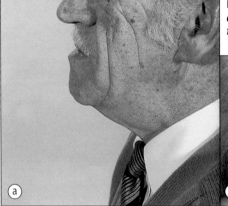

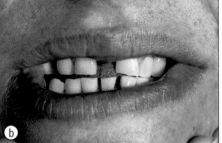

Fig. 15.35   *(a) Prognathism in acromegaly. (b) Leading to increased interdental spacing.*

gonadotrophins. They are frequently large at presentation with effects due to mass, as well as thyrotoxic features. They need to be distinguished from thyroid hormone resistance, which is usually due to mutations in exons 9 and 10 of the thyroid hormone β-receptor, and in which there is no excessive α-subunit production and no association with pituitary tumours (see Ch. 17).

OTHER PARASELLAR AND SUPRAPITUITARY LESIONS

Craniopharyngiomas

These are the commonest tumours affecting the hypothalamo-pituitary region in childhood. They may, however, present at any age.

Clinical features

- *Infancy*. Features of raised intracranial pressure and gross visual impairment
- *Childhood*. Raised pressure and short stature
- *Puberty*. Endocrine insufficiency causing delayed or arrested puberty, poor growth and DI
- *Middle/old age*. Headache, visual defects, usually also hypopituitarism

---

They are tumours arising from Rathke's pouch (**Fig. 15.37**) and are frequently cystic and solid (**Fig. 15.38**). Cysts contain cellular debris, cholesterol crystals and dark oily liquid, and β-hCG is usually detectable. They are capable of widespread extension reaching the frontal region, temporal fossae and brainstem. The solid elements frequently calcify; they are more conspicuous in childhood, but probably increase with time. Malignant transformation is exceedingly rare but the extensive spread from the hypothalamus to other critical central nervous sites means they often behave in a highly damaging fashion.

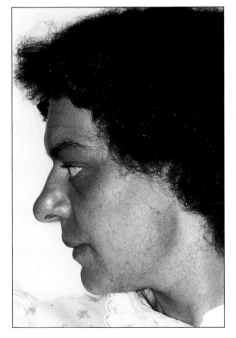

Fig. 15.36 *Hirsuties in a woman with acromegaly.*

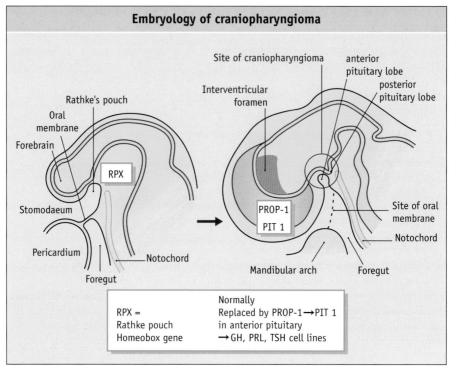

Embryology of craniopharyngioma

Site of craniopharyngioma

anterior pituitary lobe

Interventricular foramen

posterior pituitary lobe

Rathke's pouch

Oral membrane

Forebrain

RPX

Stomodaeum

PROP-1

PIT 1

Site of oral membrane

Notochord

Pericardium

Notochord

Foregut

Mandibular arch

Foregut

	Normally
RPX =	Replaced by PROP-1→PIT 1
Rathke pouch	in anterior pituitary
Homeobox gene	→GH, PRL, TSH cell lines

Fig. 15.37   *Embryology of craniopharyngioma arising from Rathke's pouch.*

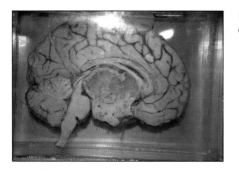

Fig. 15.38   Cystic and calcified craniopharyngioma.

Germinomas are the commonest germ cell tumours of CNS and closely resemble gonadal tumours. They usually present in young teenage girls with headache, visual loss, anterior pituitary failure especially affecting growth and diabetes insipidus, which should alert the clinician that this is not a routine pituitary tumour. Boys tend to have pineal tumours, often also with suprasellar components. Secretion of β-HCG and α-fetoprotein into blood and CSF may occur in germ cell tumours and seeding can occur down the neuraxis.

Other lesions such as optic nerve glioma and sphenoid ridge meningioma cause primarily visual disturbances, but astrocytomas and other tumours can cause hypothalamic dysfunction. Pituitary damage can follow trauma, especially in abused infants who can develop varying degrees of damage including panhypopituitarism, which is often apparent only years later when there is growth failure. Note that psychosocial deprivation can also cause GH deficiency but this often reverses rapidly on hospitalization or on being taken into care. Road traffic accidents can cause pituitary stalk section, which classically causes DI but also anterior pituitary failure. Other consequences include cortical blindness, and emotional and cognitive difficulties.

VASCULAR DISORDERS OF THE PITUITARY

Any of the following factors may lead to pituitary infarction:

- Pregnancy
- Diabetes mellitus
- Anticoagulation
- Pituitary tumours
- Cerebral aneurysms
- Coronary artery bypass grafting
- Old age

Pituitary failure can occur after vascular catastrophes such as infarction or haemorrhage. Sheehan's syndrome may follow massive ante- or postpartum haemorrhages with hypotensive shock; prompt blood transfusion should prevent this, however. Hyperplasia and hypertrophy of lactotrophs in pregnancy render the pituitary blood supply vulnerable.

Clinical symptoms occur only when more than 90% of the pituitary volume has been destroyed.

Clinical features

- Failure of lactation (hypoprolactinaemia)
- Other features of anterior pituitary failure (e.g. amenorrhoea)
- ACTH and TSH deficiency, which may declare only much later with patients classically becoming torpid, bedbound and losing all interest and initiative

Diabetes mellitus is said to enhance the risk of pituitary infarction but the incidence is very small, and this also applies to anticoagulation. Histological examination of pituitary tumours frequently reveals areas of infarction or haemorrhage of varying age that are usually symptomatically and hormonally insignificant.

Pituitary apoplexy (see p.194) may prove lethal as a result of subarachnoid haemorrhage or of easily overlooked adrenal insufficiency if the condition is not recognized. Morbidity includes ophthalmoplegia as well as pituitary deficiency – which may include complete extirpation of a hypersecreting tumour such as acromegaly. When partial deficiencies arise they do so unpredictably with, for example, ACTH or PRL deficiency but preservation of gonadotrophin secretion. This feature is typical of vascular insults causing selective losses of pituitary hormones and contrasts with the progressive pattern of growing pituitary adenomas.

Ectatic loops of carotid may occupy and expand the pituitary fossa with consequent endocrine deficiency but their recognition is much more important if surgery is planned. Coronary artery bypass grafting involves non-pulsatile flow with anticoagulated blood, which has been documented to produce major disturbances in pituitary hormone secretion and occasional early cases of pituitary apoplexy. Delayed presentation also occurs with loss of libido, secondary hypothyroidism and adrenal insufficiency, which is often indicated by persistent hyponatraemia. Imaging of the pituitary shows marked loss of volume. The same pattern can occur idiopathically in old age when the presenting feature is often orthostatic hypotension.

DEFICIENCY SYNDROMES

Any of the following hypothalamic releasing factors may be lost:

- GnRH (with anosmia: Kallman's syndrome)
- GHRH
- ACTH
- Thyrotropin-releasing hormone (TRH)
- Dopamine
- Somatostatin
- Multiple deficiencies

Deficiency of GnRH may be inherited as an isolated defect, or be due to a mutation in an adhesion molecule that leads to failure of migration of GnRH neurons from their origin in the olfactory placode to the median eminence. If there is associated anosmia it is termed Kallman's syndrome, and may also include other midline defects such as cleft lip and palate and renal tract anomalies (**Fig. 15.39**). Acquired GnRH deficiency accompanies severe weight loss especially anorexia nervosa and stress; it may be mediated by endogenous opioids and may follow excessive physical activity (usually also causing loss of body fat).

Isolated GH deficiency is rarely total, and is more often due to congenital GHRH deficiency – hence sufferers respond to exogenous GHRH, which limits its use in diagnosing GH deficiency but permits its use as a therapy (see Ch. 16). Isolated ACTH deficiency is usually acquired (presenting variously with hypoglycaemia, weight loss, hypotension and other features of cortisol deficiency). Alcohol abuse may be a factor. Most cases appear to be due to primary pituitary ACTH deficiency but there are also well-recorded cases that are apparently due to CRH deficiency. TRH deficiency is rare but may occur as an isolated acquired phenomenon. Dopamine deficiency is postulated as underlying 'idiopathic hyperprolactinaemia' but the possibility of prolactinomas too small to be visualized cannot be discounted. Somatostatin deficiency rarely presents since most pathological processes simultaneously affect GHRH. However, Alzheimer's disease is notably associated with deficiency of somatostatin amongst other neurotransmitters. Such patients often have modestly elevated GH levels though this may reflect IGF-I deficiency occasioned by their frequent though ill-explained cachexia.

Multiple hypothalamic hormone deficiencies can occur congenitally or after trauma. A common cause is cranial irradiation, which causes dose- and time-dependent GH and gonadotrophin deficiencies that are secondary to releasing factor loss, and hyperprolactinaemia due to dopamine deficiency. Hypothalamo-pituitary–adrenal and –thyroid axes may also become deficient, but usually much later after radiotherapy, which points to the need for continuing surveillance and repeated retesting over the years.

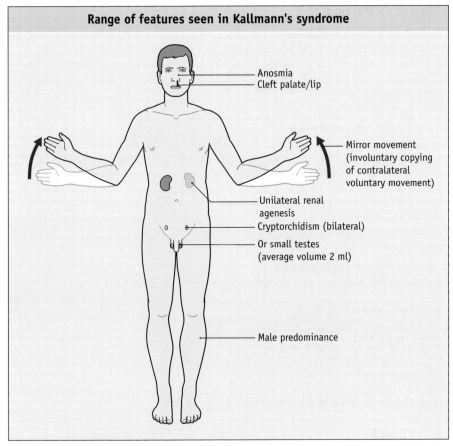

Range of features seen in Kallmann's syndrome

- Anosmia
- Cleft palate/lip
- Mirror movement (involuntary copying of contralateral voluntary movement)
- Unilateral renal agenesis
- Cryptorchidism (bilateral)
- Or small testes (average volume 2 ml)
- Male predominance

Fig. 15.39 *The range of features seen in Kallman's syndrome.*

PITUITARY ABSCESS

Pituitary abscess may arise following injury causing fracture to the base of the skull, which allows infectious agents to enter the pituitary from the nasopharynx.

Clinical features

- Moderate hyperprolactinaemia
- Diabetes insipidus
- Expanding pituitary lesion, thick-walled, lytic centre, thick pituitary stalk

Awareness of this syndrome allows transsphenoidal surgery with appropriate antibiotic cover.

OTHER CONDITIONS

Granulomatous conditions

Granulomatous conditions such as neurosarcoid and syphilis can affect the pituitary or hypothalamus. Tuberculous meningitis causes a chronic basal meningitis that often calcifies and is associated with profound pituitary failure. Idiopathic granulomatous hypophysitis has also been described.

Lymphocytic hypophysitis

Lymphocytic hypophysitis is most commonly associated with the third trimester of pregnancy or the puerperium, in association with a pituitary mass and often initially ACTH and TSH deficiency. Diabetes insipidus is sometimes also seen. In such patients it may resolve spontaneously, whereas in older women and in the few men in whom it has been recorded the disease seems more permanent and profound. Concomitant Hashimoto's disease and pernicious anaemia occurring together with limited pathological material demonstrating lymphocytic infiltration suggests an autoimmune aetiology.

Langerhans cell histiocytosis

This condition is associated with the following triad of clinical features:

Clinical features

- Punched-out skull lesions (**Fig. 15.40**)
- Exophthalmos
- DI

Anterior pituitary deficiency also occurs, especially GH deficiency. Some patients develop presenile dementia.

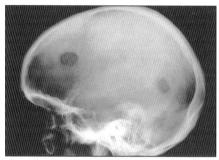

Fig. 15.40   *Skull X-ray showing punched-out lesions due to Langerhans cell histiocytosis.*

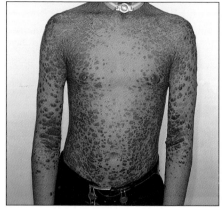

Fig. 15.41   *Cutaneous lesions of xanthoma disseminatum.*

Xanthoma disseminatum

This rare condition may present with cutaneous (**Fig. 15.41**) and mucosal xanthomatous lesions, anterior and posterior pituitary failure, deposits within the skull causing epilepsy and tracheal stenosis requiring tracheotomy.

Wegener's granulomatosis

This condition, characteristically affecting the respiratory and renal tracts, may cause pituitary involvement with mass effects and endocrine deficiency.

Metastatic disease

Metastatic disease to the hypothalamus is especially common in carcinoma of the breast and bronchus. If there is concomitant DI then this usually presages an early demise. Autopsy studies frequently reveal pituitary metastases with no clinical symptoms. However, occasionally apparently solitary metastases in the pituitary cause chiasmal compression, for instance in renal carcinoma (**Fig. 15.42**).

Iron overload

Conditions associated with iron overload (see Ch. 19) such as haemochromatosis and β-thalassaemia following multiple transfusions characteristically deposit iron in gonadotrophs causing primary pituitary gonadotrophin deficiency.

MANAGEMENT

HYPOPITUITARISM

Ideally each deficient hormone, or more frequently target organ hormones, should be replaced in as physiological a manner as possible. This is largely limited by practical considerations, however.

Adrenal insufficiency

Adrenal insufficiency, which is usually defined as an inability to respond with adequate cortisol secretion to stress, is usually treated by replacement doses of glucocorticoid. The physiological steroid hydrocortisone is preferred because its concentration can be checked by serial measurements. Conventionally, two-thirds of the total is given in the early morning to achieve a peak level approximating the time of maximum circadian secretion in normal individuals, and the remainder is given at 4–6 p.m. (because administration late at night can disturb sleep and cause polyuria). The usual regimen of 20 mg and 10 mg respectively is now

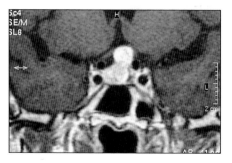

Fig. 15.42 *Renal cell metastases in the pituitary gland.*

considered excessive for many people, and carries the risk of osteoporosis and other side-effects. Some patients prefer a thrice-daily pattern, in which two small doses at lunch and tea follow the major morning dose. Prednisolone 2.5 mg twice daily, or 5 mg and 2.5 mg, may be preferred especially if given in an enteric-coated form; in the US this is also significantly cheaper than hydrocortisone. Patients on anticonvulsants may clear steroids more quickly so may need higher and more frequent doses.

- It is essential that patients understand the need to double or treble the dose for 2 to 3 days in the event of stressful illnesses, such as fever due to infection, trauma, surgery and myocardial infarction. They must take the responsibility for initiating the increase without feeling that this absolves them of the need to seek medical advice. They must clearly understand the need to secure parenteral hydrocortisone rapidly if vomiting or otherwise unable to absorb oral agents, and should keep an ampoule of hydrocortisone sodium succinate at home on standby. In addition to carrying conventional steroid cards patients benefit from a clearly worded letter as many emergency doctors seem unwisely reluctant or ignorant of the need to raise steroids appropriately. Too often a small increment is given too late but maintained chronically with the development of Cushingoid side-effects

Secondary hypothyroidism is easily dealt with using levo thyroxine, building up over weeks to a final dose of 75–200 µg daily. Obviously TSH cannot be used to monitor therapy: this should be done clinically while aiming for thyroxine levels to be in the upper normal range. Measurement of T_3 levels may be helpful. Thyroxine should not be given to ACTH-deficient patients until they have been on replacement glucocorticoid for 48 hours; this avoids the theoretical risk of precipitating an adrenal crisis.

Hypogonadism

Male patients with hypogonadism require testosterone to maintain libido, sexual function and secondary sexual characteristics, but also for general vigour, maintenance of muscle bulk and strength and prevention of osteoporosis. Oral testosterone undecanoate or sublingual testosterone preparations are rarely adequate. The main route is intramuscular, using testosterone esters usually administered every 2 weeks (the classical monthly treatment often leaves the patient with subnormal levels for 2 weeks). There has been a revival of testosterone pellet implant treatment, in which a dose of 600 mg is delivered subcutaneously every 4–6 months. Recently transdermal patches have been introduced, which were originally applied to shaved scrotal skin, but more recently to body skin. In women less than 50 years of age, hormone replacement therapy (HRT) is required, or a low dose oral contraceptive pill up to the age of 35 in cases where infertility cannot be assumed.

Growth hormone deficiency

GH is now widely available as a synthetic recombinant DNA product but this is very expensive and requires subcutaneous administration. In selected adult patients GH therapy can improve a number of the clinical features:

> **Clinical features**
>
> - Truncal obesity
> - Lack of skeletal muscle and physical strength
> - Exercise capacity
> - Adverse lipid profile
> - Lack of vitality
> - Osteoporosis
> - Reduced total body water

The dose per unit weight is much less than that required to optimize growth in children. Daily nocturnal subcutaneous injections are recommended but thrice-weekly injection is effective. Very small doses are used initially to avoid rapid overcorrection of body water, which causes joint pains and carpal tunnel syndrome. Women tend to need higher doses. A 6 month trial using physical and QOL assessment is recommended. If no clear-cut objective or subjective improvement is shown after this period then treatment should be stopped. Serum IGF-I should be monitored and GH dosage adjusted to keep it within the age-related normal range.

If there is osteoporosis, GH is given in combination with sex steroids and optimal hydrocortisone and thyroxine dosage.

DIABETES INSIPIDUS

Frank DI requires desmopressin, which is usually administered by a metered intranasal spray that provides 10 μg per squirt. A dose of 10–20 μg is administered at bedtime but a second dose may be needed in the morning. Overdosage leading to water intoxication must be avoided. This is particularly difficult in patients with hypothalamic damage to the thirst centre in addition to DI. They require a strict regimen of fluid input, adjusted appropriately in hot weather and monitored by weighing at the same time daily, or twice daily in the event of problems. Regular biochemical checks are needed and should be repeated when clinically required. Milder degrees of DI can be managed by oral DDAVP, which is especially useful in children or patients with cognitive and visual problems. In some patients medication with carbamazepine will suffice.

Postoperative DI may require intramuscular DDAVP for some days, especially following transsphenoidal surgery when nasal packs are in place. Postoperative DI is often temporary, lasting only days or weeks. Occasionally a triphasic response occurs (**Fig. 15.43**). It is advisable for patients on DDAVP after surgery to try without it every few months at a time when sudden return of polyuria will not prove inconvenient. If replacement is still needed they will experience unequivocal symptoms within 24 hours of discontinuing DDAVP.

Some patients with hypothalamic disease, rather than DI, have disturbed thirst and develop primary polydipsia. This must not be mistaken for DI as antidiuretic treatment causes water intoxication. This has been particularly recorded in neurosarcoid conditions.

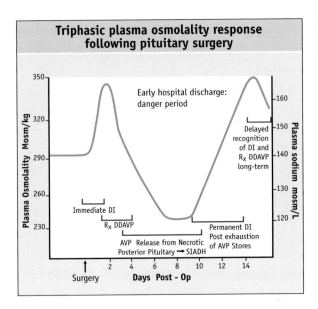

Fig. 15.43 *A triphasic plasma osmolality response following pituitary surgery.*

OTHER CAUSES OF POLYURIA

Profound polyuria after surgery for aneurysm of the anterior communicating artery, and infrequently for other intracranial conditions, may be due to cerebral salt wasting. This should not be mistaken for DI and treated with DDAVP. In fact it causes greater loss of salt than water, hence there is marked hyponatraemia, so there is no justification for confusion. Indeed it is frequently mistaken for the syndrome of inappropriate ADH secretion (SIADH) and treated by fluid restriction. However, the polyuria makes this diagnosis untenable and such management dangerous. The appropriate treatment is infusion of normal saline in quantities matching the previous, carefully measured, 24 hour urinary sodium losses. This must be continued for as long as the condition requires, and chronic cases may require oral sodium chloride supplementation. There have been suggestions that the underlying defect is excessive secretion of brain antinatriuretic peptide; if these are substantiated this may lead to the development of antagonist drugs.

Other causes of polyuria such as diabetes mellitus may occur and require appropriate treatment. Hypercalciuria is common in acromegaly, especially if there is associated hypercalcaemia from another cause; the most common of which is hyperparathyroidism due to MEN-1. Hypercalcaemia should be treated appropriately (see Ch. 14). Hypercalciuria may respond to low dose thiazide. This is also helpful in nephrogenic DI, in which, if necessary, amiloride and a prostaglandin synthetase inhibitor such as indomethacin should be added.

PITUITARY TUMOURS

Small functionless tumours causing neither mass effects nor endocrine dysfunction may be incidentally discovered during CT or MRI scans performed for other reasons. Having documented their innocuous nature no action is needed, but repeat MRI scans are recommended every 2 to 5 years unless clinical features appear.

Functionless tumours causing visual disturbance or other mass effects require surgical removal with few exceptions. The transsphenoidal approach is preferred where possible, including in those tumours with extensive suprasellar extension, when the roof of the resected tumour will be seen to descend. In contrast, tumours with eccentric lobulated extensions and most parasellar lesions are approached transcranially. However, the classical approach involving a retraction of the right frontal lobe frequently gives rise to infarction and cerebromalacia as well as serious psychological disabilities. Depending on the completeness of resection and whether there is any evidence of dural invasion (which is clinically difficult to assess) many patients require external radiotherapy, which is a skilled technique.

External radiotherapy

A suggested regimen is:

- **Maximum tumour dose** 4500 cGy
- **Maximum daily dose** 180 cGy
- **Number of fractions** 25, over 5 weeks
- **Use of three ports** Rotating through each in turn (**Fig. 15.44**)
- **Individual clear** Moulded for each patient
  Perspex mask (**Fig. 15.45**)

Radiotherapy reduces the recurrence rate strikingly. Possible long-term side effects include second tumours in the field of irradiation (gliomas often responding poorly to treatment), progressive hypopituitarism, and vasculitis particularly affecting the visual pathways. Conventional radiotherapy cannot be repeated. If tumours recur then further surgery may be

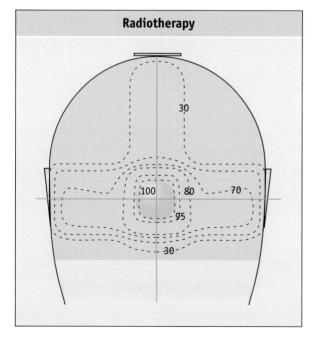

Radiotherapy

Fig. 15.44 *Radiation dosimetry using a three-port approach for external pituitary radiotherapy (from Belchetz 1986 Management of Pituitary Disease. Chapman & Hall, with permission).*

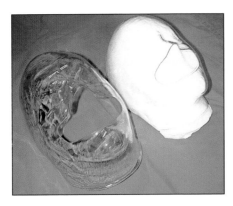

Fig. 15.45   *A Perspex mould used to ensure an accurate head position in pituitary irradiation.*

required. Newer techniques under evaluation include γ- knife stereotactic radiotherapy and photodynamic therapy.

Visual field defects improve in most patients, often completely, though in an appreciable minority they are unchanged and very rarely may worsen postoperatively. Severe headache tends to improve significantly following surgery. Pituitary function may improve after the removal of small to moderate tumours (microadenomas ≤ 10 mm maximum diameter) but with large macroadenomas there is usually no change or significant worsening of function. This implies full endocrine testing preoperatively.

A few centres recommend no steroid cover in patients with normal ACTH reserve but most suggest the following regimen:

- Hydrocortisone 100 mg i.v. with premedication
- Hydrocortisone 100 mg i.v. 8 hourly for 24–48 hours
- Hydrocortisone 50 mg i.v. 8 hourly for a further 24–48 hours
- Hydrocortisone by mouth rapidly reducing to 15 mg on waking, 5 mg at 6 p.m.

Patients should be discharged on the last dose with appropriate advice (see above).

Approximately 6 weeks after surgery stop hydrocortisone for 24 hours and check levels of ACTH and GH reserves using the ITT or glucagon stimulation test; also recheck electrolytes, PRL, and thyroid and gonadal status. If there are adequate ACTH reserves then stop hydrocortisone immediately (with no tailing of doses). If the reserves are borderline then consider stopping but advise the patient to have a standby supply to cover times of stress. Whenever possible reduce the daily hydrocortisone to 20 mg daily (see above regimen). Make adjustments to cover replacement requirements, and consider the need for GH therapy (see above). Patients will require follow-up scans, beginning within a year of surgery and 2–5 yearly thereafter. Endocrine surveillance, especially after radiotherapy, should continue indefinitely.

ACROMEGALY

The first-line treatment for most patients is transsphenoidal surgery. Cure rates with small tumours approximate 80% but reduce markedly with increasing size. The aim should be a normal IGF-I and a mean GH level over 24 hours of less than 5 mU/L (2.5 ng/ml).

In postoperative patients exceeding these values:
- Consider reoperation if the scan suggests an accessible remnant is present – but beware of early non-specific artefacts
- Consider external radiotherapy – but be aware that there may be a delay of up to 10 years before the full benefit is apparent
- Check the response to bromocriptine – in 80% of patients the GH level falls, but often only modestly
- Check the response to octreotide – 80% of patients respond, often very markedly

Medical treatment of acromegaly may suffice alone in mild cases, especially in elderly patients as in these the disease appears more indolent than in the young. As the sole treatment or as an adjuvant to surgery, radiotherapy, or both, if there is an adequate response to bromocriptine then try up to 30 mg daily or cabergoline 0.25–1 mg once to thrice weekly. If the octreotide response is adequate then use 50–100 µg subcutaneously one to three times daily. Octreotide often causes transient abdominal pain or diarrhoea for a week or so. Gall stones may develop but are seldom clinically troublesome. Watch for diabetes mellitus developing or worsening. Headache may disappear within minutes of octreotide injection. Lanreotide (another somatostatin analogue) and octreotide depot preparations are now available, which act for 7–14 days and 28 days plus respectively. Currently under trial is the use of the synthetic GH antagonist Pegvisomont, which may reduce IGF-I and improve clinical features in patients with resistant acromegaly.

PROLACTINOMA

Dopamine agonist therapy (bromocriptine, quinagolide or cabergoline) reduces PRL levels in almost all cases, often back to normal. Drugs are usually regarded as first-line therapy for most patients with micro- or macroprolactinomas for a number of reasons:
- Reversal of amenorrhoea usually occurs within months and in 90% after a year's treatment
- Fertility responds rapidly and almost as satisfactorily
- Galactorrhoea usually diminishes or disappears
- Tumours usually shrink often strikingly with improvement in visual fields
- Drugs are usually withdrawn in pregnancy but bromocriptine is safe to continue
- Pregnancy-associated tumour expansion can be rapidly reversed
- Impotence in men is usually corrected if testosterone is normalized
- Cessation of therapy allows tumour re-expansion especially after short-term treatment

Surgery may be considered in the following circumstances:
- Rapid visual deterioration
- Resistance to drugs (rare), resulting in inadequate PRL fall or tumour shrinkage
- Intolerable side-effects, such as nausea, dizziness, headache, or white hands
- A patient preference

However, surgery rarely cures macroprolactinomas and often involves hypopituitarism. The benefits of radiotherapy are delayed but may constrain tumour expansion in pregnancy.

CUSHING'S DISEASE

When a secure diagnosis has been achieved (itself a major challenge), most patients are submitted to pituitary surgery. This is a highly specialized area, however, and so surgery should be confined to the few neurosurgeons with sufficient experience and expertise. Tumours are usually small – often only a few millimetres in diameter – and may not show up on MRI or CT scanning. At transsphenoidal surgery, serial sagittal cuts through the pituitary may be needed to disclose the tumour. Sometimes nothing is found and then near-total hypophysectomy may be required. Pathological examination may not demonstrate a tumour, simply hyperplasia or indeed no obvious abnormality, even when clinical and biochemical evaluation postoperatively indicates a cure. The finding of undetectable morning cortisol within days of surgery (before the first dose of hydrocortisone) indicates a likely cure though late relapses are well recognized. Low-normal cortisol levels are associated with higher and earlier relapse rates but can be followed by long-term remissions. A clear failure to improve biochemistry can indicate the need for early further surgery. There is some dispute over whether preoperative reduction in hypercortisolaemia by adrenal-blocking drugs such as metyrapone and ketoconazole improves the perioperative course (see Ch. 18).

Bilateral adrenalectomy as primary therapy for Cushing's disease has largely been abandoned because of the risk of causing Nelson's syndrome (**Fig. 15.46**). Most 'cured' patients require corticosteroid replacement therapy for at least a year after pituitary surgery, and sometimes permanently. Radiotherapy has a role but is less often used than formerly. Rare macroadenomas are especially difficult to treat and may exceptionally metastasize.

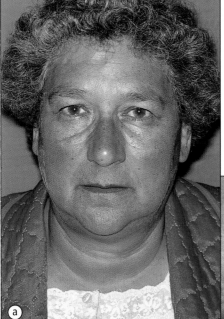
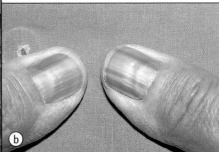

Fig. 15.46   *(a, b) Nelson's syndrome in a patient treated for Cushing's disease by bilateral adrenalectomy.*

CRANIOPHARYNGIOMAS

These require surgery for mass effects and almost invariably require anterior and posterior pituitary replacement therapy, especially after surgery. Though radical surgery is optimal for prevention of recurrence, incomplete resection is often all that can be safely achieved without damaging critical neural centres, depending on the extent of the tumour. Radiotherapy is often combined with surgery – which is usually transcranial and carries quite a high morbidity. The radiotherapy dose is generally slightly higher than with pituitary tumours but daily fractions are restricted to 180 cGy. Other problems are common including hydrocephalus requiring ventriculo-peritoneal shunting. Hyperphagia, inertia, adipsia, visual and cognitive impairments can also seriously complicate management. Recurrent cysts may be drained and ^{90}Yttrium or bleomycin instilled. These tumours are commonly aggressive and unsatisfactory to treat when, in most cases, they present early in life.

chapter 16

Endocrinological Problems in Children and Adolescents

INTRODUCTION

Growth is most rapid postnatally; its subsequent deceleration is interrupted by growth spurts that are minor in mid childhood and much greater in puberty. The main influences on growth at different phases of development are:

- *Infancy*. Nutritional factors
- *Childhood*. GH
- *Adolescence*. GH and sex steroids

Many other factors can also influence the individual growth pattern. These may be familial, genetic (including chromosome anomalies), dietary and nutritional (including intrauterine development and placental insufficiency) and the effects of concomitant disease: (including malabsorption, inflammatory, neoplastic, cardiovascular, respiratory and psychological effects). Endocrine disorders may advance or retard growth.

The neuroendocrine mechanisms determining GH and gonadotrophin secretion are summarized in Chapters 13, 15 and 19. Growth changes driven by GH are largely modulated by the changing amplitude of the GH secretory pulses – which increases from 5 to 10 years of age, then often dips just before rising markedly in the pubertal growth spurt. For all of these stages, the bulk of the GH is secreted at night. However, at the peak of pubertal growth, additional daytime secretory peaks are readily discernible (**Fig. 16.1**).

Variations in timing and level of growth between individual children are reflected in the GH dynamics. GH has both direct effects on progenitor prechondrocytes and indirect effects on the proliferative chondrocytes produced from these, prompting them to undergo clonal expansion. The latter category is mediated by IGF-I, which is produced locally from these differentiated cells and acts in an autocrine or paracrine fashion; it is also secreted by the liver and so has an additional endocrine action. IGF-I has been found bound to at least six different binding proteins (BPs), but the major circulating factor is IGF-BP3. This forms a trimeric complex together with IGF and an acid-labile subunit, which because it has a long half-life confers relative stability on IGF-I levels. Both IGF-BP3 and the acid-labile subunit concentrations are GH dependent. IGF-BP1 is much more labile; this molecule may be involved in IGF delivery to cells and is modulated by metabolic changes – particularly insulin, with which its levels are inversely correlated.

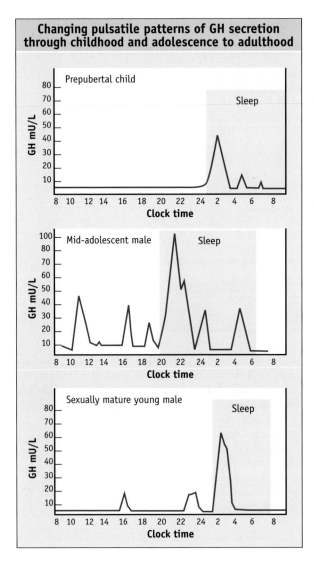

Fig. 16.1 *Changing pulsatile patterns of GH secretion in childhood and adolescence.*

The processes underlying normal puberty remain unclear, but it is known that they lead to the derepression of gonadotrophin pulsatility. In consequence, there is an increase in FSH levels, followed by one in LH levels, and nocturnal secretion of LH, which gives way to the late-pubertal 24 hour pattern of pulsatile LH and FSH secretion (**Fig. 16.2**). It seems likely that a somatic, possibly adipose tissue-related, signal is involved (leptin has been investigated as a candidate but results so far are conflicting). Hypothalamic changes may involve an alteration in the balance of inhibitory gamma amino butyric acid (GABA)-ergic and stimulatory amino acids. Some pineal involvement has also long seemed likely but remains unconfirmed.

The clinical assessment of pubertal development depends on Tanner's classification (**Figs 16.3–16.5**) (note that the preadolescent stage is 1; there is no stage 0).

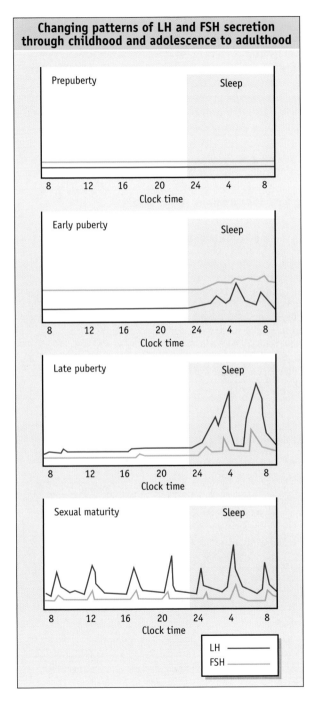

Changing patterns of LH and FSH secretion through childhood and adolescence to adulthood

Fig. 16.2 *Changing pulsatile patterns of FSH and LH secretion in childhood and adolescence.*

- The timing (*tempo*) of normal puberty varies from person to person, but its general order or pattern (*consonance*) remains consistent, so it is loss of this pattern that raises the suspicion of underlying pathology. Although there are probably differences in the regulation of puberty in the two sexes, the earlier onset in girls is more apparent than real as the earliest changes in boys (especially testicular growth of more than 4 ml) are less obvious than the early breast changes in girls. In addition, the growth spurt in girls tends to be an early event in puberty, whereas it tends to be late in boys

Fig. 16.3   Stages in pubic hair development (both sexes)

Stage 1	Preadolescent. The vellus over the pubis is no further developed than that over the abdominal wall (i.e. no pubic hair)
Stage 2	Sparse growth of long, slightly pigmented downy hair, straight or slightly curly chiefly along the labia (girls) or at the base of the penis (boys)
Stage 3	Considerably darker, coarser and more curled. The hair spreads sparsely at the junction of the pubis
Stage 4	Hair now adult in type, but area covered is still considerably smaller than in adult. No spread to medial surface of thighs
Stage 5	Adult in quantity and type with distribution of the horizontal (or classically 'feminine') pattern. Spread to medial surface of thighs but not up linea alba or elsewhere above the inverse triangle
Stage 6	Spread up linea alba, occurs late

Fig. 16.4   Stages in breast development (girls)

Stage 1	Preadolescent: elevation of papilla only
Stage 2	Breast bud stage: elevation of breast and papilla as small mound. Enlargement of areola diameter
Stage 3	Further enlargement and elevation of breast and areola, with no separation of their contours
Stage 4	Projection of areola and papilla to form a secondary mound above the level of the breast
Stage 5	Mature stage: projection of papilla only, owing to recession of the areola to the general contour of the breast

PATHOGENESIS AND PATHOLOGY

SHORT STATURE

Low birth weight

Low birth weight may be caused by any of the following factors:

- Intrauterine growth retardation
- Poor nutritional support

Fig. 16.5 Stages in developement (boys)

Stage 1 Preadolescent, testes, scrotum and penis are about the same size and proportion as in early childhood

Stage 2 Enlargement of scrotum and testes. Skin of scrotum reddens and changes in texture. Little or no enlargement of penis at this stage

Stage 3 Enlargement of penis, which is at first mainly in length. Further growth of testes and scrotum

Stage 4 Increased size of penis with growth in breadth and development of glans. Testes and scrotum larger, scrotal skin darkened

Stage 5 Genitalia adult in size and shape

- Premature birth
- Russell–Silver syndrome – the clinical features of which are low birth weight, triangular facies, asymmetry, a thin profile and clinodactyly (**Fig. 16.6**)

- The deficit in early growth is largely irremediable

Turner's syndrome

Turner's syndrome (see also Ch. 19) affects 1 in 2500–3000 live female births. Typically there is normal growth for the first 3 years. Subsequently, however, the rate of growth

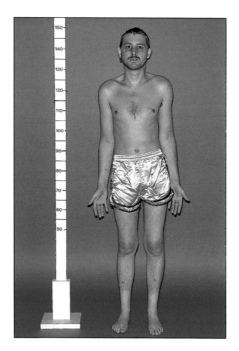

Fig. 16.6 *Russell–Silver syndrome.*

declines compared with that normally observed in prepubescence, and the pubertal growth spurt is completely absent.

Growth hormone deficiency/insufficiency/resistance

Deficiency of GH may be innate or acquired. In the former, abnormalities (e.g. large deletions) of the *GH* gene on chromosome 17 result in primary GH deficiency. This may also be caused by a mutation. For instance, pituitary aplasia may be caused by GHRH receptor mutation. Or there may be a mutation in the *Pit-1* gene (this is the transcription factor for GH, PRL and TSH cells). Bioinactive (but immunoreactive) GH polymer secretion also occurs.

Acquired GH insufficiency may be caused by:

- Idiopathic abnormality of GHRH secretion
- Tumours – such as craniopharyngioma, adenoma
- Cranial irradiation – for example from treatment of an intracranial tumour, or leukaemia
- Trauma – for example abuse, or a road traffic accident
- Histiocytosis-X
- Psychosocial factors

Some conditions are due to resistance to GH; this is seen in congenital GH resistance (called Laron syndrome), and where there is abnormality of GH receptors.

Finally, some cases may be due to a mixture of causes – as seen in some systemic diseases such as thalassaemia major, or renal or hepatic failure.

Endocrine causes

The following endocrine conditions can result in short stature:

- Hypothyroidism
- Cushing's syndrome (**Fig. 16.7**)

Bone/cartilage disorders

Several disorders of bone and cartilage can also be an underlying cause:

- Pseudohypoparathyroidism
- X-linked hypophosphataemic rickets
- Achondroplasia and other dysplasias

EXCESSIVE GROWTH

Familial cases are the most common cause of excessive growth. Obesity in children is characteristically associated with advanced skeletal growth (if associated with arrested growth it indicates a possible endocrine disorder; see above section). Precocious puberty is dealt with in the next section. Adrenal androgen excess, as seen in congenital adrenal hyperplasia (CAH) and in androgen-secreting tumours (see Ch. 18), may cause accelerated childhood growth and premature fusion of epiphyses with muscular hypertrophy (called 'pocket Hercules'). Hyperthyroidism may not be obvious in childhood and present with rapid skeletal growth. GH excess causing pituitary gigantism (dealt with in Ch. 15) can be confused with cerebral gigantism (de Soto's syndrome). Marfan's syndrome and homocystinuria may give rise to tall thin stature, a high-arched palate, pectus excavatum, arachnodactyly and dislocated lenses. Aortic root abnormalities occur in Marfan's syndrome. Klinefelter's syndrome is typically, but not always, associated with tall stature, eunuchoidal proportions and invariably small testes (see Ch. 19). The XYY karyotype was formerly considered to be associated with tall stature and an aggressive psychopathic personality; however, the latter association has since been questioned on the grounds that it was produced from selection bias of the data.

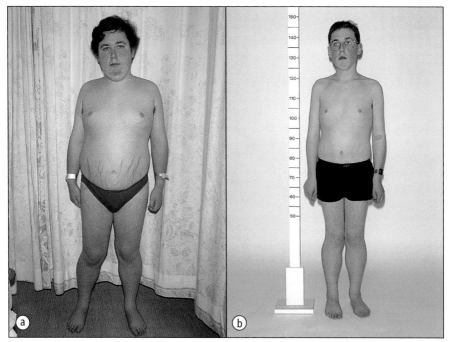

Fig. 16.7 *Growth arrest with progressive obesity in Cushing's syndrome in childhood (a) before and (b) after curative surgery.*

PRECOCIOUS PUBERTY

By far the greater number of cases of precocious puberty are girls. The cause of this condition may be idiopathic. Early puberty may also be triggered by tumours –including intracranial tumours, such as optic nerve gliomas, pineal tumours or hamartomas, and adrenal tumours, which are rare but may be malignant, and dysgerminomas, which secrete hCG (they may be pineal or hepatic). Irradiation, for instance from cancer treatment, can also be a factor.

Other possible causes include hydrocephalus and hypothyroidism, in which there may be raised FSH levels. In CAH, the androgen excess sensitizes the hypothalamus, and the subsequent corticosteroid supplement may trigger true central precocity. Finally, precocious puberty may be due to constitutively activated G protein, such as seen in testitoxicosis and McCune–Albright syndrome.

DELAYED PUBERTY

A temporary delay in puberty may be due to constitutional factors. This is much commoner in boys, and is often familial. There may be concomitant systemic disease. It may be associated with either hypothyroidism or Cushing's syndrome. An isolated GH deficiency may also be the cause. Finally, particularly in girls, it may be due to feeding/eating disorders, or to excessive exercise.

HYPOGONADOTROPHIC HYPOGONADISM

Hypogonadotrophic hypogonadism (see Chs 15 and 19) may be congenital or acquired. It may be found in fertile eunuchs with relative LH deficiency. Secondary hypogonadism is a feature of Kallman's syndrome, in association with anosmia due to agenesis of the olfactory lobes.

It may accompany hyperprolactinaemia. Pituitary or parapituitary tumours, surgery and trauma can all result in hypogonadism. The cause may also be idiopathic.

HYPERGONADOTROPHIC HYPOGONADISM

This condition may also be congenital or acquired, and its pathogenesis tends to be different for females and males.

In females, it may be caused by chromosomal disorders such as Turner's syndrome and variants of this, or gonadal dysgenesis. It may also be autoimmune in nature (possibly polyglandular syndrome). It may follow trauma or surgical castration, cytotoxic chemotherapy, or radiotherapy, or be a result of idiopathic premature ovarian failure.

In males, innate causes include Klinefelter's syndrome, anorchia, vanishing testis (partial) and Leydig cell agenesis or hypoplasia. It may also be a result of testosterone biosynthetic defects or partial insensitivity to androgens. As in females, it may be autoimmune, possibly polyglandular. It may be caused by the orchitis accompanying mumps, or tuberculosis (TB). It may alternatively be secondary to castration, trauma or surgery or torsion. Finally, it may be a result of chemotherapy or radiotherapy.

INVESTIGATION AND DIAGNOSIS

The key to evaluation of possible growth or pubertal disorders is careful clinical assessment. The standing height should be measured if the child is over 2 years, but the supine height if the age is less than 3 years, or both if the child is between the ages of 2 and 3 years. Use a careful technique with a frequently calibrated stadiometer (**Fig. 16.8**). Check also the parental height (the predicted height should be the mean of their heights plus 7 cm for a boy, or minus 7 cm for a girl, as the average height difference between the sexes is 14 cm). Where possible obtain a series of previous accurately dated height measurements. Calculate height velocities where possible: this theoretically helps define changes but short-term fluctuations and compounding inaccuracies in calculation lessen the practical value. Weight should be accurately measured and previous measurements, accurately dated, collected whenever possible.

All values should be plotted on an appropriate, updated chart (**Fig. 16.9**) – this is necessary as appreciable secular trends towards increased growth have occurred in many affluent areas of the world. Where appropriate, check the skinfold measurement with callipers, especially that on the triceps and scapular (**Fig. 16.10**). Pubertal status for pubic hair, breast or genital development should be ascertained, and in boys the testicular volume checked accurately using a Prader orchidometer. Check for features of concomitant disease – such as thyroid, adrenal, gastrointestinal, cardiac or respiratory. Check the bone age from an X-ray of the left hand/wrist, preferably by the lengthy but well-validated Tanner–Whitehouse-2 method.

ASSESSMENT OF GH SECRETION

Assessment is highly problematic because of the pulsatile nature of GH secretion, with peaks separated by long intervals with undetectable levels. There is also the variability of GH secretion at different stages of development, especially in puberty, and the ethical problems in obtaining normal children's data. The use of frequent sampling over prolonged periods up to 24 hours has been of interest but is not practical as a routine test. The consensus is to use pharmacological stimuli such as the following tests of GH reserve:

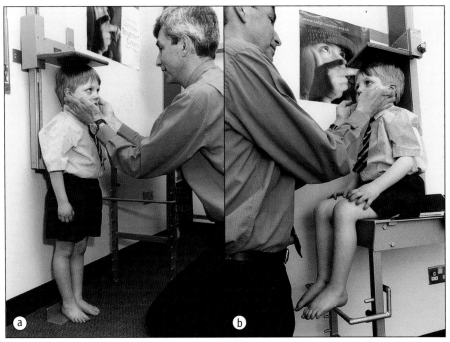

Fig. 16.8 *(a, b) Measurement of standing and sitting height with a stadiometer.*

- **ITT**   Intravenous
- **Arginine**   Infusion
- **Glucagon**   Intravenous in children (cf. adults)
- **Clonidine**   Oral

The possible hazards of hypoglycaemia discourage many clinicians from using the ITT. The specificity and sensitivity of the other tests are poor, however, whether measured against the peak GH in ITT (as the gold standard) or – worse – measured against height velocity. Some children appear to secrete insufficient GH physiologically but respond to stimulation tests. Several individuals appear to have the biochemical responses and growth patterns indicating GH insufficiency yet when retested in adult life demonstrate normal responses. They may constitute a group of developmentally delayed subjects in terms of GH secretion. Many cases of GH deficiency appear to be due to GHRH deficiency. The criteria for normality of GH response need careful and preferably local assessment.

Children with delayed puberty should be primed with sex steroids before assessment with pharmacological tests. However, there is as yet no agreement on what constitutes appropriate priming; suggestions have ranged from stilboestrol 1 mg twice daily for 48 hours before the test, in both sexes, to ethinyloestradiol 50 µg for 3 days in girls and testosterone proprionate 50 mg i.m. 3 days before the test in boys.

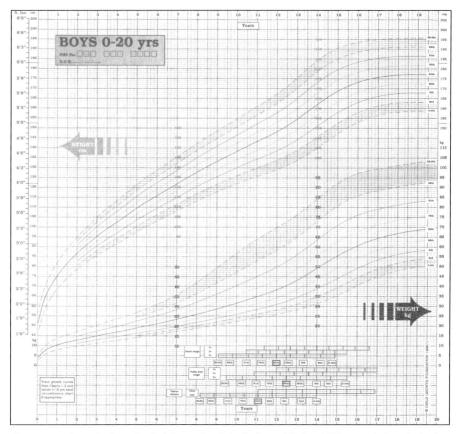

Fig. 16.9   *Growth chart for height and weight in boys (©the child Growth foundation).*

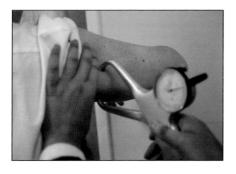

Fig. 16.10   *Measurement of skinfold thickness.*

PRECOCIOUS PUBERTY

The procedure for investigation of precocious puberty is:

- First check gonadotrophins, and sex steroids
- Check for virilizing CAH by measuring 17-hydroxy progesterone

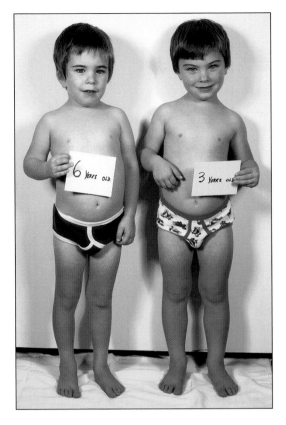

Fig. 16.11 *Growth hormone deficiency in a 6-year-old with sibling aged 3 years (from Wales et al. 1996 Pediatric Endocrinology and Growth. Mosby, with permission).*

- Check thyroid function
- In boys especially, perform MRI imaging of the head – to check for hydrocephalus and pineal or hypothalamic tumours

EXCESSIVE GROWTH

First it should be remembered that GH dynamics in normal but very tall and rapidly growing adolescents often resembles acromegaly. However, gigantism may be associated with large pituitary tumours, so in these cases a MRI scan should be performed. It may also be associated with hypopituitarism, or with mass effects on vision and intracranial pressure.

CLINICAL FEATURES AND MANAGEMENT

GROWTH HORMONE DEFICIENCY

Poor growth becomes apparent only after 6 months of age. An immature chubby appearance is typical, together with central crowding of facial features (**Fig. 16.11**). Micropenis is common in boys. GH deficiency may present with neonatal hypoglycaemia, especially if ACTH also deficient.

Management

The following procedure is suggested for management of GH deficiency:

229

- First, administer only biosynthetic GH. The daily dose is adjusted according to response; the maximum benefit is seen in the first 6 weeks
- Many patients are primarily GHRH deficient; if therapeutic benefit is shown from this then more frequent dosing is needed
- GH resistance requires IGF-I therapy
- Many children treated with GH show normal GH responses on retesting after their growth is complete

PRECOCIOUS PUBERTY

This is defined as any secondary sexual development before the age of 8 years in girls and 9 years in boys. Idiopathic central precocious puberty occurs almost exclusively in girls. Premature thelarche is breast development at the age of 5 years or less without other features of pubertal progression. In boys there may be evidence of central lesions, especially tumours, or hydrocephalus.

Management

It is important to remember that true central precocious puberty in girls may not jeopardize the final height, and a decision to treat should include behavioural and emotional considerations. The following treatment agents may be used:

- **GnRH agonists**   These are best given as long-acting implants to suppress pituitary gonadotrophins
- **Cyproterone acetate** This can help peripherally
- **Ketoconazole**   Gonadotrophin-independent changes may respond to this agent; however, its use requires monitoring of liver function, and it may impair adrenal cortisol secretion

DELAYED PUBERTY

Delayed puberty is much commoner in boys than in girls. It may follow a familial pattern – which includes the pattern of growth. It may also be secondary to a number of other disorders:

- Distinguish secondary causes such as chronic disease, or GH or multiple pituitary deficiency
- In girls, watch especially for occult or mosaic Turner's syndrome

Management

In girls the problem is more often an indication of underlying problems and efforts to find evidence of weight-related disorders are especially important (see section in Ch. 19 on primary amenorrhoea). In boys the distinction between constitutional delay in growth and development (by far the commonest situation) and hypogonadotrophic hypogonadism may be difficult. An important consideration is the adverse effects on mood, scholastic attainment and emotional development that can ensue – hence the readiness to treat this condition early. A popular approach is to use a low dose (100 mg) testosterone ester injection every 4 weeks for about 3–6 months, and then increase the dose to 250 mg every 4 weeks after the initial few months in older boys. Progress in height, weight, pubertal staging and testicular volume needs monitoring carefully. Alternative treatments include nocturnal oral testosterone undecanoate 40 mg especially in younger boys and hCG 2000 IU intramuscularly twice weekly for several months.

chapter 17

Thyroid Disorders

INTRODUCTION

The normal thyroid weighs between 15 and 25 g, and more in women than in men (**Fig. 17.1**). Enlargement due to any cause may referred to as goitre (struma in Europe) (**Fig. 17.2**). Epidemiological studies on epidemic goitre have generally used the WHO classification (**Fig. 17.3**).

Physiological enlargement of the thyroid in pregnancy, which is greater in areas of iodine deficiency, was made use of by Ancient Egyptians who tied a reed round the neck of a young woman on marriage; when the reed broke this signalled pregnancy. Although the empirical use of iodine-containing substances for the treatment of endemic goitre has long been known, the function of the normal thyroid was discovered only much more recently, considerably later than hyperthyroidism and hypothyroidism had been described clinically.

EPIDEMIOLOGY

Worldwide, endemic iodine deficiency is estimated to affect an estimated 800 million people (**Fig. 17.4**). It is largely preventable at relatively low cost but nevertheless remains a major unfulfilled public health challenge. In iodine-replete areas the major cause of thyroid disease is autoimmune disease. Extensive studies in Whickham, County Durham in the UK (by Tunbridge and colleagues) reveal a high prevalence, strikingly more so in women than in men, which increases with advancing age (**Fig. 17.5**).

PATHOLOGY AND AETIOLOGY

Autoimmune thyroid disease, mediated by both the humoral and the cellular limbs of the immune system, operates at various sites. Autoantibodies have been described against various antigens within the thyroid. However, measurement of anti-thyroglobulin antibodies is of little significance since the titre in which these are present appears to bear no relationship to any aspects of thyroid function or disease. Anti-microsomal antibodies are now more precisely designated as anti-thyroid peroxidase (anti-TPO) antibodies and correlate with the degree of lymphocytic infiltration in thyroid glands (**Fig. 17.6**).

The clearest involvement of humoral antibodies is in Graves's disease. Substances initially described as long-acting thyroid stimulator (LATS) and subsequently LATS-protector (LATS-P) in a modified system, are now recognized as immunoglobulin G (IgG) molecules, which bind to and activate the TSH receptor. A functionally opposing class of antibodies bind to and block the TSH receptor. The clearest evidence for their pathogenic role is neonatal thyroid disease (usually thyrotoxicosis), which is caused by the passive transplacental

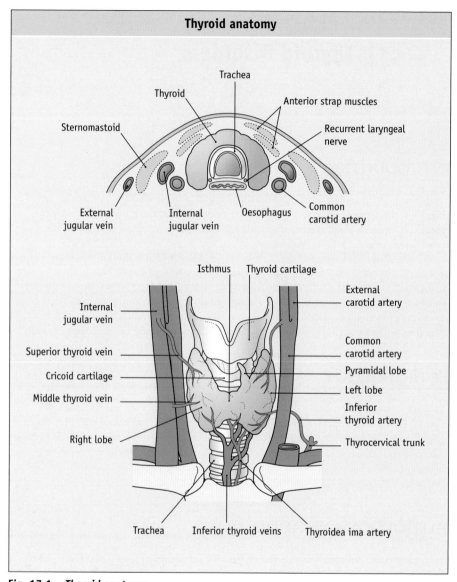

Fig. 17.1 *Thyroid anatomy.*

transfer to the fetus. This condition subsequently becomes self-limiting as the antibody is cleared from the newborn infant.

THYROID NODULARITY

Nodularity is a striking finding in many glands, and is often associated with their marked enlargement. The macroscopic appearance exhibits heterogeneity, with large abutting small nodules, fibrosis and cysts. This is reflected at a microscopic level with follicles varying in size and follicular epithelium, and in height, indicating marked variation in activity. Greater

Fig. 17.2   Causes of goitre

- Endemic goitre
- Sporadic non-toxic goitre
- Multinodular goitre
- Hashimoto's thyroiditis
- Thyrotoxicosis
- Solitary nodule
  - follicular adenoma
  - toxic adenoma
  - thyroid cancer
- Thyroiditis
- Infiltration
- Goitrogens
- Dyshormonogenesis

Fig. 17.3   WHO classification of goitre size

Class	Characteristics
0	No palpable or visible goitre
1a	Goitre detected by palpation only
1b	Goitre palpable and visible with neck extended
2	Goitre visible with neck in normal position
3	Large goitre, visible from a distance

Global distribution of iodine deficiency disorder

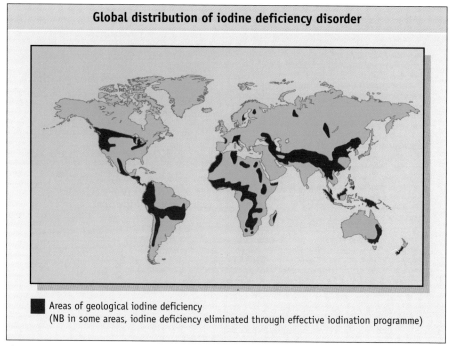

Areas of geological iodine deficiency
(NB in some areas, iodine deficiency eliminated through effective iodination programme)

Fig. 17.4   *Global distribution of iodine deficiency disorder.*

nodularity is found with increasing age and in glands affected by iodine deficiency. This probably represents waves of stimulated growth and activity followed by quiescent periods. An important feature is the relative autonomy of some nodules, which are sometimes followed by the development of hyperthyroidism. This especially occurs after iodine repletion in iodine-deficient individuals.

Fig. 17.5 Epidemiology of autoimmune disease in Whickham, Country Durham (Tunbridge et al. Clinical Endocrinology 1977; 7: 481–493, with permission)

Measure	Female prevalence	Male prevalence
Overt hyperthyroidism	19/1000	1.6/1000
Including possible hyperthyroid	27/1000	2.3/1000
Overt hypothyroid	14/1000	< 1/1000
Including possible hypothyroid	19/1000	–
TSH > 6 mU/l	75%	2.8%
Mic Abs	10.3%	2.7%
(frequency rose markedly in females > 45 years)		
Goitre	Palpable but not visible	Palpable and visible
(female 4 × male)	8.6%	6.9%

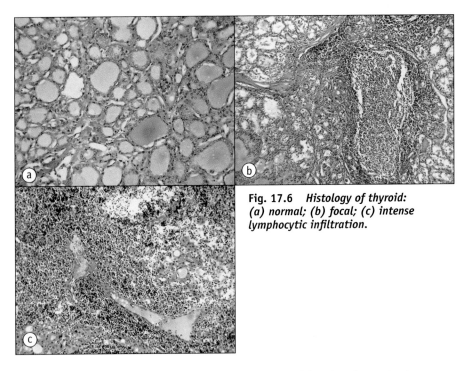

Fig. 17.6 Histology of thyroid: (a) normal; (b) focal; (c) intense lymphocytic infiltration.

Fibrous tissue may lead to deviation of local structures. Although only one dominant nodule may be clinically obvious, ultrasonography often demonstrates the widespread existence of thyroid nodules. Involvement of other growth factors or goitrogens seems likely but is not fully documented.

IODINE-INDUCED THYROID DYSFUNCTION

Exposure to increased levels of iodine can result in a variety of responses ranging from goitre and hypothyroidism to iodine-induced thyrotoxicosis (the Jod–Basedow effect). The last of

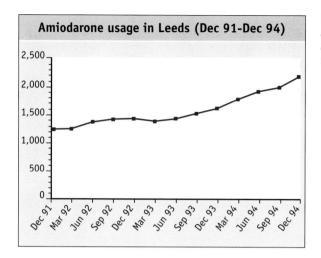

Fig. 17.7 *Increase in use of amiodarone as documented by prescription in a teaching hospital.*

Fig. 17.8   Biochemical and clinical effects of amiodarone on the thyroid

Amiodarone regularly disturbs TFTs
1. Raised total and free T_4 with normal TSH = euthyroid, do not treat as thyrotoxic
2. Raised total and free T_4 AND T_3 but suppressed TSH suggests thyrotoxic
3. Normal T_3 with suppressed TSH may be normal or sick/toxic: difficult!
4. Raised TSH may be hypothyroid even if total and free T_4 are normal: difficult!

these is classically seen when iodine prophylaxis is introduced into areas where endemic iodine-deficiency goitre exists. Thyrotoxicosis due to Graves's disease has long been treated with iodine prior to surgery; its effect is usually transient, with escape occurring on continued iodine exposure (the Wolff–Chaikoff effect). The Jod-Basedow effect can be precipitated by several iodine-containing agents including X-ray contrast media and especially amiodarone, a drug that is being used with increasing frequency in patients with supraventricular tachycardia and atrial fibrillation (**Fig. 17.7**).

Amiodarone exerts complex effects on hormone levels. Iodine constitutes 37.5% of this drug by weight and so its chronic use constitutes a major load of iodine. The drug resembles thyroid hormone in its conformation, and thereby inhibits the deiodination of thyroxine to T_3. It also has a long biological half-life.

The patterns of response to amiodarone vary. Initially the iodine load predominates, resulting in high thyroxine levels (both total and free). If the deiodination is commensurately inhibited, the outcome may be a balanced euthyroid state with normal TSH levels. If the T_3 also rises then thyrotoxicity, rather than just hyperthyroxinaemia, ensues. On discontinuation of the drug, the inhibition of deiodination may cause hypothyroidism accompanied by high TSH but normal thyroxine levels (**Fig. 17.8**).

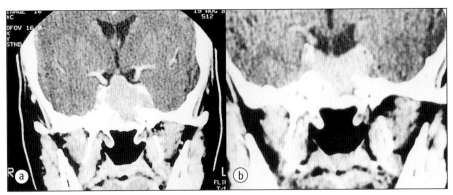

Fig. 17.9 TSH-secreting pituitary adenoma (a) before and (b) after therapy with octreotide.

THYROID HORMONE RESISTANCE AND TSH-SECRETING PITUITARY ADENOMAS

Thyroid hormone resistance is rare. The resistance is due to mutation of the thyroid hormone receptor. There are two major classes of receptors, α and β, which are variably expressed in different body tissues. The mutations so far identified have all occurred in the β receptor.

It needs to be distinguished from the rare TSH-secreting pituitary adenomas (**Fig. 17.9**), which cause thyrotoxicosis from excess TSH-secretion. These tumours characteristically cosecrete glycoprotein α subunit.

THYROID NEOPLASMS

Thyroid neoplasms display various degrees of differentiation. Benign autonomous thyroid nodules (Plummer's syndrome) may in some cases be due to point mutations in the TSH receptor that are linked to the G-protein system coupling with adenyl cyclase. Such mutations are constitutively active – that is, they do not require TSH binding for activation. Both genetic and environmental factors may be implicated.

Several oncogenes have been associated with papillary, follicular and anaplastic cancers (**Fig. 17.10**). There is also an association between thyroid autoimmunity and follicular carcinomas, and also thyroid lymphomas. Increased iodine intake raises the incidence of papillary relative to follicular carcinoma of the thyroid. The Chernobyl disaster has led to a focus on the causal role of relatively high doses of radioactivity, especially iodine radioisotopes. The infant thyroid, in contrast, is sensitive to even low levels of irradiation.

INVESTIGATION AND DIAGNOSIS

THYROID HORMONE TESTS

The widespread availability of precise measurements of thyroid hormone levels and TSH in blood at relatively low cost has transformed the ease and reliability of defining thyroid status.

Serum TSH concentration – This is the most reliable diagnostic test, although measurement of TSH alone without any estimate of thyroid hormone concentration is insufficient.

Thyroid hormones – Although these hormones are largely protein bound the major

Fig. 17.10 Oncogenes associated with papillary follicular and anaplastic thyroid cancer

Genes	Abnormality	Phenotype of thyroid tumor
Receptors with tyrosine kinase activity		
• *RET*/papillary thyroid carcinoma	Rearrangement	Papillary carcinoma (radiation-associated)
• *TRK* oncogene	Rearrangement	Papillary carcinoma
• *Met* oncogene	Over-expression	Papillary carcinoma
Intracellular signalling pathway		
• *RAS*	Point mutation	Follicular carcinoma, adenoma
Cyclic AMP pathway		
• TSH-receptor	Point mutation	Follicular carcinoma
• G-α subunit	Point mutation	Follicular carcinoma
Tumour-suppressor gene		
• *p53*	Point mutation	Anaplastic carcinoma (papillary carcinoma)
• adenomatous polyposis coli	Point mutation	Papillary carcinoma (familial)

biological effects are exerted by picomolar levels of the free hormone. These can be measured by equilibrium dialysis methods; however, these are too cumbersome for routine use.

Free and total T4 and T3 assays – Several indirect assays of free T_4 and free T_3 are commercially available. These operate satisfactorily over quite wide ranges of thyroxine-binding globulin (TBG) concentration, but artefactual readings are not uncommon. There is still a school adhering to the use of total T_4 and T_3 measurements. In this case, allowance must be made for common conditions perturbing TBG concentration such as pregnancy and use of oral contraceptives.

TRH – The TRH test involves injecting 200–500 µg of TRH intravenously and measuring the TSH before, and then 20 minutes and 60 minutes after the injection. Minor brief sensations of nausea and urethral tingling are common and rare cases of pituitary infarction or apoplexy have been associated with the test, especially in patients with acromegaly and other pituitary tumours. Also, modern TSH assays have rendered it largely obsolete.

Laboratory reference ranges apply to untreated patients needing assessment of thyroid status. Test results need careful interpretation if the patient is seriously ill (e.g. with non-thyroid illness or sick euthyroidism) or is already on treatment for thyroid disease, as other drugs may also interfere (**Fig. 17.11**).

It is often helpful to measure the level of TPO antibodies in patients with thyroid disease, especially goitre. High levels may suggest Hashimoto's thyroiditis. The titre is not an indication of thyroid function.

RADIONUCLIDE STUDIES

These are infrequently used now, but may be appropriate in some conditions. For instance, I^{123} scan and uptake is useful for confirming the presence of a single hyperfunctioning 'hot' adenoma (Plummer's disease). Conversely, thyroiditis (subacute or silent) or iodine-induced thyrotoxicosis (the Jod–Basedow phenomenon) shows negligible uptake and this information may be useful to prevent inappropriate treatment with radioiodine. Conditions associated with impaired organification, such as Pendred's syndrome and Hashimoto's thyroiditis, demonstrate high uptake that falls off rapidly instead of remaining steady after

Fig. 17.11   Conditions requiring sophisticated interpretation of thyroid function tests

Condition	Biochemical profile	Thyroid status	Explanation
Hypothyroid on T4	T_4/free T_4: high–normal or slight ↑ TSH: low–normal or slight ↓ T_3: normal	Normal	Normal tissue T_3 all derived from peripheral deiodination Pituitary deiodinase esp. selective active
Subclinical hypothyroid	T_4/free T_4: normal to low TSH: ↑ (slight)	Hypothyroid (mild)	Early thyroid failure ↓ T_4 secretion: plasma level within population range, low for individual
Severe treated thyrotoxicosis	T_4/free T_4: slightly low T_3: high normal to slightly high TSH: ↓ or low–normal	Normal	↓ intrathyroidal iodine: organification block + high turnover, delay in TSH de-suppression
Pregnancy/COC	T_4: ↑ TSH: normal	Normal	Raised TBG (free T_4 normal)
Phenytoin	T_4: ↓ TSH: normal	Normal/slight hypothyroid	T_4 displacment from TBG (free T_4 normal), ↑ hepatic clearance, possible slight impaired TSH response
Hyperemesis gravidarum	T_4: ↑↑, free T_4: ↑ T_3: ↑ TSH: ↓	Transient thyrotoxic	↑↑HCG: thyrotrophic ? some thyroiditis
Severe non-thyroid illness	T_4: ↓↓, free T_4: ↓/normal, T_3: ↓↓ TSH: normal or ↓	Unclear: normal or hypothyroid	T_4 displacement from TBG ↓↓ $T_4 \rightarrow T_3$ deiodination ? functional hypopituitarism Rx dopamine ↓ TSH
Acute Addison's	T_4: ↓/low normal TSH: ↑	Usually normal, occ. hypothyroid	↓ cortisol disinhibits TSH ? T_4 displaced from TBG if ill may be coincident true hypothyroid
Acute psychiatric illness	T_4: ↑/↓ (depends phase of illness) TSH: ↑/↓ (depends phase of illness)	Probably normal	Unclear

administration of a dose of sodium perchlorate (which competitively blocks further iodine ion uptake) (**Fig. 17.12**).

Radioiodine scans are also useful for identifying ectopic differentiated thyroid tissue in conditions such as congenital maldescent or when searching for metastases after surgery for thyroid cancer (this requires TSH stimulation to enhance uptake). Radioiodine scans and uptake measurement have been largely abandoned for the investigation of solitary thyroid nodules, however.

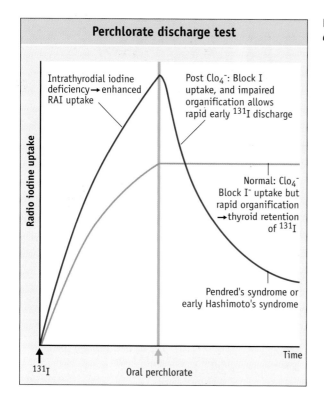

Fig. 17.12 *Perchlorate discharge test.*

Perchlorate discharge test

Intrathyrodial iodine deficiency→enhanced RAI uptake

Post Clo₄⁻: Block I uptake, and impaired organification allows rapid early ^{131}I discharge

Normal: Clo₄⁻ Block I⁻ uptake but rapid organification →thyroid retention of ^{131}I

Pendred's syndrome or early Hashimoto's syndrome

Radio iodine uptake

Time

^{131}I

Oral perchlorate

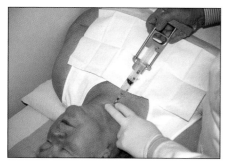

Fig. 17.13 *Thyroid aspiration using a syringe in a holder.*

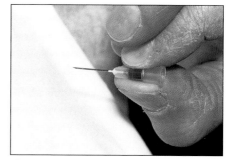

Fig. 17.14 *Thyroid aspiration using a hand-held needle.*

FINE NEEDLE ASPIRATION OF THYROID

This is used in the initial investigation in patients presenting with a solitary nodule of the thyroid. The purpose is to obtain useful specimens for cytology and if the lesion is cystic then to evacuate the fluid.

It is often performed using a 23 gauge needle attached to a 20 ml syringe held in a syringe holder. This arrangement enables controlled aspiration with one hand whilst the lump is immobilized with the other (**Fig. 17.13**). Only slight suction should be exerted to avoid undue bleeding as this can reduce the cytological value of the specimen. Gentle movements of the needle should be made up and down within the nodule while maintaining minimum negative pressure; this improves the yield of tissue. An alternative method is to use a small 21

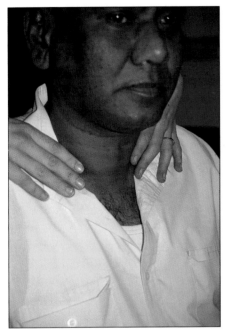

Fig. 17.15 *Palpating a goitre from behind.*

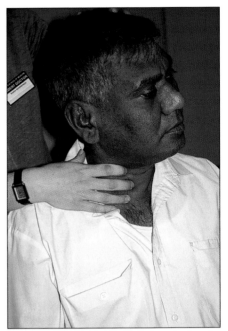

Fig. 17.16 *Tilting and turning the head to reveal a thyroid lump.*

gauge needle vibrated in and out of the lump (**Fig. 17.14**). Three aspirates are recommended. Ultrasound can help guide fine needle aspiration.

DIFFERENTIAL DIAGNOSIS

When assessing a patient for possible thyroid disease the level of thyroid hormone activity always needs to be established – that is, whether it is normal (euthyroid), deficient (hypothyroid) or excessive (hyperthyroid). This diagnosis is initially based on clinical evaluation, but the appropriate choice of thyroid function tests should always be performed in addition. It is equally mandatory to check whether the thyroid is detectably enlarged – and, if so, how big it is, where the enlargement is situated, and whether diffuse, focal or multinodular. In addition, the mobility or immobility should be assessed, especially on swallowing (provide the patient with some water to sip). Also assess the presence of any local lymphadenopathy, and tenderness or deviation of local structures, particularly the trachea. The presence of a thrill or thyroid bruit should be ascertained.

The thyroid is classically palpated as follows.

- Stand behind the patient, lightly resting the index fingers on the cricoid cartilage and feel with the middle and fore fingers on either side (**Fig. 17.15**)
- A local lateralized mass is often better examined by tilting the patient's head to the same side and rotating the head to the opposite side; this slackens the ipsilateral sternomastoid muscle enabling the mass to be revealed more extensively (**Fig. 17.16**)
- On occasion, a firm central thyroid enlargement above the sternal notch can give rise to 'Pemberton's sign'; in this, when the patient's hands are raised above the head a goitre causes a position-dependent superior vena caval obstruction, with dusky engorgement to the face and faintness due to impairment of the cranial circulation (**Fig. 17.17**)

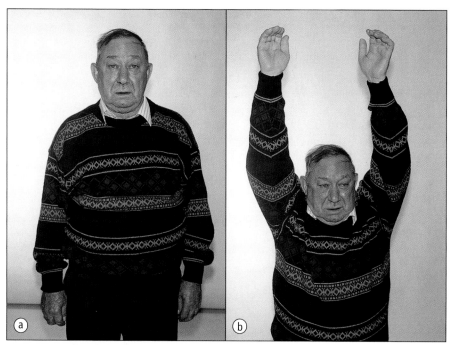

Fig. 17.17 *(a, b) Pemberton's sign.*

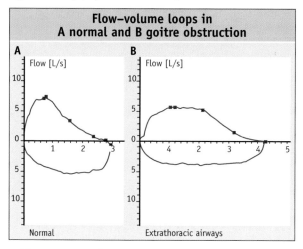

Fig. 17.18 *Flow–volume loops.*

- The extension of a goitre retrosternally is difficult to assess clinically; percussion is often recommended but is not reliable
- The most important consequence is compression rather than deviation, as the latter can only be guessed at from examining the direction and position of the trachea at the sternal notch
- An important sign is stridor, which should be elicited by asking the patient to inspire forcefully with an open mouth before expiring air forcefully. Enlarged airways and extrathoracic compression classically restrict breathing in more than breathing out. This is best demonstrated by a flow-volume loop (**Fig. 17.18**)

CLINICAL FEATURES AND MANAGEMENT

HYPOTHYROIDISM

Signs and symptoms

Symptoms:
- Cold intolerance
- Physical and mental slowing
- Tiredness and lack of energy
- Worsening memory and concentration
- Deafness, unsteadiness
- Weight gain
- Constipation
- Chest pain
- Muscle aches and rheumatism
- Pins and needles in fingers
- Heavy periods
- Infertility and miscarriages
- Lump in throat
- Dry skin, hair loss
- Psychiatric disturbance
- Voice change
- Sleepiness, snoring

Signs:
- Sluggishness in action and responses
- Facial puffiness, especially periorbital oedema
- Cold, dry, sallow skin
- Loss of hair on scalp and occasionally body (not eyebrows), rarely lanugo growth
- Goitre
- Bradycardia
- Hypertension, which is rarely marked; occasionally hypotension
- Faint heart sounds
- Myotonic tendon jerks
- Galactorrhoea

Hypothyroidism in its extreme form is clinically obvious and striking (**Fig. 17.19**). Patients display general slowness, as well as facial puffiness especially around the orbits, which lends a 'piggy' appearance. Patients may also use of layers of clothing even in warm surrounding, and have a palpable coldness to the touch, a slow pulse and very slow relaxing ankle jerks (these are best elicited by asking the patient to kneel on a chair - if this can be managed – **Fig. 17.20**). A goitre may be either absent (atrophic myxoedema) or present (Hashimoto's thyroiditis). A collar scar may betray previous thyroid surgery. However, loss of eyebrows is diagnostically useless – it is a textbook myth (**Fig. 17.21**). Rarely elderly hypothyroid patients develop hypothermic coma in cold weather, but it is difficult to distinguish clinically between hypothermia associated with thyroid failure and hypothermia that is not; TSH measurement is needed to make the diagnosis (see Ch. 14).

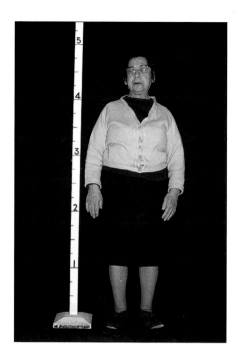

Fig. 17.19 *Gross hypothyroidism.*

Most patients with clinically significant hypothyroidism do not present with such gross features. Frequently the effects on one system predominate; as many of these features are non-specific, a high index of suspicion must be maintained to ensure recognition of this most treatable condition.

Females – In teenage girls the first sign is often a goitre and change in behaviour or personality, including becoming uncharacteristically 'good' and well behaved (**Fig. 17.22**) but also emotional and depressed, and with few other signs. In women of reproductive age the features may be similarly subtle and often relate to the reproductive system; presenting features include menorrhagia, recurrent abortions and infertility. One cause of infertility is the syndrome of hyperprolactinaemic amenorrhoea or galactorrhoea, in which the first suspicion is microprolactinoma; careful inquiry and examination may subsequently disclose goitre and features of hypothyroidism (**Fig. 17.23**). However, this syndrome is not a regular, or a predictable, consequence of hypothyroidism in women. Falling thyroid hormone levels may enhance TRH secretion from the hypothalamus – which also elevates PRL levels. Though empirical use of thyroxine in treating unexplained infertility is to be deplored, even mild hypothyroidism may warrant treatment when it is biochemically proven and this anecdotally seems to improve fertility in many cases (postpartum thyroiditis is dealt with on p. 247.)

Nervous system – The nervous system is commonly affected clinically in hypothyroidism. There may be a slowing up both physically and mentally (which is often more apparent to the family than to the patient). In the elderly these effects may become more pronounced and include sensorineural deafness, cerebellar dysfunction, especially of the vermis, causing truncal ataxia and a tendency to falls particularly in the dark. Hypothyroidism rarely causes a reversible dementia and occasionally the paradoxical hyperactivity of myxoedematous madness – this is again usually, but not exclusively, seen in the elderly. Peripheral neuropathy occurs rarely but entrapment neuropathy is common, especially that of the median nerve causing carpal tunnel syndrome.

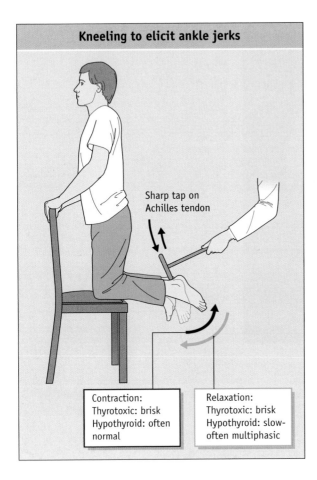

Fig. 17.20 *Kneeling to elicit ankle jerks.*

Kneeling to elicit ankle jerks

Sharp tap on Achilles tendon

Contraction:
Thyrotoxic: brisk
Hypothyroid: often normal

Relaxation:
Thyrotoxic: brisk
Hypothyroid: slow-often multiphasic

The clinically valuable sign of myotonic reflexes, mentioned earlier, may be associated with myotonia, which is dimpling of a muscle belly on being struck with a percussion hammer. Myopathy is commonly demonstrable on testing – electromyographically, histologically and most easily biochemically by the elevation of serum levels of creatine kinase and other muscle enzymes – but the clinical expression is less frequent. Myalgia is especially common when thyroid hormone levels fall rapidly in thyrotoxic patients becoming hypothyroid soon after surgery or radioiodine; this may, paradoxically, worsen transiently when thyroid hormone replacement is begun in the elderly who may then need cajoling to continue treatment. Headaches may develop very rarely in long-standing untreated hypothyroidism; these are due to the pituitary expansion or formation of a 'feedback tumour'.

Myxoedema coma is frequently a fatal complication in the elderly; it is often precipitated by a combination of cold exposure, intercurrent illness such as pneumonia and the use of sedative drugs. It may also be associated with pancreatitis (a poor prognostic feature), type 2 respiratory failure, hyper- or hypoglycaemia and hyponatraemia, the last of which is due to impaired renal water clearance.

Cardiovascular system – The cardiovascular system may be additionally susceptible to hypothyroidism in elderly patients as well as those with pre-existing heart disease. Bradycardia may be complicated by varying degrees of heartblock and arrhythmias. Blood

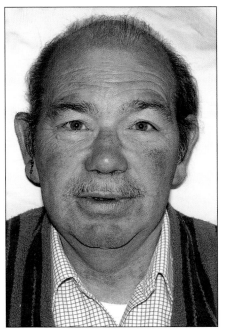

Fig. 17.21 *Good eyebrow growth in hypothyroidism.*

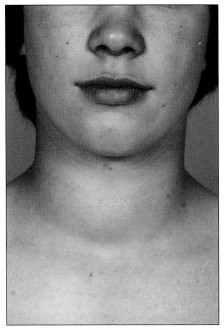

Fig. 17.22 *Occult hypothyroidism in a teenage girl.*

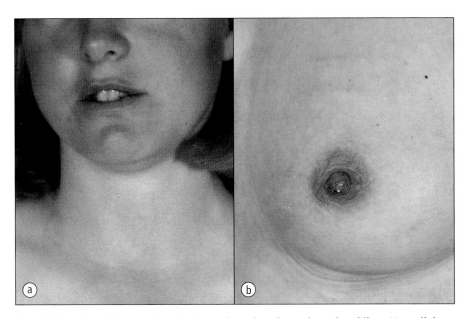

Fig. 17.23 *(a, b) Amenorrhoea/galactorrhoea in primary hypothyroidism. Note slight malar flush.*

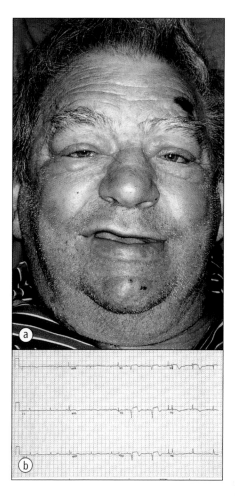

Fig. 17.24   *(a) Hypothyroidism and (b) the ECG showing low amplitude complexes and bradycardia as well as anterior myocardial infarction.*

pressure is often moderately elevated but in severe cases it may be low. Angina and myocardial ischaemia are well recognized in hypothyroidism and may be associated with hypercholesterolaemia – which indeed was used biochemically as a thyroid function test before the present generation of blood tests was developed.

The ECG often demonstrates low amplitude complexes (**Fig. 17.24**). It has been noted that angina and ECG changes, and especially T-wave flattening or inversion, may rapidly improve when thyroid replacement is started. The speed of these improvements seems to suggest metabolic rather than structural changes in the blood vessel wall. A possible mechanism is that it corrects the reduction in red blood cell 2,3-diphosphoglycerate (DPG) levels seen in hypothyroidism. This metabolite contributes to the dissociation of oxygen from haemoglobin in circumstances of raised aerobic need.

Occasionally gross hypothyroidism may complicate the course after myocardial infarction by causing hypotension and low cardiac output. In general, however, hypothyroidism, as opposed to thyrotoxicosis, does not prove to be a major problem in patients requiring surgery for other reasons.

Gastrointestinal system – In the gastrointestinal system, weight gain is prominently associated with hypothyroidism. Though increases in weight up to 10 kg are common, the

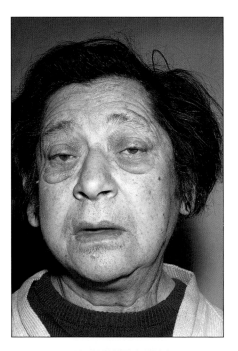

Fig. 17.25 *Periorbital oedema in hypothyroidism.*

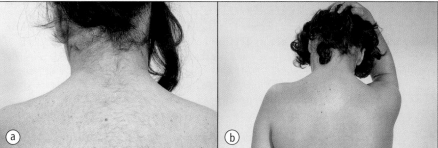

Fig. 17.26 *Increased hair growth in hypothyroidism: (a) before and (b) after treatment.*

condition does not routinely cause gross obesity. Constipation is not infrequent but perhaps more common and less recognized is a liability to 'windy distension' of the abdomen with the waistband being intermittently tight and loose. In elderly patients there may be faecal impaction and ileus.

Skin and hair – The skin is characteristically cold and dry. In severe cases myxoedema occurs, infiltration with mucopolysaccharide causing non-pitting oedema. Facial puffiness, especially periorbital oedema, is common (**Fig. 17.25**), and the skin is often sallow. This may be due to a yellow tinge conferred by β carotene. It can also be associated with anaemia – this is most commonly iron-deficiency anaemia due to menorrhagia but in about 5% of hypothyroid patients, especially elderly, it is pernicious anaemia, an autoimmune condition coexisting with hypothyroidism.

Hair loss, especially from the scalp, is commonly associated with hypothyroidism. Often the body hair is reduced. Excess hair growth may rarely accompany hypothyroidism and disappear on treatment (**Fig. 17.26**).

> ### Fig. 17.27   Post partum thyroiditis – epidemiology
>
> Exremely common (5%) in Caerphilly
> Of whom 50% clinically significant
> Usually a brief toxic phase: destructive thyroiditis
> May be followed by hypothyroidism or hypothyroid alone
> (or reverse order)
> Autoantibody status ? should be screened for
> Important cause of psychological morbidity

Other features – Huskiness may also occur but is fairly uncommon except in long-standing hypothyroidism. Typically the timbre changes, sometimes deepening, and the ability to sing is impaired; a frequent complaint is not being recognized on the telephone. Sleep apnoea, sometimes associated with excessive snoring is underdiagnosed in hypothyroidism. In myxoedema coma there may be retention of carbon dioxide.

Despite well-described accounts dating back many years, the occurrence of non-specific rheumatic complaints (including the already-mentioned features of nerve entrapment and myopathy) is often not rightly attributed to hypothyroidism, yet is common.

Postpartum thyroiditis

This condition has been estimated to occur in 1 of every 20 unselected pregnancies and is clinically significant in about half of these (**Fig. 17.27**). Many women who go on to develop the condition have raised levels of anti-TPO antibodies. The condition may have an early phase with high thyroid hormone levels and suppressed TSH. However, this phase is usually short lived, occurring 2 or 3 months' postpartum and not clinically significant. It appears to be a form of destructive thyroiditis; isotope studies show little or no thyroid uptake and the thyroid hormone pattern reflects the contents of the normal gland – that is, more T_4 than T_3. This pattern contrasts with that of a driven gland (whether by TSH or immunoglobulins), which tends to be iodine deplete because of the high turnover so that T_3 increments exceed T_4. Between 3 and 5 months' postpartum, a more pronounced phase of hypothyroidism supervenes; this can be profoundly symptomatic but is often overlooked and attributed to the tiring effects of young infants and broken sleep.

It is now recognized that most cases resolve spontaneously after a year but the condition certainly merits treatment until then. Subsequent pregnancies tend to elicit the same response, while, about 30 % of patients go on to develop permanent hypothyroidism. It is also suggested that postpartum depression and other psychological problems at this time are disproportionately found in women with positive thyroid autoantibodies, even if their formal thyroid function tests are normal.

Neonatal hypothyroidism

The typical features of neonatal hypothyroidism are prolonged neonatal jaundice, coarse dull features, protruding tongue, apathy, poor feeding and umbilical hernia. However, 50% of affected infants display none of these clinical features. The toll of untreated neonatal hypothyroidism is severe: if treatment is delayed by a year then it is estimated that the IQ loss amounts to 30 %, which would bring an average IQ down to a severely disabled 70. If thyroid hormone replacement is commenced early on (i.e. within a couple of weeks of birth) then it largely, or in mild cases completely, prevents this irreversible damage. This has led to the development of various screening programmes in different countries, most of which rely on heel-prick blood samples assayed for T_4 or TSH, or both. The causes of hypothyroidism include thyroid gland agenesis, maldescent of the gland with malfunction, dyshormonogenesis and iodine deficiency. Acquired transient hypothyroidism may result from transfer of TSH-receptor-blocking antibodies from mother to fetus across the placenta.

Management

Thyroxine   The American thyroidologist, J. H. Means, described the treatment of hypothyroidism as 'as perfect a form of therapy as any known to medicine'. Almost all cases need oral thyroxine. This is usually administered as a daily dose and, because it has an average biological half-life of about 6–7 days, the dose should not be adjusted at intervals of less than 2 weeks. By the same token it has been found acceptable to give thyroxine in a single weekly dose rather more than seven times the usual daily dose in very non-compliant patients. A further advantage of thyroxine is that it is essentially a prohormone – its conversion to T_3 providing the active agent. This controlled deiodination allows the metabolic provision to be relatively smooth.

The full replacement dose in adults usually ranges between 100 and 200 µg daily – and is partly weight related, hence men tend to need more than women although variations in requirements between individuals may be large. In otherwise fit healthy young adults it is appropriate to start with 100 µg daily. With older patients and those with cardiac disease it is advisable to start with a low dose such as 25 µg daily and raise the dose by 25 µg increments at 2–4 week intervals. Angina may prevent a full replacement dose being achieved but equally often cardiac function and angina may improve with cautious slow increases in thyroxine. Elderly patients may need a lower dosage, often only 75 µg. During pregnancy, hypothyroid women usually require more thyroxine; as in all hypothyroid patients the optimum dose leads to a TSH level in the low-normal range. This change occurs early in pregnancy and rapid reversion to the status quo follows delivery. The pregnancy-associated rise in TBG cannot account for this; it may instead be related to altered renal handling of thyroid hormones in pregnancy.

Tri-iodothyronine   The use of T_3 is limited, but it is specifically indicated in circumstances where rapid but controlled treatment of hypothyroidism is needed. It has a short half-life so requires a thrice-daily regimen. The benefit of this feature is that it enables a rapid reduction in action if adverse effects necessitate its withdrawal.

There is renewed controversy about the benefit of adding T_3 to thyroxine for routine oral therapy. Its use for myxoedema coma is another controversial therapeutic area. In North America, the widely followed advice is to load the patient with a high dose of thyroxine, but this may be partly related to the unavailability of ready supplies of T_3 for therapeutic use. It is the author's preference to use T_3, which has rapid beneficial effects on cardiac function when used in low doses (see Ch. 14). This regimen has proved safe and useful also in dealing with myxoedema coma (**Fig. 17.28**) in patients with critical cardiac disease and severe hypothyroidism. It is particularly useful in amiodarone-induced hypothyroidism where the drug cannot be withdrawn.

Biochemical monitoring of hypothyroidism   The current ready availability of accurate, sensitive and cheap thyroid hormone blood tests makes their use obligatory in the diagnosis of hypothyroidism. If the laboratory tests are all perfectly normal then there is no basis for treating symptoms with thyroxine. Early hypothyroidism can present with symptoms and raised TSH but T_4 levels still within the reference range. Debate continues about the need to treat subclinical hypothyroidism in which only the TSH is raised. If the need for treatment is not apparent, why then was the TSH measured?

When monitoring the dosage of thyroxine, one should note that the well-treated patient may have hormone levels outside the diagnostic reference range. The reason is that T_4 needs

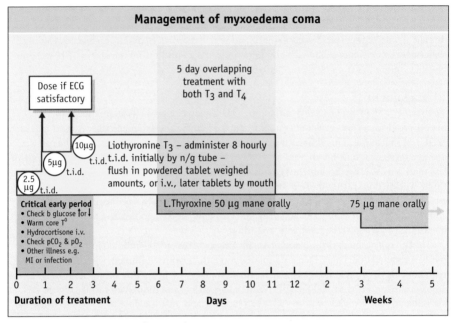

Fig. 17.28 *Management of myxoedema coma.*

to be present in slightly higher levels than in the normal individual whose T_3 is only 80 % derived from circulating T_4 (20 % being secreted directly by the thyroid). Also the presence of the relatively more powerful pituitary deiodinase (type II) enzyme tends to produce TSH levels at the lower end of normal in a person relying on thyroxine therapy to achieve euthyroidism, so slightly 'subnormal' TSH values are acceptable. However, frankly low or suppressed levels are also frequently seen in patients who are clinically euthyroid and who have perfectly normal circulating T_4 and T_3 levels. This situation seems to be more frequent since the introduction of some of the newer supersensitive TSH assays, and so it is questionable whether these patients are subtly overtreated – that is, whether they have mild iatrogenic hyperthyroidism. A major focus of concern is whether this leads to diminished bone density and increased risk of oestoporotic fracture, but the evidence here is conflicting, much greater concern having been expressed in the USA than in the UK and Europe in general.

Thyroid extract There are no grounds for using thyroid extract. This has long been rendered obsolete by the availability of precisely standardized tablets of pure thyroxine. The issue of differing bioavailability of different brands of thyroxine is not fully resolved but evidence to date suggests that any differences are minor. Patients appear to differ in their sensitivity to the precise dose of thyroxine they receive but its onset and termination of action are sufficiently slow to render implausible any biologically significant responses within a day to changes in a dose of thyroxine.

THYROID HORMONE RESISTANCE AND TSH-SECRETING PITUITARY ADENOMAS

Thyroid hormone resistance has mixed clinical and biochemical manifestations but the constant feature is an inappropriately elevated TSH secretion for the degree of thyroid hormone secretion. There is no consensus on management with thyroid hormones or analogues.

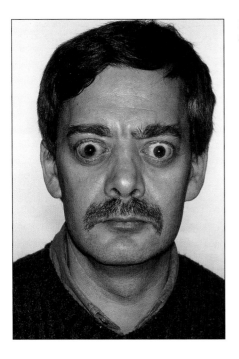

Fig. 17.29 *Florid Graves' disease in a male.*

TSH-secreting pituitary adenomas will respond to suppression by the somatostatin analogue octreotide (see **Fig. 17.9**, p.236).

THYROTOXICOSIS

Clinical features and signs

Some non-specific features may occur in hyperthyroid and hypothyroid patients alike, including tiredness, angina and hair loss. Age is a major determinant of the clinical picture. Thyrotoxicosis in childhood is uncommon and may cause accelerated growth and behavioural problems. Florid features including eye signs of Graves's disease (**Fig. 17.29**) are common in young women. The classical signs are numerous and often pathognomonic:

Uncommon and underrecognized clinical features and signs in thyrotoxicosis

- Hyperphagia leading to weight gain
- Vomiting
- Pruritus
- Thirst
- Hyperthyroid myopathy
- Myasthenia gravis
- Periodic hypokalaemic paralysis
- Apathetic thyrotoxicosis with ptosis

The hyperphagia is typically accompanied by weight loss, but occasionally may be so great as to allow weight gain. The pruritus is a feature of the thyrotoxicosis rather than a drug

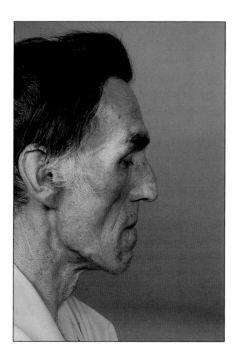

Fig. 17.30 *Apathetic thyrotoxicosis.*

reaction following its treatment. Thirst is an almost constant complaint, and is not apparently due to excessive fluid loss but rather to a resetting of hypothalamic mechanisms including vasopressin release. Hyperthyroid myopathy affects largely proximal and occasional bulbar muscles, but is not associated with elevated serum levels of muscle enzymes. Myasthenia gravis and thyrotoxicosis coexist more often than expected by chance. Periodic hypokalaemic paralysis is particularly seen in Oriental patients.

Atypical presentations of thyrotoxicosis occur most importantly in the elderly, with cardiovascular problems predominating. Elderly patients in atrial fibrillation with normal T_4 and T_3 levels but suppressed TSH often proceed to frank biochemical thyrotoxicosis. Such presentations are termed 'hidden' or 'masked' thyrotoxicosis. Anorexia is common, which distracts the investigator from recognizing the weight loss as a sign of thyrotoxicosis in these patients as they often lack eye signs or goitre. Apathetic thyrotoxicosis is the presentation most removed from the classical image, with inertia prompting thoughts of hypothyroidism, ptosis and marked weight loss suggestive of neoplastic cachexia, especially that featuring temporalis muscle wasting resulting in scaphoid temples (**Fig. 17.30**). Atrial fibrillation and severe congestive cardiac failure are the rule. Biochemical hyperthyroidism confirms the diagnosis, although values are often only moderately elevated; nevertheless the clinical response is usually very gratifying.

'Thyroid storm' represents a special and potentially lethal form of thyrotoxicosis (see Ch. 14).

Management

Management remains potentially taxing despite experience with thionamide drugs, surgery and radioiodine over a period of more than 50 years.

Medical treatment   Medication is generally used in a course of treatment usually lasting 6–18 months, or in order to achieve euthyroidism prior to ablative therapy, though it may occasionally be employed in the very long term.

The first-line drugs are carbimazole or its main metabolite methimazole, which is preferred in North America and used in equivalent doses. The initial dosage is usually 20–60 mg daily, depending on the severity of disease. It is classically administered in three divided doses, though its long half-life often allows once-daily use. The conventional pattern is to taper doses as thyrotoxicosis responds clinically and biochemically, beginning 4–6 weeks after onset of treatment. The dosage may need to be reduced to 5 or 2.5 mg daily, which is maintained for a total treatment period of 6–18 months. It is suggested that the relapse rate falls with longer courses but still is over 50% in most series, the great majority relapsing within a year of stopping therapy. A large goitre and very severe disease militate against achieving remission medically, as does an inability to gain long-term control on daily doses of 20 mg or more.

An increasingly used alternative regimen is 'block and replace' in which the initial high dose thionamide needed to achieve euthyroidism is continued. The advantages of this regimen are:

- Abolition of distressing swings in thyroid function that occur in some labile patients due to spontaneous variations in thyroid-stimulating immunoglobulins
- Stabilization of the medical condition – improving well-being
- Reduction in frequency of clinical attendance consequent upon stability being achieved
- Potential improved chance of long-term remission after a course of medical treatment, due to the dose-dependent immunomodulatory properties of carbimazole/methimazole (?plus thyroxine)

As TSH rises to the upper end of the normal range, thyroxine is added, usually at a dosage of 100 µg daily. However, the precise dosage may need individual tailoring to maintain biochemical and clinical normality.

In the early stages of treatment, β-blocking drugs provide rapid symptomatic improvement, especially for tachycardia, tremor, sweating and nervousness. Non-selective drugs such as propranolol or nadolol (used once daily, 40–80 mg) are normally preferred but selective agents such as atenolol are also beneficial. They can be discontinued when the patient improves after several weeks.

- Beta blockers are avoided in asthma or heart failure

Special circumstances

Pregnancy – Untreated thyrotoxicosis reduces fertility but once a thyrotoxic patient is pregnant then drug treatment is essential for maternal and fetal health. Carbimazole can on rare occasions cause aplasia cutis or choanal atresia in the infant. Therefore some clinicians prefer to use propylthiouracil (PTU) for treating thyrotoxicosis in pregnancy, partly also because this drug is said to cross the placenta less well. All thionamides in fact do so, hence minimal doses are used, the aim being no more than 15 mg of carbimazole or methimazole, or 150 mg PTU, daily. The short half-life of PTU necessitates several doses daily in severe disease. Fortunately, the majority of cases ameliorate in the third trimester, which allows a reduction of drug dosage to the minimum, or even occasional discontinuation. Attention to possible rapid exacerbation postpartum is essential, however. The need to minimize antithyroid drug doses rules out use of the block and replace regimen. Use of high doses of carbimazole or methimazole in pregnancy has sometimes previously led to fetal hypothyroidism and goitre – which were occasionally big enough to obstruct labour.

Treatment with antithyroid medication as described is safe and the condition poses no contraindication to pregnancy, nor any reason to delay conception. Low dose carbimazole or PTU treatment is also compatible with safe breast feeding, which should not be discouraged. Small amounts do enter the milk, but are insufficient to affect the baby's thyroid function, though prudence dictates occasional monitoring of the blood levels.

Infants born to mothers with high titres of stimulating immunoglobulins may develop transitory fetal and neonatal hyperthyroidism (even if the mother is euthyroid after thyroid surgery) (**Fig. 17.31**).

Hypersensitivity to thionamides – Minor symptoms of pruritus or rash may be tolerable with antihistamines; they subside with continued use of carbimazole or methimazole. However, any more severe involvement, arthralgia or hepatitis requires that the drug be discontinued. PTU is used much less often so its side-effects are rarely seen but they include the additional specific features of vasculitis. Other side-effects of thionamides include hair loss, gastrointestinal disturbance, headache and general malaise. The most serious is agranulocytosis.

Critical features of agranulocytosis due to thionamides

- Mild leukopenia can be an irrelevant feature of untreated thyrotoxicosis
- Agranulocytosis is rare, occurring in only about 3 in 10 000 patients treated with carbimazole
- It can occur precipitously and without warning so routine white counts may engender a false sense of security
- It is usually accompanied by a severe sore throat, fever or mouth ulcers
- All patients should be instructed to obtain a white cell count immediately if they have symptoms, and to carry a card (**Fig. 17.32**)
- A neutrophil count of $1.0 \times 10^9/L$ or less indicates a need to stop the drug at once
- All cases should be admitted to hospital and haematological and microbiological help must be obtained urgently
- Use of granulocyte-colony stimulating factor seems to speed recovery and reduce mortality

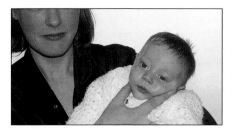

Fig. 17.31   *Neonatal hypothyroidism.*

Card giving measures to take in event of sore throat when taking carbimazole

WTA 169

THE
TEACHING
HOSPITALS

TO WHOM IT MAY CONCERN:

FROM
CONSULTANT PHYSICIAN/
ENDOCRINOLOGIST

Signed ....

Date ....

RE: This patient is on carbimazole (Neo-mercazole) for thyrotoxicosis. He/she has been told that in the event of a severe sore throat that he/she should attend the nearest hospital, bring the tablets with him/her, and ask for an urgent white cell count to be obtained. I would be grateful if this could be performed and the patient informed of the results, so that further tablets can be taken if white blood cell is normal, but no further tablets should be taken if the neurophil count is **less than 1.0 x 10^9/litre.**

In this event the patient has been asked to contact me urgently. If there are any queries please telephone me direct on any of the following numbers:

Fig. 17.32 *A card giving measures to take regarding possible development of agranulocytosis.*

Iodine-induced thyrotoxicosis – This is most commonly due to use of amiodarone (see above). High dose carbimazole should be used and maintained. If possible, and after the patient has been rendered euthyroid, surgery should be considered. Radioiodine cannot be used in this situation (**Fig. 17.33**). Potassium perchlorate has been suggested for use in conjunction with carbimazole even though it carries the risk of irreversible aplastic anaemia. Glucocorticords are recommended and β blockers can be helpful. Lithium carbonate can also on occasion be very beneficial. Treatment of this condition is therefore difficult, sometimes dangerous and often uncertain or even unsuccessful, with a fatal outcome.

Thyroid crisis (or storm) – See Ch. 14.

Surgery   Though decreasingly used, it is valuable in patients who have relapsed after a full course of antithyroid medication has been completed, or in very severely toxic patients in whom euthyroidism can only be achieved with continued high doses of drugs. It is useful in patients intolerant of medication. It is essential that all patients are rendered euthyroid by the time of surgery. Usually thionamide therapy alone suffices, but some surgeons still prefer administration with iodine for 10–14 days beforehand to reduce the vascularity. The surgical goal is to leave a remnant of an eighth to a quarter of the original gland – usually about 8 g. An experienced surgeon is required to obtain negligible mortality and low morbidity.

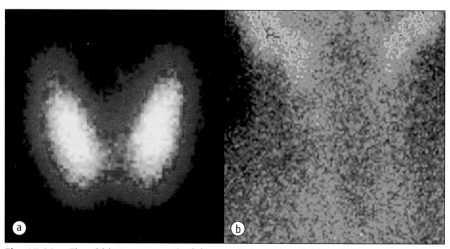

Fig. 17.33   *Thyroid isotope scans in (a) normal thyroid and (b) amiodarone-induced thyrotoxicosis*

Postoperative complications of subtotal thyroidectomy include:

- Haematoma with possibility of asphyxia (very rare)
- Recurrent laryngeal damage, which may be transient (uncommon) or permanent (rare)
- Hypocalcaemia with tetany, which may be transient (common) or permanent (uncommon)
- Hypothyroidism, which may be transient (common) or permanent (immediately uncommon, eventually common)
- Problems with scarring, including keloid (variable, e.g. racial influences) and infection (rare)
- Recurrent thyrotoxicosis (rare)

Radioiodine   The simplicity, confirmed safety and efficacy of this modality of treatment promote its growing popularity. There is no evidence of increased risk of carcinoma or leukaemia after its use, nor of teratogenicity, although women of childbearing age are recommended to avoid pregnancy for at least 4 months following its use.

Regulations differ widely between countries concerning what measures are needed following its administration and for how long, in order to safeguard others from risk of contamination. Complex calculations based on estimates of goitre size and handling of tracer doses of radioiodine fail to provide any reliable guidelines for dosimetry. There is a trade-off between failure to control some patients for long periods following low doses of ^{131}I and the rapid development of permanent hypothyroidism following high doses, but this generalization conceals the wide variety and unpredictability of individual responses. Hypothyroidism is easily and cheaply treated and is the near-inevitable long-term consequence of successful radioiodine treatment of thyrotoxicosis. Many physicians aim to

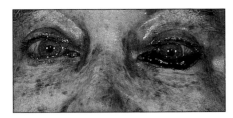

Fig. 17.34 *Inflammatory phase of Graves' ophthalmopathy.*

ablate the thyroid with relatively high doses, and the ensuing hypothyroidism can be rapidly developing and very symptomatic, with especially myalgia, cold intolerance and bloating, but these symptoms are rapidly reversible. Delayed hypothyroidism appears insidiously, therefore it is mandatory to follow all patients treated with radioiodine until they are permanently and fully established on thyroxine. Most patients receive between 185 Mbq (5 mci) to 740 Mbq (20 mci), although multiple doses or higher doses are needed more often for patients with multinodular goitre. Older patients and those with nodular goitre are less liable to hypothyroidism.

Although patients can proceed straight to radioiodine, many clinicians prefer to render patients euthyroid first with a few weeks to months of thionamide therapy, which is stopped several days before radioiodine. This reduces the severity of the flare-up of increased thyroid hormone output that is seen in some patients at a week after treatment. This uncommonly causes symptoms, occasionally a local inflammatory response in the neck and very rarely it has been associated with thyroid crisis. Patients may benefit from β blockers over this period and some require a brief restarting of carbimazole – which should be delayed until about a week after radioiodine. Use of carbimazole pre- and post-treatment might reduce the effectiveness of radioiodine but this does not constitute a major problem. There is suggestive evidence that active ophthalmopathy (see below) may be acutely worsened by radioiodine, which is a relative contraindication for its use. However, this deterioration can be largely aborted by prophylactic or, if symptomatic, early short-term prednisolone therapy. There is a reluctance by many to treat children with radioiodine, though it is now used in younger people than previously.

Extrathyroidal manifestations of Graves' disease

Thyroid-associated ophthalmopathy (TAO) occurs frequently but mildly so requires no attention in most patients. However, in a minority of patients it may be severe enough to compromise the vision.

The aetiology is thought to be autoimmune, although the antigen(s) are as yet unknown; attention is currently focused on the orbital fibroblasts, with secondary effects mediated by cytokines affecting the extraocular muscles and fat with accumulation of glycosaminoglycans. This ocular involvement commonly accompanies thyrotoxicosis but it may also occur in isolation, precede thyroid dysfunction by many years, occur long after thyroid ablation, or occasionally occur with Hashimoto's disease. The course of disease involves an early, often rapidly developing, phase with much inflammation evident (**Fig. 17.34**), followed by a much slower long-lasting spontaneous improvement with disappearance of the inflammation but usually incomplete resolution of ocular symptoms and signs (Rundle's curve). These phases have been classically summarized by the mnemonic 'NO-SPECS' (**Fig. 17.35**).

(Fig. 17.35) NO-SPECS classification of Graves' ophthalmopathy			
Class	**Mnemonic**	**Severity score***		
		1	2	3
0 = N	No signs or symptoms			
1 = O	Only signs			
2 = S	Soft tissue involvement	Minimal	Moderate	Severe
3 = P	Proptosis	20–23 mm	23–27mm	>27 mm
4 = E	Extraocular muscle involvement	Infrequent diplopia	Frequent diplopia	Constant diplopia
5 = C	Corneal involvement	Slight stippling	Marked stippling	Ulceration
6 = S	Sight loss	20/25–20/40	20/45–20/100	<20/100

*Ophthalmic Index = the sum of the severity scores for categories 2–6 (SPECS)

The course of the various features should be serially documented, including Hess charting of eye movements, intraocular pressure measurement in forward gaze and upgaze (when typically increased), checks on visual acuity, visual fields and colour vision using Ishihara charts. Intraorbital anatomy can be displayed by CT scanning (ensuring the lens dose is minimized) and more safely and usefully by MRI. Factors that aggravate the disease include cigarette smoking, radioiodine therapy, male sex and uncontrolled thyroid disease, especially raised TSH levels. Markedly asymmetrical involvement frequently occurs, which is possibly due to differences between the bone capacity of the orbits (**Fig. 17.36**). Though cosmetically unattractive, proptosis (also called exophthalmos) may act as a safety valve by allowing forward decompression. Tight orbits lead to more marked pressure effects manifesting as unbalanced ocular movement disorders with distressing diplopia (**Fig. 17.37**), or most seriously optic nerve compression at the orbital apex by the swollen bellies of the extraocular muscles. *Management*   Local measures include methylcellulose eyedrops and the fitting of prisms to glasses to correct diplopia. Propping the head up with pillows at night might help. Lagophthalmos (incomplete lid closure) risks corneal damage so hair should be kept away especially in sleep. During the 'wet' early inflammatory stages, immunosuppressive measures are appropriate; these include the use of corticosteroids – either oral prednisolone starting at a high dosage and tapering rapidly, or beginning with i.v. pulses of methylprednisolone. However, long-term use causes iatrogenic Cushing's syndrome without any benefit (**Fig. 17.38**). Azathioprine and occasionally cyclosporine may help.

There is a revival of popularity for the use of orbital radiotherapy at this stage of management. Diplopia may become fixed with fibrosis developing later in disease, and surgery is undertaken only when the situation is stabilized. Visual loss is rare but is an emergency and may require orbital decompression; surgical techniques are still evolving and aim to enhance cosmetic results with minimal diplopia whilst saving and restoring compromised vision.

Dermopathy and acropachy

These almost invariably occur in association with, but much less commonly than, TAO. Skin infiltration with glycosaminoglycans is often termed 'pretibial myxoedema' but it is not restricted to this site (**Fig. 17.39**). Acropachy simulates clubbing of the terminal phalanges (**Fig. 17.40**) but is asymptomatic. Typically there is a lacey appearance of the periosteum on X-ray.

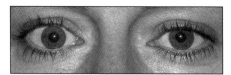

Fig. 17.36 *Asymmetrical eye signs in Graves' disease.*

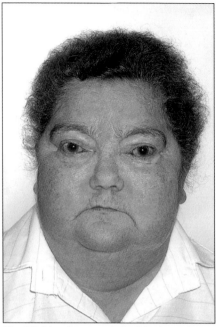

Fig. 17.38 *Iatrogenic Cushing's syndrome caused by use of corticosteroids for TAO.*

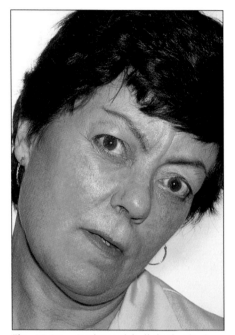

Fig. 17.37 *Patient with diplopia tipping the head to minimize double vision.*

Management   Treatment of dermopathy may need local application of corticosteroids, often under occlusive cover, or intradermal injections of triamcinolone. Azathioprine and plasmapharesis have also been used.

THYROIDITIS

Clinical features

Thyroiditis may present acutely or subacutely, such as in de Quervain's thyroiditis, which is presumed in most cases to be caused by a virus (e.g. Coxsackie, mumps), but the precise cause is often unidentified. It causes swelling, pain, inflammation and is associated with destructive release of prestored thyroid hormone giving a brief illness with systemic malaise, local neck symptoms and features of thyrotoxicosis. Levels of T_4 tend to rise more than T_3 in serum and there is virtually no uptake on isotope scans. There may be a transient rise in thyroid antibody levels and subsequent transient hypothyroidism but the expectation is for full recovery within months.

The same pattern, including findings on investigation, has been reported without the local neck discomfort and termed 'silent thyroiditis'. A similar evanescent toxic phase may be part

259

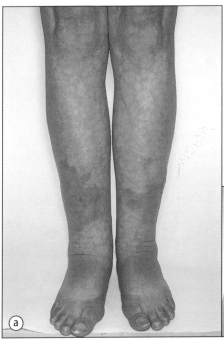

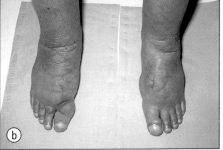

Fig. 17.39 *(a) typical appearence and (b) 'elephantiasis' variety.*

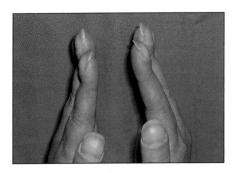

Fig. 17.40 *Thyroid acropachy.*

of the postpartum thyroiditis (see above). Hashimoto's thyroiditis can also present with a brief toxic phase. It can also mimic subacute thyroiditis but be more protracted, requiring steroids (see above).

Riedel's thyroiditis is a rare condition with fibrous tissue often found in the neck beyond the confines of the thyroid gland. It may be associated with fibrosis distantly e.g. retroperitoneally. Sometimes there are high TPO antibody levels but the aetiology is unclear.

Management

Symptomatic treatment with simple analgesics, including aspirin and β blockers may be useful. Hashimoto's thyroiditis responds rapidly to small doses of carbimazole, but care is needed to stop treatment early when hypothyroidism develops. Treatment of Riedel's thyroiditis involves radical surgery, thyroxine replacement and often corticosteroids.

GOITRE
Management
The management of goitre depends on accurate diagnosis and in particular identification of neoplastic growth, abnormality of thyroid function and significant compressive symptoms.

Endemic goitre, defined as that occurring in a region with greater than 10 % incidence of goitre in children aged 6–12 years, is principally due to iodine deficiency. This is measured by urinary iodine excretion: populations with median values of less than 15 mg/L have a goitre prevalence of over 30 %. These goitres are initially diffuse and tend to multinodularity with age. The sequelae can be avoided by iodine supplementation; this is targeted at the young, especially infants and pregnant women but in women ideally started before pregnancy. Older subjects are not treated as their partly autonomous nodular goitres predispose to the development of thyrotoxicosis with iodine treatment. In many areas, such as Zaire, dietary goitrogens from cassava (and elsewhere many members of the Brassica family) contribute to endemic goitre.

Where no obvious cause is found (sporadic goitre) treatment may not be needed unless there are pressure symptoms, cosmetic considerations or suspicion of malignancy. Therapeutic approaches include: exogenous thyroxine; radioiodine (large doses are needed) and surgery. The last of these is especially indicated if possible neoplasia or retrosternal extension is a major issue.

Multinodular goitre is largely approached in the same way as sporadic goitre. There is an increased liability to bleeding into a nodule, hence surgery is needed more often. Compression, rather than just tracheal deviation, should be established through imaging with CT or MR scanning and physiological measurements, including flow-volume loop and forced inspiratory volume (FIV_1) versus forced expiratory volume (FEV_1). Incipient stridor requires urgent investigation, including checks of vocal cords prior to surgery. A multinodular goitre may have a single dominant nodule requiring specific investigation in its own right.

Because Hashimoto's thyroiditis may masquerade as simple goitre, all cases of goitre should be investigated, and tests of thyroid function and anti-TPO antibodies should be performed (**Fig. 17.41**). Thyroxine therapy may shrink even fibrous variants and long-standing nodular Hashimoto goitres. Occasionally, though, corticosteroids or surgery, or both, are also needed.

Thyrotoxicosis can be quite occult, presenting with a goitre and few other features. A bruit is very suggestive of thyrotoxicosis (**Fig. 17.42**). Goitre and hyperthyroidism are very rarely caused by TSH-secreting pituitary adenomas (**Fig. 17.43**). Goitre, usually nodular, often occurs in acromegaly and not infrequently is hyperfunctioning. Goitre may be associated with toxic features in partial thyroid hormone resistance.

Solitary nodules of the thyroid   These need investigating for possible cancer, though most are benign. The initial investigation in euthyroid subjects is fine needle aspiration. Thyroid scintigraphy is largely unhelpful as most single nodules are 'cold' (i.e. do not take up the tracer) while 80% are benign. Ultrasonography can be helpful, however, especially with cysts and also frequently when an apparently solitary nodule is part of a multinodular goitre. Cytology is sufficiently reliable to allow significantly fewer unnecessary operations to be performed while preventing the occurrence of unacceptable rates of false negatives.

Toxic adenoma (Plummer's disease) is well treated by radioiodine or surgery (following medical induction of euthyroidism) (**Fig. 17.44**). In euthyroid subjects, nodules yielding follicular structures must be treated as potential cancers and submitted for surgery, though most prove to be benign adenomas (see below).

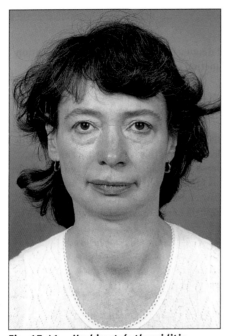

Fig. 17.41   *Hashimoto's thyroiditis.*

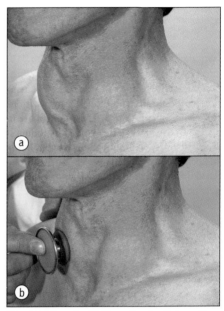

Fig. 17.42   *(a, b) Vascular bruit in goitre.*

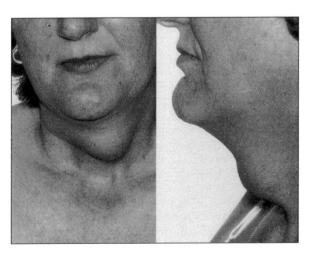

Fig. 17.43   *Recurrent goitre due to TSH-secreting pituitary adenoma.*

THYROID CANCER

Thyroid cancer is uncommon, affecting only 1 in 1000 people per year. It tends to affect young people and generally has a good prognosis. Thyroid follicular epithelium gives rise to two types of differentiated carcinoma – papillary and follicular – and the rare anaplastic variant.

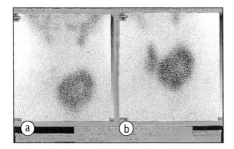

Fig. 17.44 *Plummer's disease – a hot nodule (a) pre-treatment, (b) after ^{131}I treatment, allowing normal lobe to take up isotope.*

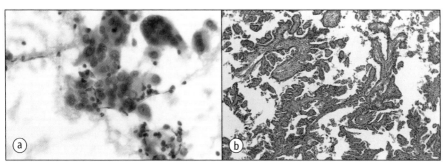

Fig. 17.45 *(a, b) Cytology and pathology of papillary carcinoma of thyroid.*

Papillary carcinoma

This is the commonest type, especially in iodine-replete areas, where it comprises 80 % of cases, compared with 60–70 % in iodine-deficient areas.

Clinical features Typical nuclear changes, and in about half of cases calcified psammoma bodies, bestow readily recognizable cytological and histological features (**Fig. 17.45**). Tumour spread is typically to regional lymph nodes and occasionally to the lung. It occurs in young age groups, including children subjected to prior irradiation. Certain features, including occurrence at age less than 40 years, a single tumour mass less than 2 cm in diameter, no evidence of local or distant spread and no history of irradiation, confer very good prognosis.

Treatment There is controversy over how radical surgery should be, and the place of postoperative ablation. In experienced hands (the only ones to be entrusted with this surgery), radical surgery is acceptable and associated with only minimal risks of recurrent laryngeal and parathyroid damage.

Follicular carcinoma

This type constitutes 10–30% of differentiated thyroid cancer (depending on the iodine availability in the population).

Clinical features This type occurs in an older age group than the papillary type. It is also more aggressive, and spreads haematogenously, especially to the lung and bone but occasionally to the brain, liver and skin.

There are no characteristic cytological features differentiating follicular adenoma from carcinoma. That distinction relies on either evidence of distant metastases or histological evidence of venous invasion or breeching of the capsule.

Treatment Near-total thyroidectomy followed by radioiodine ablation is recommended.

All patients with differentiated carcinoma require TSH-suppressing T_4 therapy (whenever practical) and serial thyroglobulin measurements after surgery. Elevated thyroglobulin levels are a warning of recurrence, which necessitates T_4 cessation for 6 weeks to allow TSH levels to rise and then whole-body ^{131}I scanning using 2–5 mci. An excessive dose 'stuns' the residual tumour tissue, preventing uptake of any therapeutic dose that may then be required. The use of recombinant biosynthetic TSH is undergoing evaluation for enhancing radioiodine uptake without requiring discontinuation of thyroxine with its attendant symptoms.

Anaplastic carcinoma

This typically occurs in the elderly presenting as a rapidly growing hard mass, probably arising from a differentiated tumour by p53 mutations. The outlook is bleak.

Treatment   Radiotherapy offers short-lived palliation. Occasionally patients survive for 2–3 years after chemotherapy.

Medullary carcinoma of thyroid

This carcinoma arises from the C cells. Most are sporadic, but about a fifth are part of MEN-2a or 2b, or familial medullary carcinoma kindreds, in which there is a germline mutation in the *ret* proto-oncogene (see Ch. 23). These tumours characteristically secrete calcitonin and often other peptides and amines. They can also cause ectopic ACTH production. With lesser degrees of differentiation, carcinoembryonic antigen (CEA) is increasingly secreted (see also Ch. 23).

Treatment   Because local lymph node spread occurs early, radical surgery and lymph node clearance are required. Chemotherapy and radiotherapy are also used, but often with little benefit.

RARE CAUSES OF GOITRE

These include amyloidosis, sarcoidosis and other infiltrative disorders. Goitrogens are most commonly drugs (e.g. iodine-induced goitre occurs with amiodarone and also frequently with lithium). Lithium usually causes hypothyroidism when associated with thyroid disorders, but can also lead to thyrotoxicosis. Less obvious causes include kelp ingestion and conversely iodine deficiency induced as part of a strict allergy-excluding regimen (Fig. 17.46). Dyshormongenesis is rare; the commonest form is Pendred's syndrome, in which a defect of organification is associated with deafness.

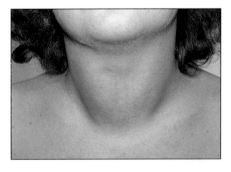

Fig. 17.46 *Iodine-induced goitre resulting from limited food intake in a patient with 'total allergy' syndrome.*

chapter 18

Adrenal Disorders

INTRODUCTION

Destruction or removal of both adrenal glands is incompatible with health and in stressful illness usually proves fatal.

- The outer layer of the adrenal glands, the steroid-synthesizing cortex, secretes three major hormones: cortisol, aldosterone and androgens

Cortisol is essential for survival. Basal amounts are required to maintain vascular tone and enable water excretion to occur, but the body needs to secrete larger amounts in order to cope with a wide variety of physical stresses.

Aldosterone is the main regulator of sodium homeostasis and also extracellular potassium (which can become dangerously high in its absence). The large doses of hydrocortisone given to treat adrenally insufficient patients in stressful illness also cater for any mineralocorticosteroid requirement.

Adrenal androgens are increasingly secreted from the age of about 6–7 years (the adrenarche) and seem to be involved in the development of secondary sexual hair. A major adrenal product, in quantitative terms, is dehydroepiandrosterone (DHA) together with its sulphate (DHAS). The circulating concentrations of these products show a variable but often profound age-related drop. There is much speculation but little solid evidence for the role of this decrease in the ageing process.

- The inner adrenal layer, the medulla, produces catecholamines – especially noradrenaline (norepinephrine) and adrenaline (epinephrine)

The medulla is regulated by postganglionic sympathetic nerves and responds rapidly to a variety of stresses including trauma, myocardial infarction, sepsis and hypoglycaemia. These medullary responses are not essential for survival.

REGULATION OF CORTISOL SYNTHESIS AND SECRETION
(Fig. 18.1)
Adrenocorticotrophic hormone (ACTH) secreted from the anterior pituitary is the immediate drive for cortisol production and release. ACTH is released in pulses that rapidly also lead to pulses of cortisol. The frequency (especially) and amplitude of ACTH pulses influence the pattern of cortisol secretion, as follows:

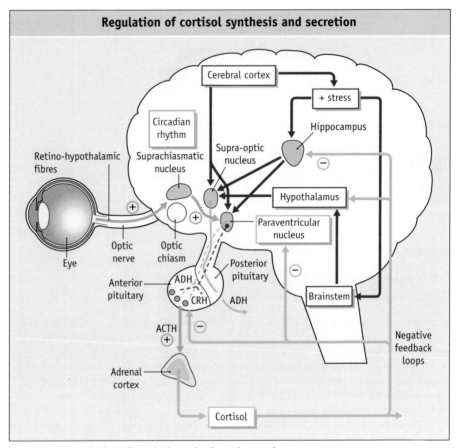

Fig. 18.1 *Regulation of cortisol synthesis and secretion.*

- The main influences on cortisol production are the circadian rhythm, negative feedback and stress
- The cortisol level usually peaks between 8 and 9 a.m., the nadir occurs at midnight, then levels rise again from about 3 a.m. (**Fig. 18.2**)
- The sensitivity of the negative feedback loop determines the overall cortisol secretion
- Stress-induced ACTH/cortisol hypersecretion overrides other influences in normal people

REGULATION OF ALDOSTERONE SECRETION (Fig. 18.3)

The predominant influence on aldosterone secretion is renin from the juxtaglomerular apparatus in the proximal renal tubules. Renin secretion increases with decreased renal perfusion, which is sensed by the macula densa, and acts on circulating plasma renin substrate released from the liver. This forms angiotensin I (a decapeptide), which

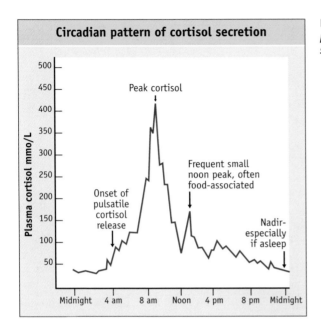

Fig. 18.2 *Circadian pattern of cortisol secretion.*

angiotensin-converting enzyme (ACE) converts to angiotensin II (an octapeptide). Angiotensin II leads to vasoconstriction and aldosterone secretion.

An increase in potassium concentration leads to aldosterone secretion both directly and also secondarily via renin. ACTH is also a minor secretory influence on aldosterone secretion. Other influences include β-adrenergic stimulation of renin, and that of serotonin on aldosterone.

REGULATION OF ADRENAL ANDROGENS

Androstenedione, DHA and DHAS are all influenced by ACTH. Other possible factors include adrenal blood flow and a hypothesized adrenal androgen-stimulating hormone.

- The main virilizing effects are due to peripheral conversion to testosterone and dihydrotestosterone
- Increased production is seen in uncontrolled CAH, with 21-hydroxylase and 11β-hydroxylase deficiency
- There is a postulated relationship to PCOS

PRODUCTION OF CATECHOLAMINES

Circulating noradrenaline (norepinephrine) is mainly derived from the sympathetic nerves by a 'spillover' phenomenon. Increased levels are secreted by phaeochromocytomas of both adrenal and extra-adrenal origin. Circulating adrenaline (epinephrine) is largely adrenal in origin as it is synthesized from noradrenaline (norepinephrine) by the enzyme phenylethanolamine-N-methyl transferase (PNMT), which is mainly confined to adrenal medulla (though some brain nuclei also contain PNMT). Adrenal PNMT is activated by high

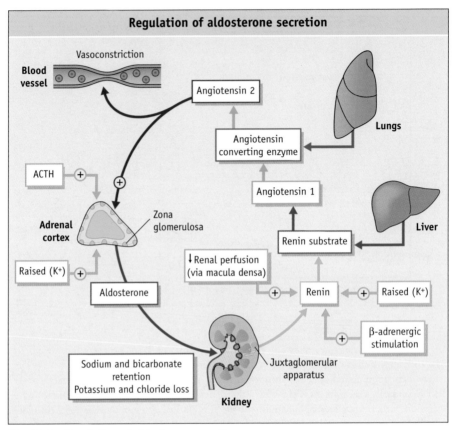

Fig. 18.3   *Regulation of aldosterone secretion.*

ambient cortisol concentrations, which are achieved by venous drainage of the adrenal cortex via the adrenal medulla. Normal adrenomedullary control is exerted by the sympathetic nervous system via cholinergic neurons that mediate reflex changes (e.g. when standing). These changes are lost with phaeochromocytomas.

PATHOGENESIS AND PATHOLOGY

ADRENAL CORTEX

Cushing's syndrome

There are many aetiological factors in Cushing's syndrome. They include various tumours and hyperplasias, receptor defects and iatrogenic factors.

Pituitary-dependent ACTH excess (Cushing's disease) may be caused by microadenoma, macroadenoma or corticotrophic hyperplasia. Macronodular hyperplasia is a variant of Cushing's disease that is independent of ACTH.

Ectopic ACTH production may be either due to a very malignant tumour, such as small-cell carcinoma of the lung, or caused by a benign bronchial carcinoid tumour. Tumours in numerous other sites have also been recorded – including those in the thymus or pancreatic

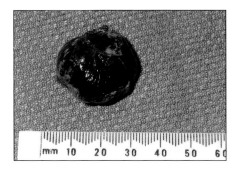

Fig. 18.4 *Black adenoma of adrenal associated with Cushing's syndrome.*

islets, phaeochromocytomas, and medullary carcinomas in the thyroid gland, ovary or liver. Ectopic CRH production may also occur either with or without ectopic ACTH. Other tumours include adrenal adenomas, such as 'black' adenoma (**Fig. 18.4**), and subclinical incidentalomas. Adrenal carcinomas may occur either with or without virilization, feminization, or mineralocorticoid excess.

In addition, Cushing's syndrome is sometimes caused by micronodular pigmented adrenal hyperplasia, or by aberrant receptors on the adrenal cortex (e.g. GIP, or the β adrenoceptor).

Iatrogenic causes include oral or injected, but infrequently inhaled or cutaneous glucocorticoids, and rarely ACTH injections. There is also an alcoholic pseudo-Cushing's syndrome.

Mineralocorticoid excess syndromes

Hyperaldosteronism may be either primary or secondary. The primary type might be due to any of the following:
- Adenoma (Conn's syndrome)
- Hyperplasia of zona glomerulosa
- Glucocorticoid-remediable hyperaldosteronism
- Carcinoma – either adrenal or ovarian
  Secondary hyperaldosteronism may be caused by:
- Sodium depletion or hypovolaemia
- Congestive cardiac failure
- Nephrotic syndrome
- Cirrhosis with ascites
- Salt-losing nephropathy or enteropathy
- Diuretic abuse
- Renal artery stenosis
- Malignant hypertension
- Renin-producing tumour
- Bartter's syndrome

Pseudohyperaldosteronism may be caused by Liddle's syndrome. There are also other excess mineralocorticoid syndromes that do not involve aldosterone. These are listed in **Fig. 18.5**.

Congenital adrenal hyperplasia

CAH encompasses a group of congenital corticosteroid defects that are due to mutations in the various enzymes involved in corticosteroid biosynthesis. The consequent cortisol deficiency triggers increased secretion of ACTH, and aldosterone deficiency may also occur leading to increased renin production. The enzymatic deficiencies result in biosynthesis being

Fig. 18.5   Excess mineralocorticoid conditions not due to aldosterone

Congenital forms	CAH: — 11β-hydroxylase deficiency leading to DOC increase — 17α-hydroxylase deficiency — 11β-hydroxysteroid dehydrogenase deficiency (11β-HSD) leading to failure of renal cortisol to cortisone conversion, allowing cortisol to act as a mineralocorticoid
Acquired types	From consuming excess liquorice From administration of carbenoxolone From administration of exogenous mineralocorticoids (e.g. fluorinated corticosteroids, oral or cutaneous) DOC/corticosteroid-producing tumours Cushing's syndrome, especially ectopic ACTH production

diverted along alternative pathways, with the consequence that biologically active precursors (androgens or mineralocorticoids) accumulate. For each step in the biosynthesis pathway the degree of effect may vary, which results in turn in variations in the clinical severity, the age at clinical onset and the phenotypic pattern.

The commonest defect is 21-hydroxylase deficiency, which accounts for more than 95% of cases of CAH. In the UK the incidence of classical cases is about 1 in 12 000. However, marked ethnic variations are seen. For instance, in the isolated Yupik eskimos there is a founder effect (where the incidence is about 1 in 500). Non-classical 21-hydroxylase deficiency is probably much commoner, with an incidence of about 1 in 100 in UK and a higher incidence in Ashkenazic Jews. The gene for 21-hydroxylase comprises an active gene (CYP21) and an inactive pseudogene, duplicated in tandem, that are located on chromosome 6 in close association with the human leukocyte antigen (HLA) histocompatibility genes. Many mutations have been described in the CYP21 gene, and these often correlate with the phenotypic expression.

Adrenal tumours

Small tumours are frequently incidentally found on ultrasound, CT or MR scanning of the abdomen for other reasons. They are discussed further below. In contrast, adrenal carcinomas are rare, but are particularly suspected when there is a large tumour more than 4 cm in diameter.

Phaeochromocytomas may either occur sporadically or as part of familial syndromes, especially MEN-2a or b, when abnormalities in the RET oncogene are commonly found. Familial incidence of phaeochromocytomas is also increased in neurofibromatosis type I and in von Hippel-Lindau syndrome (see Ch. 23).

Corticosteroid deficiency syndromes

There are a number of aetiological factors in primary adrenocortical failure (i.e. Addison's disease), including infectious agents, tumours, hyper- or hypoplasia and apoplexy.

In the autoimmune types, adrenal antibodies are detectable in 70–80% of cases. Infections that are associated with adrenocortical failure include tuberculosis, in which there is often detectable calcification that may lead to adrenal enlargement. Primary adrenal insufficiency is the commonest endocrinopathy associated with AIDS, and cryptococcus, coccidiomycosis and cytomegalovirus infections have all been observed in this condition. Associated fungal infections such as histoplasmosis may occur in south and midwest USA. In Waterhouse–Friedrichsen syndrome, there is a specific association with meningococcal or pneumococcal septicaemia.

Adrenocortical failure in amyloidosis may be either primary or secondary. It may furthermore be associated with other sites – for instance the heart or kidney. Sarcoidosis may also be a factor.

Congenital causes include adrenoleukodystrophy. This is an X-linked condition, resulting in disordered very-long-chain fatty acid metabolism. CAH (see above) or congenital adrenal hypoplasia may also cause adrenocortical failure.

In cancer, metastases in the adrenals are common. However, they only rarely lead to hypofunction as this requires the loss of more than 90% of the adrenal mass.

In apoplexy, sudden haemorrhagic destruction is seen, and there may be associated anticoagulation or trauma. Other possible causes are haemochromatosis and Allgrove's syndrome, in which there is isolated glucocorticoid deficiency, alacrima and achalasia.

Secondary adrenocortical failure

ACTH deficiency may be caused by any of the following:

- Diseases of the hypothalamo-pituitary axis (see Ch. 15)
- Iatrogenic – from rapid discontinuation of exogenous glucocorticoids
- Isolated ACTH (or occasionally isolated CRH) deficiency

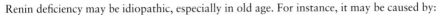

- These conditions are usually associated with relatively normal aldosterone secretion

Renin deficiency may be idiopathic, especially in old age. For instance, it may be caused by:
- Drugs that inhibit renin release, including beta blockers and prostaglandin synthetase inhibitors
- Nephropathy resulting from diabetes mellitus

ADRENAL MEDULLA

Catecholamine-secreting tumours are most frequently adrenomedullary phaeochromocytomas, consisting of chromaffin tissue, which is named after its typical histochemical reaction. Extra-adrenal phaeochromocytomas occur much less frequently; they are termed paragangliomas and the sites where they occur include the sympathetic chain, the carotid body, the mediastinum (including intracardiac tissue), the organ of Zuckerkandl and the urinary bladder.

- A rough 'rule of 10s' has been applied to phaeochromocytomas:
  — 10% are extra-adrenal
  — 10% are malignant
  — 10% are familial

The amount and chemical composition of phaeochromocytomas are partly related to the tumour size. Most produce noradrenaline (norepinephrine), often with adrenaline (epinephrine), some are pure adrenaline (epinephrine) producers whereas a third group produce only noradrenaline (norepinephrine). Phaeochromocytomas may also secrete a range of bioactive peptides including metenkephalin, ACTH, calcitonin gene-related peptide, chromogranin and adrenomedullin, a hypotensive polypeptide.

INVESTIGATION AND DIAGNOSIS

CUSHING'S SYNDROME

Cushing's syndrome arises from exposure to inappropriately high levels of cortisol secretion or, in the case of iatrogenic disease, supraphysiological levels of glucocorticoids. The first task in investigation is to establish the presence of the syndrome. This precedes the frequently very difficult task of differential diagnosis for this condition.

Establishment of Cushing's syndrome rests on the following:

- Raised 24 hour urine free cortisol
- Failure to suppress 9 a.m. plasma cortisol after overnight dexamethasone 1mg administered at 11 p.m.
- Failure to suppress urine cortisol and plasma cortisol after low dose dexamethasone
- Loss of circadian rhythm, especially the midnight drop in the cortisol level
- Failure of cortisol to rise in response to stress

- Note that there are several problems and caveats to the above, however. First, the urine free cortisol is not invariably raised (e.g. because of incomplete collection or variation in metabolism of cortisol). The overnight and low dose dexamethasone suppression tests lack sensitivity and specificity. Although the overnight test is simple to perform, each centre needs to establish its own normal range. The low dose and high dose dexamethasone tests (**Fig. 18.6**) require meticulous attention to detail. Cyclical Cushing's syndrome occurs more frequently than is commonly appreciated, therefore normal results in the face of a high index of clinical suspicion should prompt repeat investigations

Fig. 18.6 Dexamethasone suppression tests

Low dose tests: 0.5 mg dexamethasone 6 hourly (2 mg/day):

9 a.m.	Plasma cortisol – dex 2 + 0	
preceding:	dexamethasone 0.5 mg at 9 a.m.	⎫
	dexamethasone 0.5 mg at 3 p.m.	⎬ 24 hour urine: dex 2, day 1 free
	dexamethasone 0.5 mg at 9 p.m.	⎭ cortisol
	dexamethasone 0.5 mg at 3 a.m.	
9 a.m.	Plasma cortisol – dex 2 + 24 h	
preceding:	dexamethasone 0.5 mg at 9 a.m.	⎫
	dexamethasone 0.5 mg at 3 p.m.	⎬ 24 hour urine: dex 2, day 2 free
	dexamethasone 0.5 mg at 9 p.m.	⎭ cortisol
	dexamethasone 0.5 mg at 3 a.m.	
9 a.m.	Plasma cortisol – dex 2 + 48 h	

High dose tests: 2 mg dexamethasone 6 hourly (8 mg/day):

9 a.m.	Plasma cortisol – dex 8 + 0	
preceding:	dexamethasone 2 mg at 9 a.m.	⎫
	dexamethasone 2 mg at 3 p.m.	⎬ 24 hour urine: dex 8, day 1 free
	dexamethasone 2 mg at 9 p.m.	⎭ cortisol
	dexamethasone 2 mg at 3 a.m.	
9 a.m.	Plasma cortisol – dex 8 + 24 h	
preceding:	dexamethasone 2 mg at 9 a.m.	⎫
	dexamethasone 2 mg at 3 p.m.	⎬ 24 hour urine: dex 8, day 2 free
	dexamethasone 2 mg at 9 p.m.	⎭ cortisol
	dexamethasone 2 mg at 3 a.m.	
9 a.m.	Plasma cortisol – dex 8 + 48 h	

CUSHING'S DISEASE

Plasma ACTH is measurable and may be in the 'normal' range or variably elevated.

Partial suppression of cortisol after dexamethasone administration is characteristic but not invariable. The majority of cases show exaggerated cortisol and ACTH rises after CRH. The majority of cases also show more than 40% increase in cortisol and ACTH after DDAVP 10 μg i.v. The plasma ionic potassium level is usually normal, in contrast to ectopic ACTH secretion but hypokalaemic alkalosis can be seen in severe Cushing's disease. Pituitary imaging may be negative and does not exclude a pituitary cause. MRI is a better technique for revealing microadenomas (**Fig. 18.7**). Adrenal imaging may be normal, hyperplastic or macronodular (**Fig. 18.8**). Inferior petrosal sinus sampling for ACTH after CRH shows an increased central:peripheral ratio (see Ch. 15).

- No simple test is invariably accurate. Pituitary macroadenomas lead to more severe disease (see Ch. 15)

ECTOPIC ACTH SECRETION

In ectopic ACTH secretion the biochemical imbalance is usually severe, with high plasma and urinary cortisol levels. The plasma ACTH is usually elevated and is often markedly

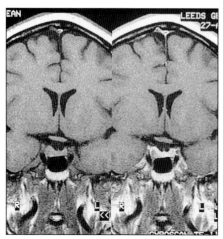

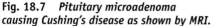

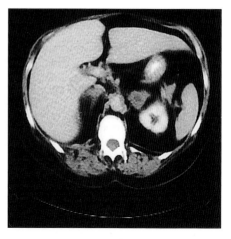

Fig. 18.7   *Pituitary microadenoma causing Cushing's disease as shown by MRI.*

Fig. 18.8   *Macronodular adrenal morphology in Cushing's disease.*

increased. There are also often increases in levels of pro-opiomelanocortin (POMC) precursors. Hypokalaemic alkalosis is common.

The site may be obvious – for instance small-cell carcinoma of the lung. However, if it is not then follow this procedure:

- Check the thorax for bronchial carcinoid or thymoma by spiral CT scanning (tumours are often less than 1 cm in diameter)
- Check the pancreas by dynamic CT or MRI
- Check the thyroid gland, as medullary cancer can lead to ectopic ACTH
- Check the adrenal glands, as non-catecholamine-secreting phaeochromocytoma leads to ectopic ACTH. Also there may be adrenal metastases from an ectopic ACTH-producing primary tumour
- Perform an octreotide scan as this may disclose an occult source of ACTH secretion
- Peripheral venous sampling may identify the source of secretion

ADRENAL ADENOMA

Adrenal adenomas are usually less than 4 cm in diameter, but are nevertheless demonstrable by CT or MRI. An isotope scan of the adrenals may show unilateral uptake. Also, a 'black adenoma' that is due to lipofuscin deposition will occasionally be found.

The ACTH level is generally suppressed, and there is usually isolated cortisol hypersecretion. Incidentally discovered adenomas may lead to mild cortisol hypersecretion.

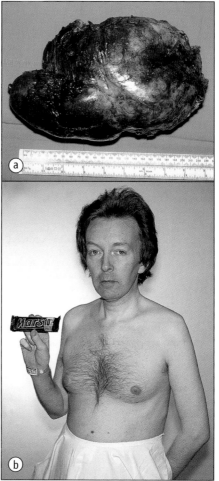

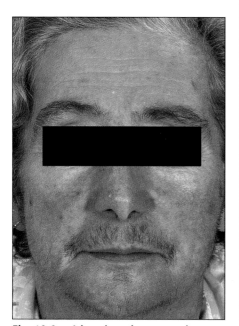

Fig. 18.9   *Adrenal carcinoma causing virilization and Cushing's syndrome.*

Fig. 18.10   *(a, b) Adrenal carcinoma causing feminization and Cushing's syndrome. Patient also suffered hypoglycaemia which he reversed using Mars bars.*

ADRENAL CARCINOMA

These are usually larger than adenomas, as their inefficient steroidogenesis means that features of hormone excess are seen only when the tumour mass has grown sufficiently large. There is a characteristic appearance on the CT or MRI but, in contrast to adenomas, there is often no uptake on an isotope scan.

As above, the ACTH level is usually suppressed. In addition, with this type of tumour there are often raised levels of DHAS.

There may also be associated virilization (**Fig. 18.9**) or feminization (**Fig. 18.10**).

PRIMARY HYPERALDOSTERONISM

This should be suspected in cases of refractory hypertension, especially if there is a decreased level of ionic potassium (hypokalaemia), although this may often be accentuated by the use of diuretics.

Check the level of plasma aldosterone with simultaneous plasma renin (or plasma renin activity, PRA) measurement, taking care to transport specimens for PRA rapidly at room temperature and centrifuge the blood and store the plasma frozen, rather than at 4°C, as at this temperature the conversion of prorenin to renin is accelerated. In cases falling into a diagnostically grey area, it is helpful to calculate the ratio of aldosterone to plasma renin (activity).

In differential diagnosis of primary hyperaldosterinoma, it is useful to check the 8 a.m. aldosterone, PRA and cortisol levels whilst the patient is supine, then repeat these measurements at noon whilst the patient is in an erect posture. If the 8 a.m. aldosterone value is greater than the noon value then this suggests that the cause is an adenoma (Conn's syndrome). The plasma cortisol measurement is used to check the pattern of ACTH secretion; it can occasionally increase later in the day (e.g. from stress) and increases the midday measurement of aldosterone from a Conn's adenoma – which is responsive to ACTH stimulation. In contrast, if the 8 a.m. supine level is less than that of the 12 noon erect aldosterone, this suggests that adrenal hyperplasia is the cause.

In glucocorticoid-remediable hyperaldosteronism, dexamethasone suppression for 5 days normalizes the ionic potassium level, lowers the BP and corrects the aldosterone/PRA abnormalities. It may also be advantageous to check for this with an isotope-labelled cholesterol adrenal scan under dexamethasone suppression, but in any case it is advisable to check adrenal morphology by MRI, as this is regarded as preferable to CT scanning. If glucocorticoid-remediable hyperaldosteronism is suspected then you should also check for a chimeric gene by southern blotting; in this condition the ACTH-responsive gene promoter of the 11β-hydroxylase gene becomes attached to the aldosterone synthase gene.

A summary of biochemical abnormalities in CAH is shown in **Fig. 18.11**.

GLUCOCORTICOID DEFICIENCY

Adrenal crisis is dealt with in Chapter 14, which details the process and priorities involved in diagnosis and management. The crucial issues are prompt appropriate treatment prior to definitive diagnosis and realization that in extreme stress the failing adrenal glands may manage to produce a plasma cortisol level that is in the 'normal' range but is wholly inadequate for the clinical situation.

HYPOADRENALISM

If the 8–9 a.m. plasma cortisol level is less than 180 nmol/L this suggests adrenal insufficiency; no further investigation is needed if the cause if obvious (e.g. pituitary surgery, or adrenalectomy). Later in the day, especially in the evening, low values can be normal, so this is of no diagnostic value.

Hyponatraemia, hyperkalaemia and prerenal uraemia are common but not invariable in the early stages of decompensation. Plasma ACTH increases early on in primary hypoadrenalism and so provides useful retrospective evidence; send an EDTA specimen kept on ice rapidly to the laboratory. Mild to moderate hypercalcaemia is commonly found and in hypocortisolism is due to vitamin D hypersensitivity. Hypoglycaemia is especially common in neonates and children but can also occur in adults. The tetracosactrin (Synacthen) test gives useful, rapid results but is not infallible. In this test, a 250 µg dose is injected intramuscularly, and the plasma cortisol level is measured prior to and 30 minutes after the injection. The peak cortisol level should be at least 600 nmol/L. The use of the test in secondary hypoadrenalism is contentious because of frequent false positive responses. In acutely ill patients it is best to defer the test; then, when the situation is clinically stable, hydrocortisone should be temporarily replaced by dexamethasone because this does not cross-react in the cortisol assay so the patient remains safely treated while the adrenal

Fig. 18.11 Biochemical abnormalities in CAH (classic)

	Cortisol	Aldosterone	PRA	17OH-progesterone	11-deoxycortisol	Androstenedione	DHA	Testosterone
21-hydroxylase deficiency	↓	↓	↑	↑↑	Slight ↑[a]	↑	↑	↑
11β-hydroxylase deficiency	↓	↓	↓[b]	Slight ↑	↑↑	↑	↑	↑
3β-hydroxysteroid dehydrogenase deficiency	↓	↓	↑	↓	↓	↓	↑	↓
17α-hydroxylase deficiency	↓	↓	↓[b]	↓	↓	↓	↓	↓
20,22-desmolase deficiency	↓	↓	↑	↓	↓	↓	↓	↓

[a] Peripheral conversion can cause increased 11-deoxycortisol in 21-hydroxylase deficiency.
[b] Due to DOC secretion, a precursor with mineralocorticoid properties.
NB: All ACTH-driven precursors display marked circadian variation; diagnosis is clearest in early morning samples or 60 minutes after stimulation by tetracosactrin (Synacthen) 250 µg i.m.

response to ACTH stimulation is tested. Patients with positive adrenal antibody status often have a subnormal cortisol response to ACTH before they are frankly hypoadrenal.

To assess mineralocorticoid status the aldosterone and plasma renin activity should be measured. Chest X-ray and tuberculin reactivity should also be undertaken as TB rates are rising worldwide. CT or MRI of the adrenal glands can be helpful. In autoimmune conditions the adrenals become small, whereas fungal infections such as histoplasmosis enlarge the adrenals, and in TB there is calcification. The appearance of adrenal apoplexy may also be recognized.

Increased TSH is frequent in acute hypoadrenalism and requires rechecking after steroid replacement as its production may return to normal leaving no long-term evidence of thyroid dysfunction. One should consider also the possibility of other autoimmune conditions such as hypoparathyroidism, true thyroid disorder, diabetes mellitus and gonadal failure, even in the absence of clinical triggers such as vitiligo, alopecia or mucocutaneous candidiasis.

PHAEOCHROMOCYTOMAS

Investigation of the possibility of phaeochromocytoma involves testing for elevated catecholamine secretion. If the levels are borderline then occasionally it is helpful to document autonomous secretion that is not regulated by the autonomic nervous system – particularly using the ganglion-blocking agent pentolinium or the α-adrenoreceptor agonist clonidine.

Currently the favoured approach is to measure urinary free catecholamines over a timed period of collection – for instance 24 hours, 12 hours or some other period – especially a period including a clinical crisis when enhanced output would be expected. These measurements have been facilitated by the use of electrochemical detection coupled to HPLC. Another frequently used measure is the level of urinary metanephrines and normetanephrines; this has a very similar sensitivity and diagnostic specificity, but there are somewhat greater problems from drug interference, particularly labetalol. Specimens need to be acidified; this is usually done by adding an aliquot of hydrochloric acid to the bottle prior to collection. Because catecholamine secretion from phaeochromocytomas may be episodic, it is often recommended that you make two or three separate collections. Measurement of vanillylmandelic acid (VMA) is less reliable and more prone to interference.

If the plasma catecholamine levels are measured then intermittent peaks of secretion may be missed, so samples are best collected during a clinical episode. A recent proposition is the measurement of plasma metanephrine and normetanephrine. It may be useful to investigate the effect of the ganglion-blocking agent pentolinium; in a normal gland there will be a fall in plasma levels in response to stress, whereas the secretion from tumours is independent of neural input. Similar results may be found following administration of clonidine, and a modification of this uses urinary catecholamines instead.

Provocative tests of catecholamines are rarely indicated, but the secretogogues tyramine, histamine, glucagon and naloxone have been used. Since the end point in these tests is the release of catecholamines, α- and β-adrenergic blockade is needed prior to the test to blunt the pressor responses.

Localization

Adrenal phaeochromocytomas are usually readily demonstrable by CT or MRI scanning. The much-quoted risk of CT contrast media precipitating a crisis is in practice vanishingly rare, especially if the patient is receiving α-adrenergic blockade. MR scans have slightly better discriminatory value and can more often point to a metabolically active tumour. The search for extra-adrenal tumours or metastases may be difficult but is facilitated by the use of a MIBG scan, since this agent is selectively taken up by chromaffin tissue (**Fig. 18.12**). On

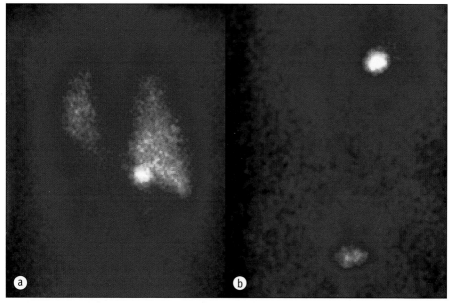

Fig. 18.12 *(a, b) MIBG scan of phaeochromocytoma.*

rare occasions there is still a place for selective venous sampling to confirm the source of catecholamine secretion.

CLINICAL FEATURES AND MANAGEMENT

CUSHING'S SYNDROME

The clinical features emphasized in many textbook descriptions are mostly non-specific and thus diagnostically unhelpful. For instance, the following features are common to both Cushing's and non-Cushing's patients:

- Central obesity and 'buffalo hump'
- Non-livid striae
- Hypertension
- Diabetes mellitus
- Menstrual disturbance

The most useful features derive from the catabolic and antianabolic effects of cortisol excess, especially on protein synthesis. The stereotype 'lemon on sticks' is often appropriate but tends to overemphasize the importance of central obesity (**Figs 18.13, 18.14**) though it can be detected even if the BMI is normal (**Fig. 18.15**). One of the commonest misconceptions with respect to possible cases of Cushing's syndrome is gross obesity (**Fig. 18.16**); in fact, in florid ectopic ACTH secretion the catabolic effects are excessive resulting in weight *loss*, dependent oedema and weakness, to which the mineralocorticoid action of high cortisol levels makes a contribution from hypokalaemia. Other manifestations include diabetes mellitus and pigmentation due to the intrinsic melanocyte-stimulating action of ACTH (**Fig. 18.17**). Addisonian-type pigmentation of skin or nails is particularly suggestive of high ACTH levels.

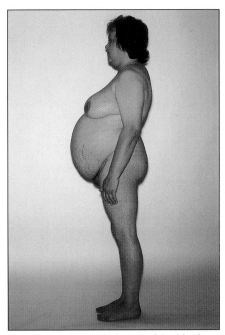

Fig. 18.13   *Typical picture of Cushing's habitus.*

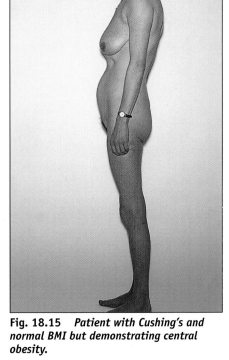

Fig. 18.15   *Patient with Cushing's and normal BMI but demonstrating central obesity.*

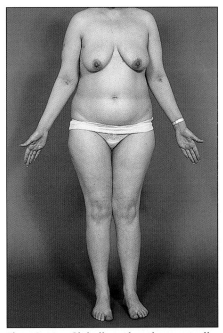

Fig. 18.14   *Globally rather than centrally obese Cushingoid patient.*

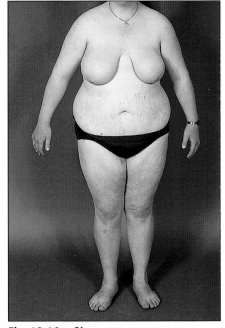

Fig. 18.16   *Obese young woman developing fine striae but no evidence of Cushing's syndrome.*

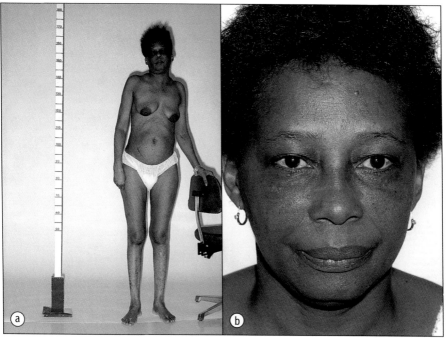

Fig. 18.17 *Afro-Caribbean patient with ectopic ACTH secretion causing skin darkening (a), which is lost after curative surgery (b).*

Diagnostically valuable clinical features

- Thin skin, measuring 1.0 mm or less over the dorsum of hand (i.e. half the normal thickness) (**Fig. 18.18**)
- Skin atrophy leading to ecchymoses – spontaneous or easy bruising is particularly suggestive
  (**Fig. 18.19**)
- Skin atrophy leading to poor wound healing after minor trauma (**Fig. 18.20**)
- Striae resulting from skin atrophy – these are broad and livid compared with the frequent fine striae in simple obesity (**Fig. 18.21**)
- Pigmentation of skin (addisonian-type) and nails (**Fig. 18.22**)
- Proximal muscle wasting (**Fig. 18.23**) and weakness (**Fig. 18.24**)
- Rapid onset vertebral crush fractures leading to kyphosis, rib crowding, height loss, multiple and often asymptomatic fractures of the ribs and the pelvis
- Conjunctival oedema – resulting in increased light reflex, and pseudocrying (**Fig. 18.25**)
- Severe mental disturbance (60% or more), including psychotic depression and paranoia
- Late onset hirsutes, or scalp hair loss (**Fig. 18.26**)
- Facial mooning (**Fig. 18.27**)
- Growth arrest in children

- The presence of striae *per se* not diagnostic, nor does their absence exclude Cushing's syndrome

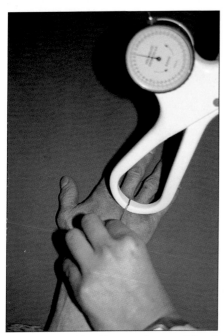

Fig. 18.18   *Thin skin over dorsum of hand measured by callipers.*

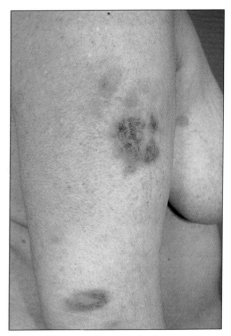

Fig. 18.19   *Spontaneous bruising in patient not showing gross Cushingoid features.*

Management

This constitutes amongst the most challenging problems in clinical endocrinology; the difficulty lies in when to suspect and how to investigate and attribute appropriate weight to the results, as no single test is 100% reliable. Most established cases have pituitary-dependent Cushing's disease (see Ch. 15).

The recognition of a primary adrenal tumour as being responsible is usually made in a straightforward manner from the biochemistry, including usually undetectable ACTH and imaging of the adrenals, which besides demonstrating the existence of the tumour may display suppression of the contralateral adrenal. The presence of metastases in the lungs and liver confirms the presence of carcinoma. Very rarely, low grade ectopic ACTH-secreting tumours metastasize predominantly to one adrenal gland; this causes unilateral swelling and stimulation (by local or paracrine action). A solitary adrenal tumour, if large (i.e. more than 4 cm in diameter), has a significantly increased risk of malignancy even if no metastases are apparent at diagnosis. Adrenal carcinomas have a propensity to secrete androgens or oestrogen, or both, as well as cortisol.

The initial therapy is adrenal blockade (**Fig. 18.28**). Most experience has been obtained with metyrapone, which inhibits the 11ß-hydroxylase enzyme system. Doses often need to be

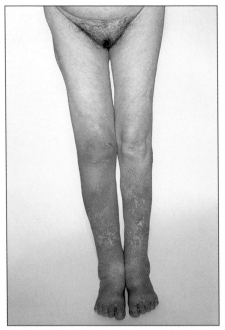

Fig. 18.20 *Poorly healing atrophic skin in Cushing's syndrome.*

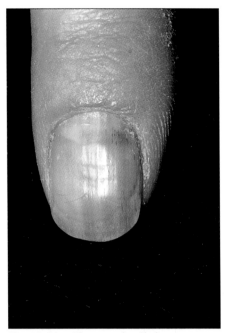

Fig. 18.22 *Pigmented nails in severe ACTH-dependent Cushing's disease.*

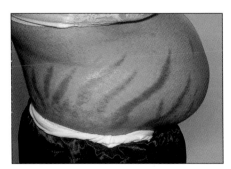

Fig. 18.21 *Livid, broad striae found in Cushing's syndrome.*

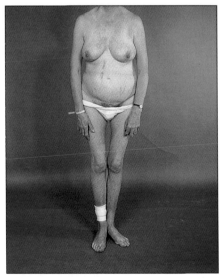

Fig. 18.23 *Proximal muscle wasting in Cushing's disease.*

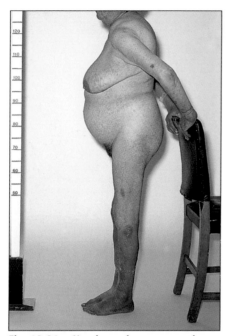

Fig. 18.24   Muscle weakness preventing the patient from standing unaided.

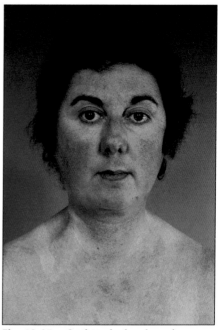

Fig. 18.25   Conjunctival oedema in Cushing's syndrome.

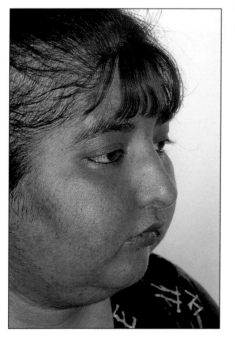

Fig. 18.26   Hirsutes and scalp hair loss in Cushing's syndrome.

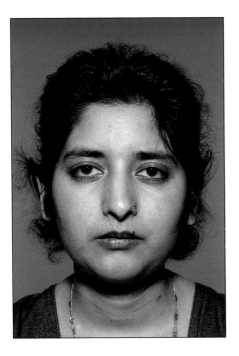

Fig. 18.27 *Same patient as Fig. 18.26, after treatment.*

titrated up, starting with 250 mg 8 hourly and increasing to 750 mg five times daily (i.e. 4 hourly but omitting the midsleep dose). Plasma cortisol day curves need to be repeated to assess response to therapy. Often it is easiest to 'block and replace' – adding a little dexamethasone, usually 0.25 to 0.5 mg on waking – and checking that plasma cortisol suppression is maintained but hypoadrenalism is averted.

After several weeks there should be metabolic and tissue improvement, which enables surgery to be performed more safely. Small benign tumours are now routinely removed by laparoscopic surgery. Adrenal carcinoma may also benefit from surgery though this will not usually prove curative. In this condition, adjunctive treatment with the adrenal-blocking drug mitotane (*o,p*-DDD) may be tried as this also has adrenolytic, cytotoxic effects on the adrenal tissue. Plasma cholesterol tends to rise as a consequence, but this responds to conventional therapy. If only the purest available *o,p*-DDD is used this helps to diminish side-effects, especially neuromuscular problems which are thought to be due to impurities in older preparations. Surgery is curative with benign adenomas (**Fig. 18.29**) but postoperative hydrocortisone supplementation is essential and it may be an exceedingly slow process to wean the patient off it altogether. The life expectancy with adrenal carcinomas varies from less than 1 to a few years.

ECTOPIC ACTH PRODUCTION

Management
- Block adrenal steroid biosynthesis. The choice of drugs includes metyrapone, ketoconazole, *o,p*-DDD and trilostane
- Treat any complications (see below)
- If possible identify the source (see previous section); especially check the thorax, pancreas and thyroid

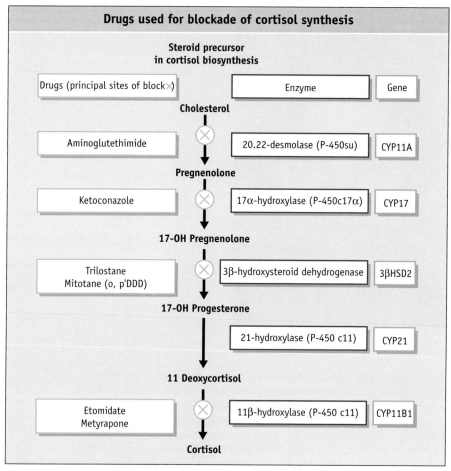

Fig. 18.28 *Adrenal blockade for Cushing's syndrome.*

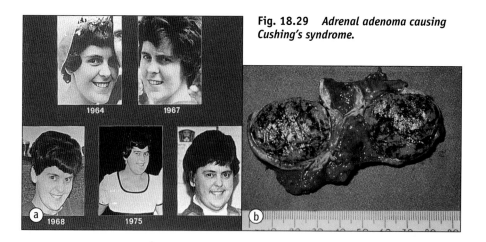

Fig. 18.29 *Adrenal adenoma causing Cushing's syndrome.*

- If possible remove the source – if surgically feasible after optimal metabolic correction
- If there is an occult source then block the adrenals and consider a repeat search after 6 months
- If there is metastatic disease then consider chemo/radiotherapy as appropriate
- If further localization studies are negative then consider bilateral adrenalectomy and replacement therapy
- If a primary source appears (e.g. growth of lung carcinoma) after adrenalectomy then consider resection
- Some tumours respond to octreotide. Octreotide binding is under investigation as means of targeting chemotherapy

---

- Complications include:
  — opportunistic infections (such as that by Pneumocystis carinii – treat with trimethoxazole)
  — diabetes mellitus (note that the insulin requirement falls and may disappear with adrenal blockade)
  — malnutrition due to protein catabolism
  — hypokalaemia
  — heart failure
  — osteoporotic fractures
  — psychological disturbance

PRIMARY HYPERALDOSTERONISM

Management

In primary Conn's adenoma, spironolactone is used to replenish ionic potassium levels and normalize the PRA. After this, resect – preferably laparoscopically.

In bilateral hyperplasia, spironolactone is used at a dosage of up to 400 mg/day. An alternative is amiloride.

In glucocorticoid-remediable hyperaldosteronism, use the minimal required dose of dexamethasone.

CONGENITAL ADRENAL HYPERPLASIA

Clinical features

21-hydroxylase deficiency:
- *Chronic salt wasting.* Severe deficiency of cortisol and aldosterone; females tend to present with ambiguous genitalia at birth, and males with poor weight gain, acute illness after 2–3 weeks or a salt-losing crisis
- *Classic simple virilization.* Less severe deficiency of cortisol, aldosterone levels normal/high, early childhood androgen excess leads to accelerated growth and advanced bone age with virilization (**Fig. 18.30**)
- *Non-classical.* Mild androgen excess, with normal cortisol and aldosterone, may present with acne (often late) and may mimic PCOS and cause infertility

11β-hydroxylase deficiency:
- *Classic.* Female sexual ambiguity at birth, virilization in childhood (both sexes), hypertension in later childhood with or without hypokalaemia
- *Non-classical.* Adult hypertension, virilization and infertility

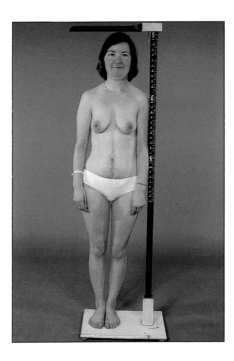

Fig. 18.30   *Classic simple virilization in CAH.*

Management

Management depends on the interrelated factors of severity of enzyme defect, clinical presentation and age of patient in each of the enzyme disorders.

In adults use minimal doses of glucocorticoid, but individual requirements vary. (For infants and children see Ch. 16.) Dexamethasone is often recommended but often leads to Cushingoid side-effects as textbook equivalents are often inappropriate and dexamethasone has a long half-life. Prednisolone, given in a reverse pattern to that of the androgen rhythm, is sometimes recommended on theoretical grounds, as administration of more of the drug on retiring should inhibit the circadian peak in androgens, and late-night steroid use may disturb sleep.

- If using prednisolone it is difficult to measure endogenous cortisol production as most cortisol assays show a 30% cross-reaction with prednisolone

Hydrocortisone, either in small divided doses or once in the morning (30–40 mg), is often the best choice. Control may be improved by adding fludrocortisone even if the patient is not frankly losing salt. In women the menstrual cycle, testosterone or androstenedione levels, or both, should be monitored. Also, monitoring of plasma renin activity helps in the assessment of the fludrocortisone dose.

In uncontrolled males increased testosterone may be adrenal in origin. Note whether LH or FSH is suppressed, as if this is the case then testicular atrophy and impaired spermatogenesis may occur. Occasionally in such males, ectopic adrenal tissue 'resting' in the testicles enlarges, mimicking a tumour.

- Patients need written instructions about handling stress including varying the steroid dosage

HYPOADRENALISM

Clinical features

Primary adrenal failure (Addison's disease) needs to be distinguished from secondary adrenal failure both clinically and therapeutically.

Primary adrenal failure   In primary adrenal failure the onset is usually gradual. However, in rare circumstances there is sudden adrenal destruction due to adrenal apoplexy, embolism, adrenal vein thrombosis, septicaemia (Waterhouse–Friderichsen syndrome) or bilateral surgical adrenalectomy.

A triphasic pattern may be discerned in the clinical features, especially in retrospect:

Clinical features of primary adrenal failure

- *Phase 1*. Few/no symptoms, non-specific malaise, pigmentation, associated disorders, including diabetes mellitus (worsening control), vitiligo, hypoparathyroidism and premature ovarian failure
- *Phase 2*. Gradually worsening symptoms including:
  — lethargy and weakness (invariable)
  — weight loss (invariable) (**Fig. 18.31**)
  — increasing pigmentation over exposed areas, or areas of pressure such as on the dorsum and knuckles of the hand (**Fig. 18.32**), palms (**Fig. 18.33**), face, buccal surface (**Fig. 18.34**), under pressure areas (**Fig. 18.35**) and recent scars
  — hypotension, lowering of postural BP, and dizziness
  — anorexia, nausea, especially in the morning, and vomiting
  — diarrhoea, and sometimes steatorrhoea
  — loss of axillary, pubic and body hair (especially in women)
  — personality change: often withdrawal, depression and occasional paranoia
  — muscle and joint aches and pains
- *Phase 3*. Decompensation: adrenal crisis, often precipitated by ostensibly mild intercurrent infection or other illness leading to:
  — prostration from vomiting and diarrhoea
  — hyponatraemia, hyperkalaemia, and sometimes hypercalcaemia and hypoglycaemia
  — profound circulatory collapse with severe hypotension
  — prerenal then renal impairment, and oliguria or anuria
  — severe abdominal pain with or without guarding mimicking surgical catastrophe
  — may be precipitated by drugs such as pethidine and morphine

Secondary adrenal failure   This is due to ACTH deficiency occurring in pituitary-related disorders, or often on withdrawal of exogenous corticosteroids (oral, topical, and occasionally inhaled). The secretion of aldosterone is usually intact so salt and water loss are much less conspicuous than in Addison's disease, though there may be hyponatraemia (there is often inappropriate ADH secretion) and hypoglycaemia. Hyperkalaemia and features of

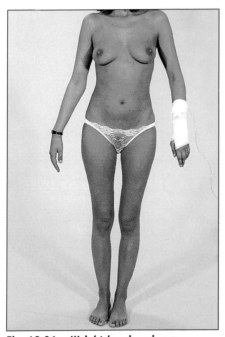

Fig. 18.31   Weight loss in primary adrenal failure.

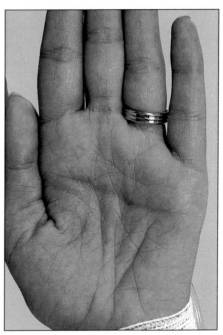

Fig. 18.33   Increasing pigmentation on the palm in primary adrenal failure.

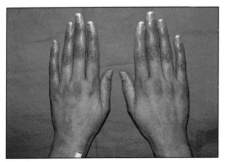

Fig. 18.32   Increasing pigmentation on the dorsum of the hands in primary adrenal failure.

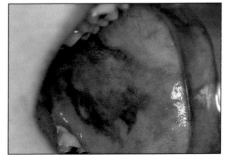

Fig. 18.34   Buccal pigmentation in primary adrenal failure.

prerenal failure are uncommon. The skin shows an abnormal pallor owing to ACTH deficiency; this is in contrast to the increased pigmentation seen in Addison's disease. Weight gain in hypopituitarism is common (compare the weight loss in Addison's disease).

Management

A procedure for routine corticosteroid replacement in adults is:

- First assess the response to the dose by multiple blood or salivary cortisol measurements throughout the day
- The previously used average dose of 30 mg of hydrocortisone was probably excessive for most people. Therefore, begin with a dosage of either 15 mg on waking and 5 mg at 6 p.m., or if preferred 10 mg on waking, 5 mg at noon and 5 mg at 6 p.m.

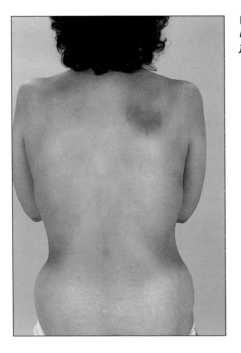

Fig. 18.35 *Increasing pigmentation under pressure areas in primary adrenal failure.*

- If mineralocorticoids are deficient then replace them with a single daily dose of fludrocortisone. Often 50–100 µg suffices, but some patients may need more; check the PRA to determine the amount needed

  - Give written advice on increasing the above dose during stress (**Fig. 18.36**)
  - Advise on wearing a Medic Alert bracelet or necklace (or equivalent) (**Fig. 18.37**)
  - Advise the patient to keep hydrocortisone sodium succinate (as 100 mg ampoules) at home

(For adrenal crisis see Ch. 14.)

PHAEOCHROMOCYTOMA

Clinical features

Phaeochromocytomas are a rare cause of hypertension, accounting for about 0.1% of cases. Though hypertension is found in most cases, the pattern is variable, ranging from persistent to paroxysmal surges rising from either basal normal or raised levels. Hypotension is also well recognized – usually following hypertensive episodes but very rarely as the sole disturbance of BP. The frequency of paroxysms and other clinical features varies from patient to patient, but their pattern tends to be fairly reproducible in any one patient. Phaeochromocytoma should be considered in patients with the following triad of symptoms:

Letter advising patients about increasing steroids during stress

THE GENERAL INFIRMARY

THE TEACHING HOSPITALS

DEPARTMENT OF ENDOCRINOLOGY

Fax:

Enquiries to: Dr Secretary

Direct line/Ext:

Our Ref:

Your Ref:

Date:

Patient I.D.:

STEROID TREATMENT:

DATE COMMENCED:

In the event of any illness/infection you must **DOUBLE** your daily steroid dose **FOR THREE DAYS.**

In the event of vomiting or being unable to swallow your steroid medication you must **SEEK MEDICAL ADVICE EARLY** since you will require a steroid injection.

Please show this sheet to any medical attendant.

Dr John Brown
Consultant Physician/Endocrinologist

Fig. 18.36 *Written advice on increasing steroid dose during stress.*

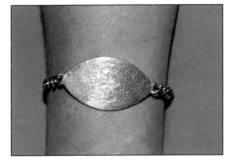

Fig. 18.37 *A Medic Alert bracelet.*

Clinical features

- Hypertension – particularly if refractory or of early onset
- Headaches
- Sweating

A positive family history of phaeochromocytoma is another feature prompting investigation. Investigation for phaeochromocytoma should also be considered in patients with onset of hypertension at a young age or who prove to be refractory to routine therapeutic measures.

Dramatic hypertension during routine anaesthesia and surgery is a well-recognized mode of presentation. Phaeochromocytoma may be associated with hyperglycaemia, hypercalcaemia and lactic acidosis. Some patients mimic the hypermetabolic state of thyrotoxicosis with tremor, palpitations and weight loss. Paroxysms may be associated with marked pallor (or much more rarely flushing) and a sense of 'angor animi' or 'impending doom'. Cardiovascular complications include myocardial infarction, heart failure, shock and myocarditis and even cardiomyopathy – both dilated and hypertrophic. Gut problems range from constipation (possibly caused by opiate peptides) to abdominal pain and mesenteric infarction. The possibility of phaeochromocytoma in the context of 'adrenal incidentaloma' – frequently discovered by abdominal ultrasound performed for unconnected reasons – is serious enough to merit urinary measurements in these patients, especially if they are hypertensive. An example recently seen was a woman who steadfastly denied all symptoms until finally on being directly asked she mentioned having suffered 'drenching sweats' for years but had considered them unimportant. Review of her old hospital notes disclosed an overnight stay 15 years previously following a drug overdose – while still sedated her BP record had shown marked lability. This chart was kept in the notes but not acted upon at the time (**Fig. 18.38**).

Management

If the possibility of phaeochromocytoma is considered on credible grounds, this constitutes a rare instance where treatment should precede definitive diagnosis. This is because untreated patients are at risk from sudden death from a hypertensive crisis or other complications. It is therefore prudent to introduce adrenergic-blocking drugs immediately but carefully, and under close supervision. Too rapid an introduction may be harmful as this dilates the precapillary arterioles, so exposing an ischaemic and permeable capillary bed to a sudden inflow of blood. The consequence may be rapid extravasation causing serious or even lethal hypovolaemia. At an early stage a short-acting and reversible agent such as doxazosin or prazosin is appropriate. As the plasma volume increases there may be a need for planned infusions of expanding fluids or blood transfusion. Calcium-channel-blocking agents such as nifedipine have also been advocated in less severely hypertensive patients.

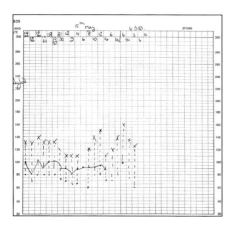

Fig. 18.38 *BP chart of a patient with phaeochromocytoma.*

When the diagnosis is confirmed many authorities continue to advocate switching to the non-competitive α_1- and α_2-adrenoceptor-blocking agent phenoxybenzamine, which alkylates the receptors. The initial dose is usually 10 mg once or twice daily, which should be gradually titrated up according to the BP and clinical response – some patients require several hundred milligrams daily. The side-effects of postural hypotension and nasal congestion are common, however, and transfusions may be needed if marked dilutional

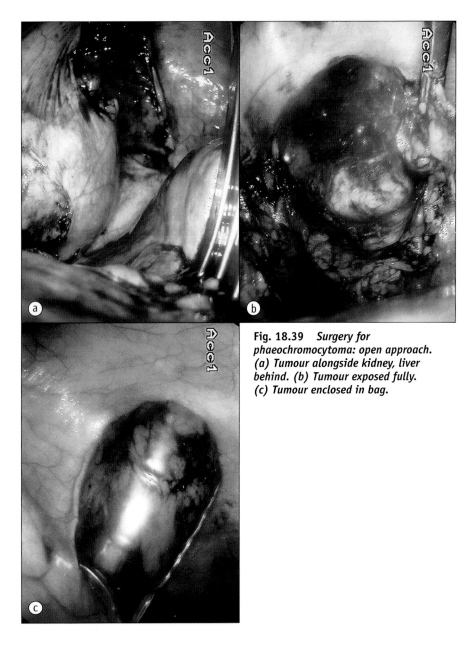

Fig. 18.39   Surgery for phaeochromocytoma: open approach. (a) Tumour alongside kidney, liver behind. (b) Tumour exposed fully. (c) Tumour enclosed in bag.

changes occur. The now very old regimen devised by Ross involves intravenous infusions of phenoxybenzamine 1 mg /kg, repeated over three successive days – the last being the preoperative day. This ensures optimal conditions for anaesthesia and surgery and is still used by the authors. Phenoxybenzamine therapy often evokes reflex tachycardia, which may require β-adrenergic blockade – but this should never be introduced without prior effective α-adrenergic blockade.

The surgery of phaeochromocytoma lies firmly in the province of an experienced team of physician, surgeon and anaesthetist. Benzodiazepines are preferred for premedication. Surges of BP require sodium nitroprusside or phentolamine in intravenous boluses, and tachycardia responds to small doses of β blockers such as propranolol or esmolol.

The operative approach depends on the experience and preference of the surgeon. Although laparoscopic surgery has been strongly advocated, this is opposed by some clinicians because of the absolute need to be able to control blood vessels without fail; also the pneumoperitoneum induced in laparoscopic surgery can evoke a sudden release of catecholamines. For these reasons the open approach is thus still widely practised (**Fig.18.39**).

- Postoperative complications include hypovolaemia, hypoglycaemia and hypotension

Malignant phaeochromocytomas are probably underdiagnosed. MIBG is valuable (see **Fig.18.12, p. 279**), and not only in diagnosis; in specialized centres high doses of MIBG labelled with I-131 have proved valuable if rarely curative. The drug α-methyltyrosine has been used to replace synthesis of natural catecholamines by false transmitter analogues; this gives a degree of clinical control in some patients with malignant tumours.

Patients at risk of heritable phaeochromocytomas are more prone to develop bilateral disease. However, the second tumour may appear only after an interval of many years. There is therefore a strong case for removing each adrenal gland individually as required whilst maintaining careful clinical and biochemical surveillance over the long term.

chapter 19

Reproductive Endocrinology

INTRODUCTION

Endocrine regulation is involved at virtually every step in the anatomical and physiological processes, in both sexes, that culminate in the fertilization of gametes and the subsequent pre- and postnatal development of a new individual. These processes support functions that have attained importance in addition to simply ensuring fecundity. If endocrine regulation is disordered, therefore, the implications are not limited to concerns of infertility, but include social, psychological and systemic health dimensions.

A number of critical events are related to reproductive function over the life span:

Definition of reproductive stages

- *Sex determination*. Genetically driven differentiation of bipotential gonads to testes or ovary
- *Sexual differentiation*. Endocrine-driven development of male internal and external genitalia
- *Puberty*. Reactivation of the hypothalamo-pituitary–gonadal axis leading to fertility and secondary sexual characteristics
- *Reproductive phase*. Fertility and sexual behaviour
- *Postreproductive phase*. Male/female contrasts, and decreases in fertility and gonadal hormones

SEX DETERMINATION

The basic programme of development leads to the female phenotype, as seen in agonadal 46,XY individuals as well as in the normal 46,XX female karyotype. The principal signal to trigger testis formation is from the *SRY* gene on the pseudoautosomal region of the Y chromosome. *SRY* interacts with other genes including X-linked and autosomal genes (**Fig. 19.1**).

SEX DIFFERENTIATION

Jost's experiments in fetal rabbits demonstrated the active role of the testes (**Fig. 19.2**). The differentiated testis directs masculine development away from the constitutive female programme via two hormones (**Fig. 19.3**):

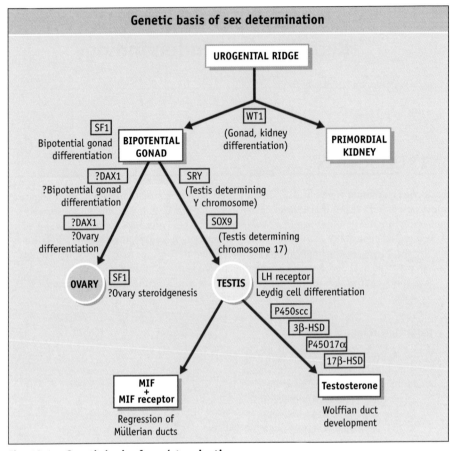

Fig. 19.1   *Genetic basis of sex determination.*

- First, antimüllerian hormone released from the Sertoli cells leads to regression of müllerian structures
- This is followed shortly after by testosterone from the Leydig cells, which promotes wolffian duct development – a paracrine (i.e. local) event

The later events of prostatic and phallic development and scrotal fusion are androgen dependent. These require the presence of dihydrotestosterone (DHT), which is generated from testosterone in the fetal circulation by 5α-reductase located in the relevant tissues (**Fig. 19.4**).

PUBERTY

The termination of childhood sexual quiescence (which sets in after a few months of postnatal life) is characterized by the reactivation of the hypothalamo-pituitary–gonadal

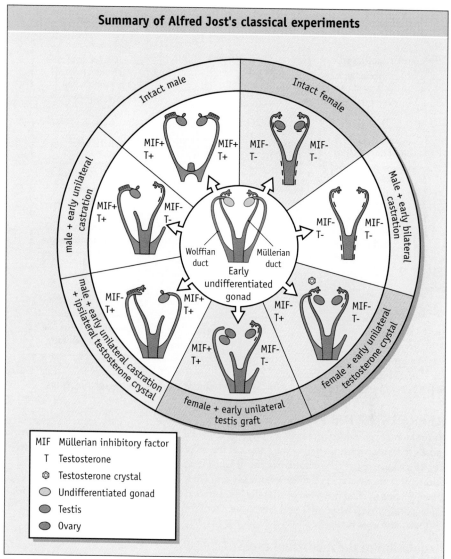

Summary of Alfred Jost's classical experiments

Intact male

Intact female

MIF+ T+

MIF+ T+

MIF- T-

MIF- T-

male + early unilateral castration

MIF+ T+

MIF- T-

Male + early bilateral castration

MIF- T-

MIF- T-

Wolffian duct

Müllerian duct

Early undifferentiated gonad

male + early unilateral + ipsilateral testosterone crystal

MIF+ T+

MIF+ T+

MIF- T+

MIF- T-

MIF+ T+

MIF- T-

female + early unilateral testosterone crystal

female + early unilateral testis graft

MIF	Müllerian inhibitory factor
T	Testosterone
⊚	Testosterone crystal
◯	Undifferentiated gonad
●	Testis
●	Ovary

Fig. 19.2 *Summary of Jost's experimental demonstration of factors influencing sexual differentiation.*

axis. This is dependent in part on signals related to size, weight and body composition. The mediators are unknown but may include changes in pineal activity, loss of inhibitors (which in experimental circumstances can be antagonized by excitatory amino acids and analogues of glutamic acid) and possibly leptin. Initially an increase in FSH secretion occurs, then the nocturnal LH level increases and finally the LH secretion exceeds that of FSH as puberty proceeds. These secretions are pulsatile rather than continuous (see below). The underlying mechanisms determining the timing of puberty remain obscure.

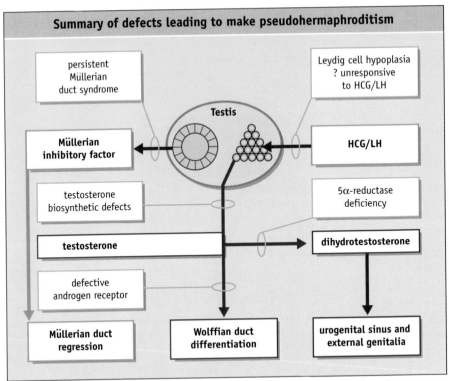

Fig. 19.3   *Induction of male pattern of development by dual testicular functions.*

REPRODUCTIVE PHASE

Regulation of reproductive function in both sexes is controlled by the activity of a neuronal pulse generator, which is sited in the region of the arcuate nucleus of the hypothalamus (see Ch. 15). This triggers the pulsatile release of GnRH, which in turn leads to the pulsatile release of both pituitary gonadotrophins: LH and FSH. LH and FSH are heterodimeric glycoproteins sharing common α subunits but different β subunits. They are essentially the same in both sexes. Molecular polymorphism arises from a variation in sialylation leading to different half-lives in serum.

Regulation of the menstrual cycle (Fig. 19.5)

The key event in the female cycle is pulsatile release of GnRH, which primes pituitary secretion of FSH and LH. The steps of the menstrual cycle are as follows:

- FSH enables a dominant follicle in the ovary to be selected; this recruits granulosa cells secreting estradiol (E_2), which is formed by aromatization of testosterone from the theca cells
- E_2 initially has a negative feedback effect, especially on FSH production, but as follicular development proceeds the level of E_2 increases (despite FSH production decreasing) because of an increase in the number of FSH receptors
- When E_2 reaches a sufficient level for a long enough time, a positive feedback effect occurs – that is, a transient but very marked release of LH (and a minor increase in FSH)

(continued)
- This LH surge leads, after 36–48 hours, to ovulation from the primed follicle. The ruptured Graafian follicle then luteinizes to form a body called the corpus luteum, which is prompted by the LH pulse to release progesterone (and E_2)
- The corpus luteum has only a finite life, undergoing demise after about 14 days. The subsequent decrease in progesterone and E_2 levels leads to spasm of the uterine spiral arteries and shedding of the endometrium (menstruation). The decrease in E_2 also leads to an increase in FSH levels and hence the start of a new cycle

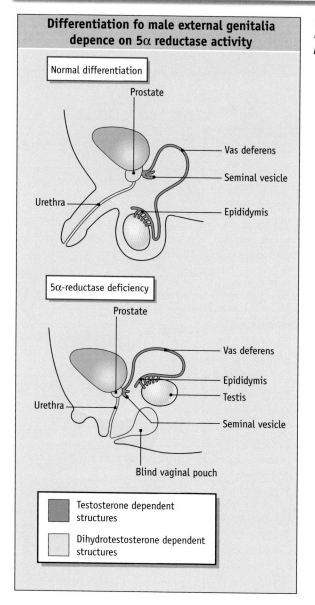

Differentiation fo male external genitalia depence on 5α reductase activity

Fig. 19.4 *Development of male external genitalia and prostate by DHT.*

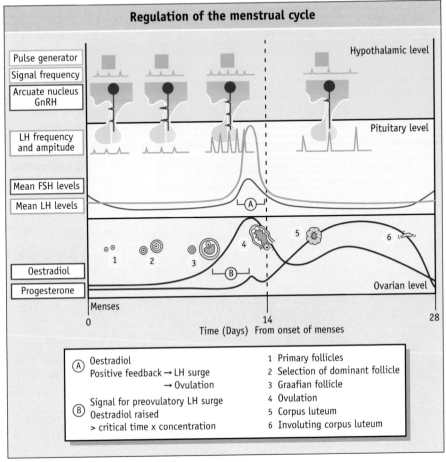

Regulation of the menstrual cycle

| | Hypothalamic level |

Pulse generator
Signal frequency
Arcuate nucleus GnRH

Pituitary level

LH frequency and ampitude

Mean FSH levels
Mean LH levels

Oestradiol
Progesterone

Ovarian level

Menses

0   14   28
Time (Days) From onset of menses

Ⓐ Oestradiol Positive feedback → LH surge → Ovulation	1 Primary follicles 2 Selection of dominant follicle 3 Graafian follicle
Ⓑ Signal for preovulatory LH surge Oestradiol raised > critical time x concentration	4 Ovulation 5 Corpus luteum 6 Involuting corpus luteum

Fig. 19.5 *Regulation of the menstrual cycle.*

Regulation of testicular function (Fig. 19.6)

As with the female axis, the function of the testis depends on pulsatile release of GnRH. However, there are no physiological positive feedback events in males, and thus no cycles. The key hormonal effects are:

- Testosterone exerts a negative feedback, principally at the hypothalamic level, by slowing the pulse generator. Testosterone effects are partly mediated by conversions to DHT and to E_2
- Inhibin, a heterodimeric glycoprotein from the Sertoli cells, selectively inhibits FSH secretion
- FSH has a prime role in spermatogenesis, acting via the Sertoli cells (**Fig. 19.7**)
- LH plays a prime role in testosterone synthesis by the Leydig cells (**Fig. 19.8**)

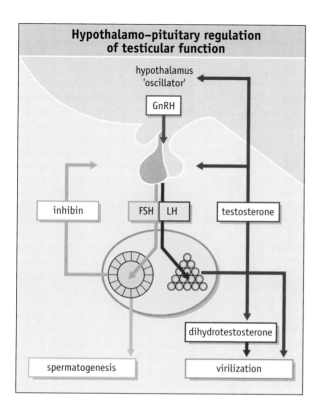

Fig. 19.6 *Regulation of testicular function.*

Intratesticular testosterone is important for spermatogenesis, while testosterone secretion results in the production of some secondary sex hair (partial), bone and muscle (male habitus), and in libido. Testosterone conversion to DHT is required for facial hair growth, scalp balding and the male escutcheon of abdominal hair growth up to the umbilicus. DHT is also needed for phallic growth (including during the neonatal period), and prostate growth and function (**Fig. 19.9**).

LATE REPRODUCTIVE PHASE

Menopause

The mean age of the menopause is about 52 – showing no significant secular trend, in contrast with the much-increased female life span observed in the last 100 years (**Fig. 19.10**). The actual age in any individual is largely genetically determined, often replicating familial patterns. When it occurs at less than 45 years it is regarded as an early menopause. Fertility in women begins to decline from their 30s onwards, and sharply decreases from the age of 40. This is associated with decreased numbers of ovarian follicles because of atresia (**Fig. 19.11**). An early signal of premenopause is an increased level of FSH, which is due to loss of ovarian inhibin.

The years of declining ovarian function (the climacteric) can be subdivided into several phases:

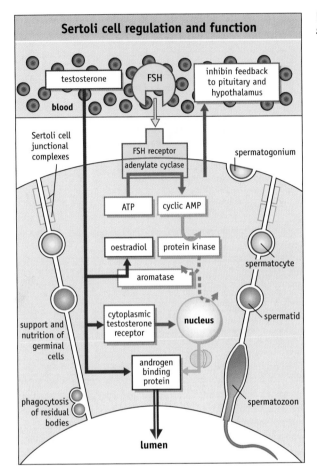

Fig. 19.7   *Role of FSH in spermatogenesis.*

- *The premenopause.* This is characterized by increased anovulatory cycles
- *The menopausal transition.* The premenopause later merges with the menopausal transition, with its erratic often heavy cycles and an endocrine profile swinging between the patterns of the reproductive and the menopausal spans of life
- *The menopause.* This is technically defined as amenorrhoea for 6 months or more – that is, it has to be at a retrospectively determined age

In the menopause, loss of E_2 disinhibits FSH and LH leading to elevated pulsatile levels of both hormones. Pulse generator activity synchronizes classical menopausal vasomotor events (hot flushes) (**Fig. 19.12**). Decreased E_2 secretion leads to accelerated bone resorption

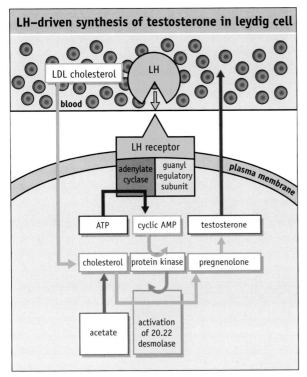

Fig. 19.8   *Role of LH in testosterone synthesis.*

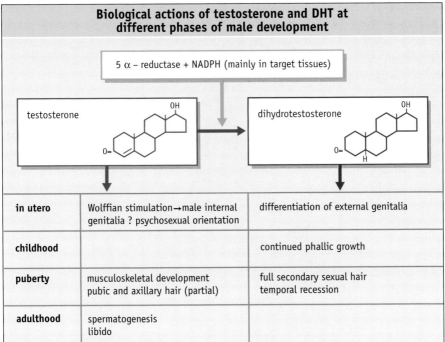

Fig. 19.9   *Roles of DHT.*

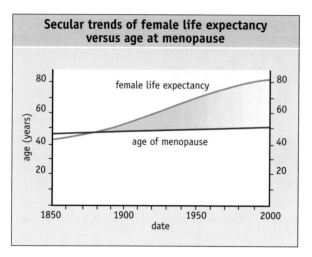

Fig. 19.10 *Secular trend in female life span versus age at menopause.*

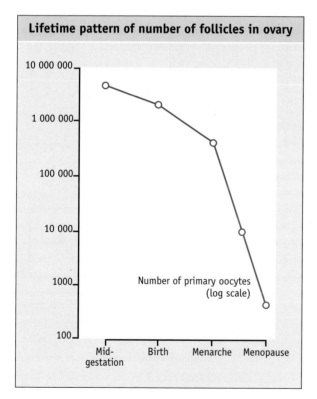

Fig. 19.11 *Life-time pattern of follicle numbers in the ovary.*

(**Fig 19.13**). This decrease is associated with increased cardiovascular risk factors such as increased LDL-cholesterol and decreased HDL-cholesterol.

The postmenopausal ovary continues to secrete some androstenedione, which converts to estrone and thence to some estradiol peripherally.

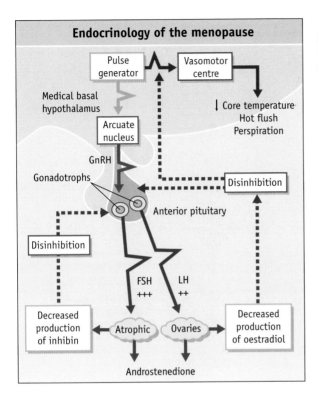

Fig. 19.12 *Pulse-generator drive of menopausal vasomotor phenomena.*

Andropause

Age-related testicular failure in men is much less clearly defined than the menopause in women. Testicular senescence is often gradual and the age of onset is variable. Thus male fertility may be preserved in some octogenarian men. The biologically active free testosterone level may fall with no change in the normal total testosterone level, owing to increased sex-hormone-binding globulin (SHBG) concentration. The gonadotrophin levels increase variably, with FSH usually increasing more than LH. Gynaecomastia is common in older men (see below). Erectile dysfunction becomes increasingly common with increasing age; its cause is multifactorial (see next section).

PATHOGENESIS AND PATHOLOGY

AMENORRHOEA AND OLIGOMENORRHOEA

Many pathological disorders can lead to various degrees of menstrual dysfunction ranging from primary amenorrhoea to secondary amenorrhoea (defined as no periods for more than 6 months), oligomenorrhoea (a cycle length more than 6 weeks) or anovulatory cycles. In many circumstances there is oestrogen deficiency and hypogonadism, and sometimes androgen excess, but often no endocrine abnormality is immediately obvious.

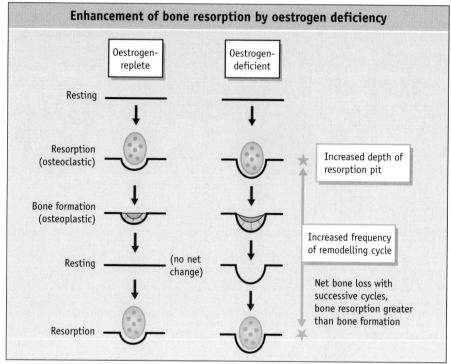

Fig. 19.13 *Effect of diminished E₂ secretion enhancing bone resorption.*

Causes of amenorrhoea

A number of anatomical anomalies may cause amenorrhoea, including:

- Müllerian failure–androgen insensitivity syndromes (46,XY individuals)
- Vaginal/müllerian failure in 46,XX individuals
- Virilization in vitro leading to labial fusion
- Imperforate hymen
- Asherman's syndrome – after surgery, parturition or abortion, or infection

Gonadal failure may also be a cause – for instance gonadal dysgenesis as seen in Turner's syndrome, mosaicism and 46,XY dysgenesis. There may be premature ovarian failure, which can be familial, autoimmune or due to a resistant ovary. Gonadal failure may also occur after chemotherapy or irradiation therapy.

Amenorrhoea can be due to PCOS – which comprises a heterogeneous group of conditions, and is characterized by ultrasound.

A number of hypothalamo-pituitary disorders are also potential causes, including:

- GnRH deficiency – such as Kallman's syndrome
- Craniopharyngioma
- Anorexia or weight-related disorders
- Radiotherapy
- Gonadotrophin deficiency – such as seen in pituitary tumours, apoplexy, surgery, and Sheehan's syndrome
- Iron overload
- Hyperprolactinaemia – as seen in prolactinoma, functionless tumours (stalk compression) and as a result of some drug treatments
- Hypothyroidism

HIRSUTISM AND VIRILIZATION

In idiopathic hirsuties there is no endocrine abnormality but excess hair occurring in a male distribution is seen. Hirsutism may also be due to PCOS, the aetiology of which is unclear, although hypothalamic, adrenal and ovarian factors are known to contribute.

Virilization may be seen with hirsuties and acne, and with scalp hair loss, clitoromegaly, muscular male habitus or a deep voice. Its causes include:

- CAH (21-hydroxylase and 11β-hydroxylase deficiencies)
- Androgen-secreting ovarian and adrenal tumours
- Ovarian hyperthecosis
- Cushing's syndrome

MALE HYPOGONADISM

Primary gonadal failure

Primary gonadal failure may occur after trauma such as castration, vascular damage, surgery, or torsion of the testis. Drugs including chemotherapeutic agents, especially alkylating agents, antiandrogens and inhibitors of testosterone synthesis, can also result in this. Radiation therapy tends to lead to seminiferous rather than Leydig cell damage.

Congenital causes include chromosomal disorders such as Klinefelter's syndrome (both the 47,XXY karyotype and the variants with additional X chromosomes). It can also be due to cryptorchidism, or to varicocele.

Primary gonadal failure may occur as a consequence of infections or inflammation. Examples include mumps, granulomas, autoimmune disease and iron overload. A number of systemic diseases such as paraplegia, renal failure, cirrhosis and thyrotoxicosis may also be the cause.

Secondary gonadal failure

Secondary gonadal failure may occur as a consequence of pituitary tumours, including the after-effects of surgery for these, and pituitary irradiation. Hyperprolactinaemia – from any cause – may also underlie such failure. A number of hypothalamic disorders are potential causes, including craniopharyngioma, isolated gonadotrophin deficiency and Kallman's syndrome.

GYNAECOMASTIA

Gynaecomastia is the most specific feature of feminization in males, often accompanying hypogonadism. Its aetiology may be physiological, whether neonatal, pubertal, or senescent.

There may be an androgen deficiency, as a result or either primary or secondary hypogonadism, or biosynthetic defects. Alternatively there may be androgen resistance, in which the androgen insensitivity can be either complete or incomplete. Another possible cause is excessive oestrogen production, as may be seen in adrenal carcinoma, and testicular tumours involving the Leydig or Sertoli cells, or to a tumour producing hCG – for instance in the testis, lung or colon.

Drugs such as oestrogens, oestrogen receptor stimulants, antiandrogens such as spironolactone, and cytotoxic drugs can all cause gonadal failure. Other possible causes include:

- Hyperprolactinaemia, or acromegaly
- Thyrotoxicosis
- Liver disease including cirrhosis
- Renal disease, or haemodialysis°
- Starvation and refeeding

309

INTERSEX STATES

Female pseudohermaphroditism

This may be caused by:

- CAH (21-hydroxylase deficiency, 11β-hydroxylase deficiency, or 3β-hydroxysteroid dehydrogenase deficiency)
- Aromatase deficiency
- Intrauterine androgen exposure from administered drugs such as progestogens, or from maternal virilizing tumours

Male pseudohermaphroditism

This may be caused by:

- Biosynthetic defects of testosterone
- An LH receptor defect
- Androgen insensitivity syndromes
- 5α-reductase deficiency
- XY gonadal dysgenesis, or mixed gonadal dysgenesis

True hermaphroditism

In this condition there is simultaneous possession of ovarian and testicular tissue.

INFERTILITY

Assessment of the causes of infertility suggests that about a third of cases are due to female factors, in 30–40% both partners have contributory problems and in the remainder male factors alone are responsible. More than one factor is quite commonly present in an individual. Unexplained infertility still accounts for nearly a third of the total.

Female factors include:

- *Ovulatory difficulties.* Hypothalamic, pituitary and ovarian factors may all be involved
- *Luteal phase defects.* These may be short phases or inadequate progesterone levels
- *Barriers to sperm.* These may be anatomical (vaginal, uterine or tubal), cervical hostility, a result of infections, or immunological
- *Systemic illness.* Possibilities include thyroid disease, diabetes, and hepatic, renal, or cardiac disease

Male factors include:

- *Impaired spermatogenesis*:
— which is idiopathic in most cases
    — chromosomal abnormalities such as Klinefelter's syndrome and variants
    — varicocele
    — infections such as mumps, tuberculosis, sexually transmitted diseases
    — chemotherapy or irradiation
    — autoimmune
- *Obstruction*:
    — epididymis, including Young's syndrome (associated with chronic chest disease)
    — blocked vas, or absent vas (as in cystic fibrosis)

Other possible causes of infertility include hypothalamo-pituitary disorders associated with hypogonadism, and syndromes of GnRH deficiency including Kallman's syndrome. Also pituitary and parapituitary tumours can lead to FSH or LH deficiency with or without hyperprolactinaemia.

DISORDERS OF LIBIDO AND SEXUAL FUNCTION

Psychological factors figure prominently – if not as primary causes then often as secondary complications. The major endocrine factor is testosterone, though the impact of low testosterone varies widely between individuals. Hyperprolactinaemia can impair libido and potency independently of testosterone, though normal values of both hormones are required for optimal function. Testosterone probably plays an important role in female libido also.

Erectile dysfunction

The cause of this is often multifactorial. Possible aetiological factors include:

- Arteriosclerotic disease – including diabetes, smoking and hypertension
- Incompetent venous valves
- Neuropathy, as seen in diabetes, or paraplegia
- Endocrinopathies such as primary or secondary hypogonadism, hyperprolactinaemia and/or thyrotoxicosis
- Drugs such as alcohol, marijuana, opiates, hypotensive and psychotropic agents
- Systemic illness such as cardiac, pulmonary, renal and hepatic disease
- Psychological factors
- Peyronie disease

MISCELLANEOUS DISORDERS

Menorrhagia

Menorrhagia is a major complaint; it occurs very often in women with an erratic cycle at perimenopause, when it is not uncommonly associated with fibroids. It is also clearly associated with hypothyroidism and this should be checked for. Less common associations are with end-stage renal failure and anticoagulation.

Spontaneous abortion

There is increasing frequency of spontaneous abortion with increasing maternal age; such abortions in women older than 35 years are associated with chromosomal abnormalities in the fetus. It may also be associated with untreated thyrotoxicosis or with hypothyroidism, necessitating tight management of thyroid hormone levels in pregnancy.

Catamenial disorders

Premenstrual tension or syndrome varies with the ovarian cycle; it develops in the luteal phase and finishes at the end of this phase. Its aetiology remains unclear. Several medical conditions may worsen; for instance, there is often premenstrual exacerbation of migraine, and also commonly of epilepsy.

INVESTIGATION AND DIAGNOSIS

PRIMARY AMENORRHOEA

First, measure the level of gonadotrophins, to distinguish whether there is primary or secondary hypogonadism. Furthermore disturbed thyroid function, especially hypothyroidism, may delay menarche yet be quite unsuspected so this possibility needs to be checked biochemically.

It is also essential to assess the karyotype – especially if the patient is short or dysmorphic – to detect the presence of Turner's syndrome, mosaics and variants. Bone age, as an index of developmental status, is a mandatory investigation. Important information may also be obtained by pelvic ultrasound, including determination of whether ovarian tissue is present and its morphology, and similarly for the uterus.

Chronic illness such as malabsorption – especially if this causes low body weight – may delay the onset of periods. Hyperprolactinaemia may rarely cause primary amenorrhoea, and androgen excess due to PCOS or CAH is another rare cause, requiring measurement of both testosterone and SHBG.

SECONDARY AMENORRHOEA

As above, measure the gonadotrophins to distinguish primary from secondary hypogonadism, and also PRL, as hyperprolactinaemia is the commonest pituitary cause of secondary amenorrhoea (20% of total).

Assay of testosterone and SHBG allows most cases of PCOS to be diagnosed – this is the most important cause of secondary amenorrhoea. Bone densitometry is advisable as it is important to check for this clinically important effect of long-standing hypo-oestrogenism. Pelvic ultrasound helps confirm PCOS and is useful if ovarian failure or tumour is suspected.

A pituitary MR or CT scan should be performed if there is significant hyperprolactinaemia (> 1000 mU/L) present. Lesser elevations of this hormone are most commonly due to microprolactinomas, but a stalk effect from non-functioning pituitary adenomas or craniopharyngiomas can cause similar elevations in PRL.

HIRSUTISM AND VIRILIZATION

Virilization is usually associated with a plasma testosterone level greater than 5 nmol/L. SHBG decreases with obesity, so patients with PCOS often have high normal testosterone levels but low SHBG, which leads to markedly increased free testosterone levels.

The ratio of LH to FSH is often increased in PCOS but this is not invariable. LH and FSH levels are often, though not invariably, suppressed with virilizing states. An elevated level of 17-hydroxy progesterone, especially in a morning specimen, indicates late onset or poorly controlled CAH. If there is doubt the 17-hydroxy progesterone level should be measured after ACTH stimulation (see Ch. 18). Increased DHA and DHAS levels suggest adrenal androgen excess.

Pelvic ultrasound is important in the assessment of ovarian morphology, and also endometrial thickness. MR or CT of the adrenals is indicated if adrenal tumour or Cushing's syndrome is suspected.

MALE HYPOGONADISM

Gonadotrophin assay is necessary to distinguish primary from secondary hypogonadism. It is necessary to measure both testosterone and SHBG (the latter is occasionally increased with normal testosterone, leading to decreased free testosterone).

Karyotype assessment is needed in primary hypogonadism to diagnose Klinefelter's syndrome and its variants with extra X chromosomes, or mosaics.

Liver function tests should be performed and may need appropriate investigations if specific causes such as haemochromatosis are suspected. It is prudent to perform thyroid function tests also.

PRL excess is an important cause in men as it is usually due to a macroadenoma of the pituitary. Indeed it is advisable to perform MR or CT of the pituitary region if there is secondary hypogonadism, especially if acquired in middle age.

GYNAECOMASTIA

Blood tests that are commonly indicated include those for:
- Gonadotrophins
- Testosterone and SHBG
- Estradiol-17β
- Thyroid function, PRL and liver function

Scrotal ultrasound is important as a feminizing testicular tumour may be impalpably small. It is also helpful to check for tumour markers (e.g. hCG-β and α-fetoprotein).

INFERTILITY

Both partners need consideration, and often a postcoital test should be included.

Women

Blood tests that need to be performed include those for:
- Gonadotrophins
- Day 21 progesterone (or several measurements if there is a short luteal phase)
- PRL and thyroid function
- Testosterone and SHBG

Pelvic ultrasound may be informative but more often laparoscopy is preferable, and can also be linked to assessment of tubal patency.

Men

Seminal analysis is indicated to assess sperm density, volume, motility and morphology. Assessment of sperm antibodies is often necessary.

The important blood tests are those for:
- Gonadotrophins
- Testosterone and SHBG
- PRL

Some researchers suspect undiagnosed CAH is an underdiagnosed cause of male infertility. The level of 17-hydroxy progesterone should be measured (using a morning specimen) if this possibility is under consideration.

Karyotype assessment, sometimes requiring G banding, may be diagnostic. Testicular biopsy with or without scrotal exploration may also rarely be indicated.

Scrotal ultrasound or thermography is important in the assessment of varicocele.

MALE SEXUAL DYSFUNCTION

Screening blood tests that should be considered include those for:
- Testosterone and SHBG
- Gonadotrophins (unexplained high FSH is common) and PRL
- Plasma glucose
- Thyroid, liver and renal function
- γ-GT
- Mean red cell volume (especially if alcohol abuse is suspected)

CLINICAL FEATURES AND MANAGEMENT

TURNER'S SYNDROME

Management

GH, oxandrolone and oestrogens have all been used to promote growth.

Clinical features

- Short stature
- Sexual infantilism
- Small jaw, with a carp-like mouth
- Epicanthic folds, or ptosis
- Multiple lentigenes (**Fig. 19.14**)
- Congenital lymphoedema (which may prompt early diagnosis)
- Wide carrying angle (cubitus valgus) (**Fig. 19.15**), a short fourth metacarpal (50%)
- Broad chest, widely spaced nipples, and a webbed neck (25–40%) (**Fig. 19.16**)
- Hypertension with or without coarctation of the aorta, aortic stenosis and bicuspid aortic valve
- Renal abnormalities including horseshoe kidney
- Deafness – including otitis media, sensorineural
- Impaired spatial orientation
- Propensity to autoimmune thyroid disease, rheumatoid arthritis, or inflammatory bowel disease
- Hyperlipidaemia and osteoporosis – which is secondary to hypo-oestrogenaemia
- 45,X0/46,XX mosaics – who may be of normal height and menstruate, but are rarely fertile
- Deletions of the second X chromosome – leading to shortness and streak gonads, but few Turner features (**Fig. 19.17**)
- Pure gonadal dysgenesis (45,XX or 45,XY) – manifesting as streak gonads, and various degrees of masculinization

---

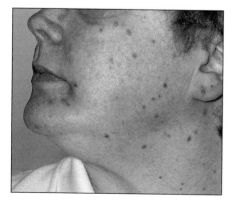

Fig. 19.14   *Turner's syndrome showing multiple lentigenes.*

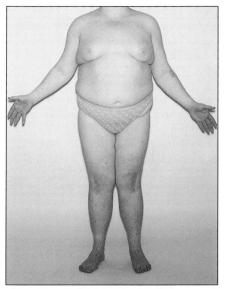

Fig. 19.15 *Wide carrying angle in Turner's syndrome.*

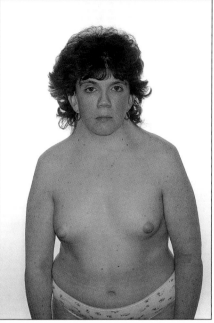

Fig. 19.16 *Turner's syndrome: broad chest, widely spaced nipples and a webbed neck.*

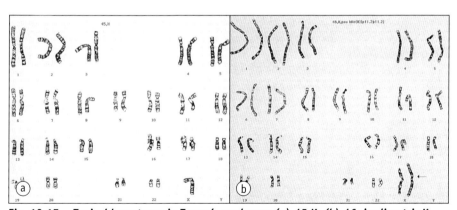

Fig. 19.17 *Typical karyotypes in Turner's syndrome: (a) 45,X; (b) 46, isodicentric X.*

Early use of these has been recommended because of the early appearance of growth retardation (under 10 years of age).

Oestrogen is required to induce puberty and continue long term to avoid osteoporosis. However, premature, excessive oestrogen may compromise the ultimate height. Also, it needs to be introduced at a low dose so as to avoid abnormal breast development. Oestrogen in adult life is helpful to control lipid abnormalities

Congenital abnormalities such as coarctation of the aorta and renal tract need to be identified. Surveillance is also required to detect any development of thyroid disease, diabetes or rheumatoid arthritis. Colonic cancer may also be more prevalent in Turner's syndrome.

The BP needs lifelong monitoring and treatment as necessary. Ongoing assessment of hearing is also important.

PREMATURE OVARIAN FAILURE

Premature ovarian failure may follow a familial pattern. Alternatively, it may be autoimmune, and is sometimes associated with conditions such as thyroid or adrenal dysfunction, or vitiligo. It may follow surgery, radiotherapy, or chemotherapy. If associated with normal ovarian morphology it may be resistant ovary syndrome.

Management

Oestrogen replacement therapy is required promptly on diagnosis (see above). Sporadic, unpredictable ovulation (and hence fertility) can occur. The occurrence of rebound fertility after use of oral contraception is unproven, however.

Fertility may also be achieved by embryo donation in an in vitro fertilization (IVF) setting.

HYPOGONADOTROPHIC HYPOGONADISM

This is most commonly seen in women in association with weight loss or anorexia nervosa. It may also be associated with excessive physical training or psychogenic stress. Idiopathic hypogonadotrophic hypogonadism has no associated features.

Clinical features

- Extreme weight loss that may be associated with lanugo hair growth (**Fig. 19.18**)
- Kallman's syndrome – with associated anosmia
- Hyperprolactinaemia (see Ch. 15)
- Hypothalamo-pituitary dysfunction (see Ch. 15)

Management

Psychogenic, anorexic and exercise induced require HRT, and dietary and psychological help.

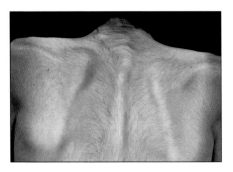

Fig. 19.18   *Lanugo hair growth in anorexia nervosa.*

Organic disease needs appropriate hormone replacement. Hyperprolactinaemia requires dopamine agonist therapy (e.g. with bromocriptine, cabergoline, etc.).

Infertility is usually managed by use of exogenous gonadotrophins. GnRH deficiency may be treated by pulsatile GnRH to achieve pregnancy. This reduces the chance of multiple pregnancy but is more inconvenient than the use of exogenous gonadotrophins.

POLYCYSTIC OVARIAN SYNDROME

PCOS is common, has a wide range of features and may be familial. It may also be associated with various underlying conditions causing testosterone excess. A clinical grading of hirsuties has been described by Ferriman (**Fig. 19.19**).

Clinical features

- *Hirsutism*. This commonly starts at about the age of menarche
- *Obesity*. This is common but not invariable (**Fig. 19.20**)
- *Reduced fertility*. This includes anovulation, oligomenorrhoea and amenorrhoea
- *Increased miscarriage rate*. This is possibly related to increased LH and obesity
- *Insulin resistance*. This is common; there may be hyperlipidaemia with or without acanthosis nigricans
- *High non-cyclical oestrogen levels*. The risk of endometrial and breast cancer is increased here

---

Management

Local measures such as hair plucking or electrolysis may help, and do not aggravate hirsuties. Hirsutism worsens with obesity (because of peripheral androstenedione conversion to testosterone).

Antiandrogen therapy – low or high dose cyproterone acetate (which is also progestogenic) – may be used in combination with ethinylestradiol. Spironolactone may also be useful. However, if used alone it may cause polymenorrhoea.

- Spironolactone is not licensed for use in the UK because of findings of carcinogenicity in rats.

The addition of a non-androgenic oral contraceptive helps hirsutism and cycle control.

- Note, however, that some available appropriate combined oral contraceptives are associated with an increased risk of venous thrombosis

---

317

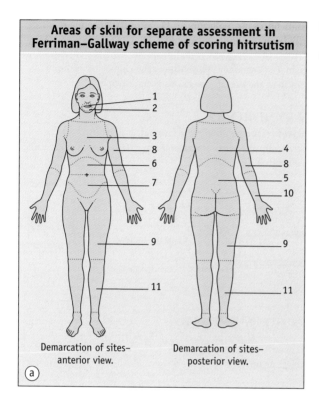

Areas of skin for separate assessment in Ferriman–Gallway scheme of scoring hitrsutism

Demarcation of sites– anterior view.

Demarcation of sites– posterior view.

(a)

Fig. 19.19
(a, b) Ferriman-Galwey grading of hirsuties.

VIRILIZATION

This may be associated with polycystic ovaries (see above).

Clinical features

- *Hirsutism*. This is often more severe than in PCOS or idiopathic hirsuties, and may develop later in life, rarely 'early'
- *Male habitus*. Affecting musculature, while deepening of the voice may occur
- *Scalp hair loss*. Occurs in a marked male pattern (**Fig. 19.21**)
- *Anovulation and amenorrhoea*. This is the rule
- *Clitoromegaly*. This is also common (**Fig. 19.22**)
- *Skin*. This will usually be thick and greasy, but if associated with cortisol excess (Cushing's syndrome) then it is often thin
- *Stromal hyperthecosis*. May be found in postmenopausal women (**Fig. 19.23**)

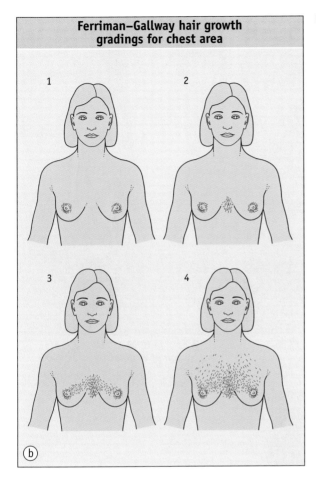

Fig. 19.19 *(b)*

MALE HYPOGONADISM

Clinical features

- Delayed puberty – if constitutional (often familial), there may be short stature
- Prolonged failure may cause excessive limb growth before epiphyseal fusion
- Eunuchoid features include span exceeding height by more than 5 cm (**Fig. 19.24**)
- Reduced testicular volume (**Fig. 19.25**)
- Reduced secondary sexual hair growth – including facial, pubic, axillary and body hair
- Reduced temporal hair recession (**Fig. 19.26**)
- Finely creased skin, especially on the upper lip (**Fig. 19.27**)
- Reduced muscle mass and strength
- Reduced bone mass and density leading to fragility fractures (**Fig. 19.28**)
- Impotence and erectile dysfunction
- Infertility

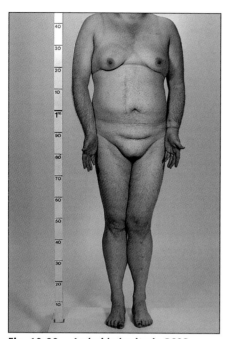

Fig. 19.20   *Android obesity in PCOS.*

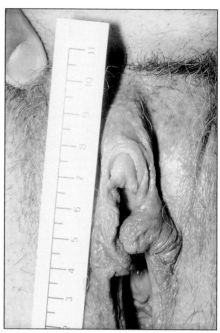

Fig. 19.22   *Clitoral enlargement – a cardinal sign of virilization.*

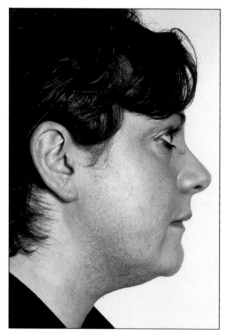

Fig. 19.21   *Scalp hair loss and hirsuties caused by virilizing adrenal adenoma.*

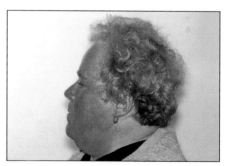

Fig. 19.23   *Virilization in postmenopausal woman due to stromal hyperthecosis.*

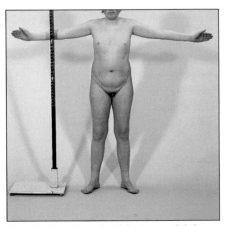

Fig. 19.24   *Eunuchoid features with long limbs giving a span greater than the height.*

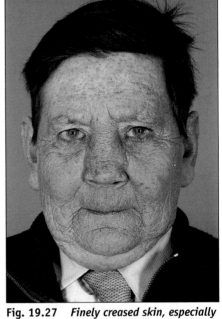

Fig. 19.27   *Finely creased skin, especially on the upper lip, in hypogonadism.*

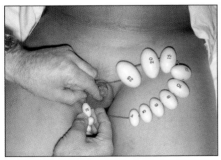

Fig. 19.25   *Reduced testicular volume assessed by a Prader orchidometer.*

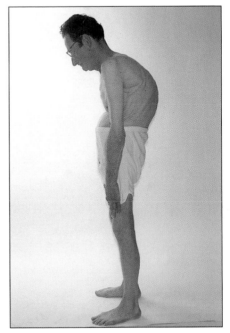

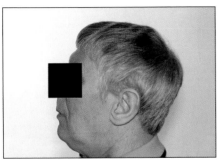

Fig. 19.26   *Reduced temporal hair loss in hypogonadal male.*

Fig. 19.28   *Osteoporotic fracture in a hypogonadal male.*

In Klinefelter's syndrome, much phenotypic variation is seen, including an essentially normal phenotype except for small testes (**Fig. 19.29**). Typically patients are tall, eunuchoidal, with gynaecomastia and features of hypogonadism. Testosterone levels may be normal postpubertally but then fall in subsequent years. Klinefelter's syndrome is associated with varicose veins, chronic chest disease, osteoporosis and quite frequently thyroid dysfunction. Patients may have psychosocial difficulties and reduced IQ. Confirmed reports of spontaneous fertility are exceedingly rare, with the possible exception of mosaics. Osteoporosis may manifest prepubertally and become clinically important later in life.

Management

Delay in growth and development warrants androgen therapy for 10–25 weeks. The therapeutic options include nocturnal oral testosterone undecanoate, intramuscular testosterone esters (starting low dose) and hCG injection.

In long-term hypogonadism androgen replacement can be provided by the following regimens:

- *Oral testosterone undecanoate.* This often needs frequent dosing, up to four times daily.
- *Testosterone esters by deep intramuscular injection.* This is usually needed every 2 weeks (**Fig. 19.30**)
- *Testosterone patches.* These may be applied to body skin, or scrotal skin
- *Testosterone pellet implants.* For example, three 200 mg pellets 4–6 monthly (**Fig. 19.31**)

- It is advisable to monitor prostate specific antigen (PSA) if using testosterone in men over 50 years old

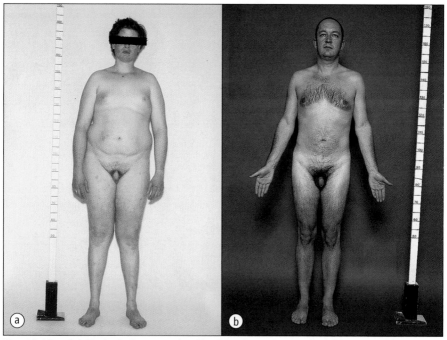

Fig. 19.29   *(a) Typical phenotype in Klinefelter's syndrome with (b) an atypically normal male phenotype.*

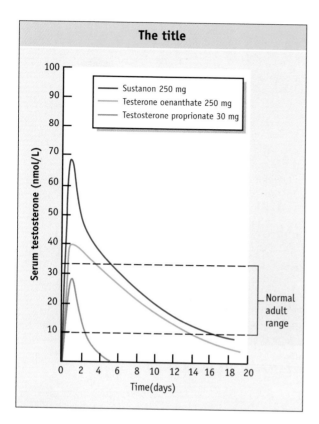

Fig. 19.30 *Testosterone levels following intramuscular injection of testosterone ester preparations.*

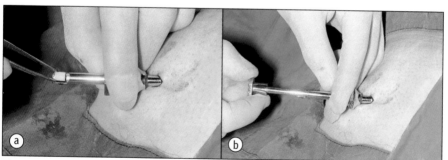

Fig. 19.31 *(a, b) Implantation of testosterone pellets using a trocar and cannula.*

GYNAECOMASTIA (Fig. 19.32)

Management
- First deal with any underlying factors such as testicular or other tumours, thyrotoxicosis, or drugs
- Correct testosterone deficiency if this is present
- Consider the use of an antioestrogen such as tamoxifen, especially if there is tenderness of the breast or nipples
- Consider plastic surgery

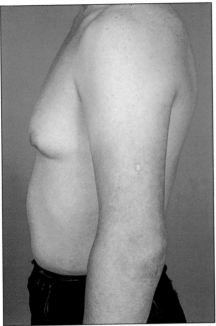

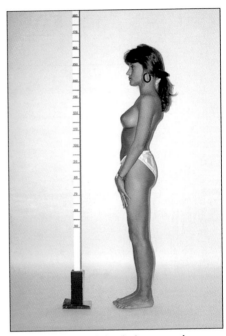

Fig. 19.32   Gynaecomastia (palpate to define disc of breast tissue separate from fatty tissue).

Fig. 19.33   Feminized phenotype in complete androgen insensitivity.

ANDROGEN INSENSITIVITY

Complete androgen insensitivity causes a female phenotype in 46,XY individuals (**Fig. 19.33**). These patients are often tall, with rudimentary nipples, absent secondary sexual hair and a blind vaginal pouch. Inguinal or labial testes are present, which may present as hernia in childhood. However, more often there is a later presentation because of primary amenorrhoea.

Partial androgen insensitivity encompasses a wide range from mild to complete virilization.

Clinical features

- In the more severe forms, androgynous external genitalia, hypospadias, gynaecomastia and partial labial fusion are found
- In contrast, the mildest forms present only with azoospermia, causing infertility
- Female orientation is clearest in the complete form

5α-reductase deficiency leads to fetal lack of DHT and sexual ambiguity. At puberty increased secretion of testosterone leads to acquisition of male habitus (the phenotype having previously been female) (**Fig. 19.34**). Some DHT formation at puberty leads to partial phallic

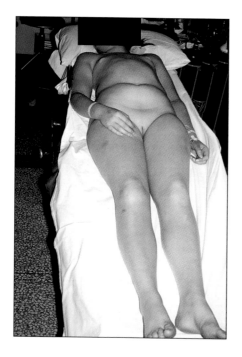

Fig. 19.34 *Incomplete but still feminized phenotype in a patient with androgen insensitivity.*

enlargement; the testes enlarge and descend with partial spermatogenesis as these are testosterone-dependent processes. Gender identity often switches from female to male at puberty with remarkably little difficulty.

Management

Gonadal tumour formation in the testes necessitates gonadectomy by the time of puberty.

Oestrogen replacement is indicated to develop female characteristics and avoid osteoporosis. Adults with 5α-reductase deficiency may virilize more fully with high dose testosterone.

- Careful counselling is necessary together with an appropriately timed discussion of the underlying pathophysiology

INFERTILITY

Management

Management of infertility lies mainly outside the scope of this volume but brief accounts of some therapeutic approaches are given below.

Hyperprolactinaemia in women   (See Ch. 15.)

Polycystic ovarian syndrome   A procedure for management is:

- The first line is antioestrogen therapy, e.g. clomiphene 50–150 mg/day for 5 days
- Weight loss improves the ovulation rate in obese PCOS patients. This improvement may be due to a decrease in insulin resistance, which may also be helped by administering metformin

- Exogenous gonadotrophins may be necessary
- Prior use of GnRH agonists may help by:
  — reducing the risk of spontaneous premature ovulation of an immature follicle
  — reducing the potentially oocyte-damaging influence of excess LH levels

- Some patients may require IVF

Hypogonadotrophic/hypogonadal men   A procedure for management is:
- If there is hyperprolactinaemia then normalize with dopamine agonists

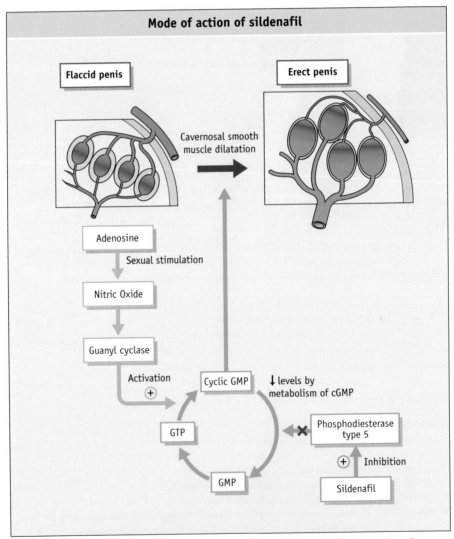

Fig. 19.35 *Mode of action of Sildenafil by inhibition of phosphodiesterase type 5.*

- Use intramuscular hCG 2000 IU twice weekly to normalize testosterone secretion
- Monitor seminal ejaculate for spermatogenesis
- Most patients need additional FSH, e.g. three times a week intramuscularly, or daily subcutaneous injection
- When FSH is added monitor the hCG dosage to prevent excess estradiol production
- Hypothalamic GnRH deficiency responds to pulsatile GnRH given in a 90–120 minute injection. However, this can be impractical especially if there is a long treatment requirement
- Fertility can be achieved with very low sperm density

- For other aspects of infertility treatment especially that including IVF, gamete intrafallopian transfer (GIFT) protocols, intracytoplasmic sperm injection (ICSI) and treatment of antisperm antibodies, reference to specialist texts is advised

---

SEXUAL DYSFUNCTION

Management

The following are general pointers:

- Loss of libido may be related to testosterone deficiency and corrected by replacement
- Hyperprolactinaemia also often causes lack of libido and impotence. In this case, correction of the hyperprolactinaemia usually benefits the problem
- If not, check that the testosterone level is normal; if it is low then add testosterone also
- Erectile failure in diabetes and most other causes responds to Sildenafil; this acts as a specific inhibitor of phosphodiesterase type 5 (**Fig. 19.35**). However, it is contraindicated if nitrates or amyl nitrite is being used
- Testosterone deficiency may significantly impair libido in women; this is particularly seen following oophorectomy
- Testosterone implants (low dose) are often helpful with few side-effects

---

- In most cases of sexual dysfunction, including lack or loss of libido, erectile dysfunction, and premature ejaculation or its failure, psychological problems may be the primary cause. Even if not, they usually significantly add to and may perpetuate problems and hence always need consideration, sympathetic and skilful handling

chapter 20

Calcium Disorders and Metabolic Bone Diseases

INTRODUCTION

Because calcium plays major roles in determining neuromuscular excitability, the body must regulate the extracellular ionic calcium concentration closely, and maintain the strength and morphology of the skeleton, in which more than 98% of the body's calcium is found. Calcium also constitutes a major intracellular signalling system connected with the generation of inositol triphosphate.

These separate but connected processes involve important fluxes of calcium in and out of the gastrointestinal tract, kidney and bone as well as across cell membranes and between intracellular compartments.

The main regulatory influences on calcium metabolism are:

- Parathyroid hormone
- Vitamin D metabolites
- Calcitonin
- Calcium-sensing receptor
- Magnesium
- Phosphate

Parathyroid hormone

The actions of PTH are illustrated in **Fig. 20.1**. They include:
- Increasing the renal distal tubular reabsorption of calcium
- Increasing the resorption of calcium from bone
- Enhancing the renal synthesis of 1,25-dihydroxy vitamin D, leading to increased absorption of calcium from the gut
- An anabolic action on bone (low, intermittent levels)

Influences on parathyroid secretion

The influences on parathyroid secretion are illustrated in **Fig. 20.2**. The major influence is the serum ionized calcium concentration, and a short negative feedback effect is mediated by calcium-sensing receptors. Other major influences include the following:

- Parathyroid secretion is enhanced by 1,25-dihydroxy vitamin D
- Parathyroid secretion is enhanced by hyperphosphataemia (mainly via a reciprocal lowering of the calcium concentration)
- Parathyroid secretion is inhibited by hypomagnesaemia

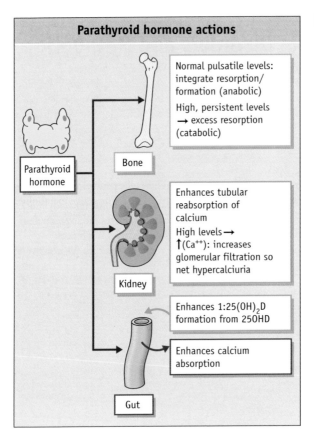

Fig. 20.1   *Actions of PTH.*

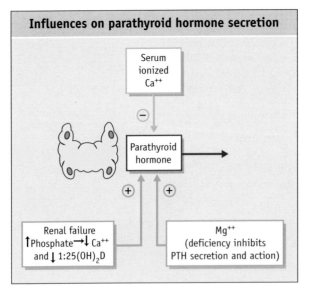

Fig. 20.2   *Influences on PTH secretion.*

Vitamin D sources

Skin production from provitamin D_3 takes place under the influence of ultraviolet (UV) light (especially UVB, with a wavelength of 290–315 nm). Its production is thus decreased at high latitudes owing to the limited availability of UVB light in winter. It is also decreased in subjects with dark skin (because of the higher levels of melanin), and by the use of skin blockers, and in old age. Dietary sources of vitamin D include: yeast and plants (D_2), fatty fish and cod liver oil (D_3). The UK recommended dietary intake is likely to be an underestimate; 600–800 units in an adult (15–20 mg) is probably necessary. Sources containing vitamin D_2 and D_3 are metabolically equivalent.

Vitamin D metabolism (Fig. 20.3)

Vitamin D is converted in the liver to 25-hydroxy vitamin D. This is the main circulating form of vitamin D, and its measurement therefore gives the vitamin D status. The active metabolite, 1,25-dihydroxy vitamin D, is produced from this form in the kidneys. Its conversion is critically regulated, and an alternative pathway leads to the formation of inactive 24,25-dihydroxy vitamin D.

Major influences on vitamin D production include the following:

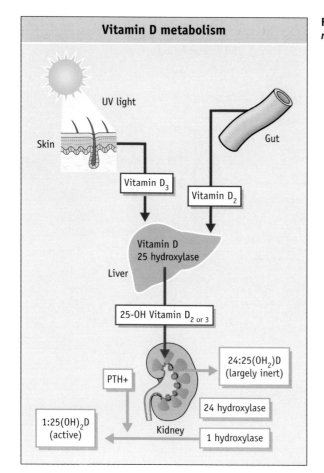

Vitamin D metabolism

Skin — UV light — Gut

Vitamin D_3

Vitamin D_2

Vitamin D 25 hydroxylase

Liver

25-OH Vitamin $D_{2\ or\ 3}$

PTH+

24:25(OH_2)D (largely inert)

24 hydroxylase

1:25(OH)$_2$D (active)

Kidney

1 hydroxylase

Fig. 20.3 *Vitamin D metabolism.*

- It is enhanced by PTH
- It is enhanced by decreased phosphate
- It is enhanced by decreased calcium

There is unregulated 1α-hydroxylase activity in granulomas (such as sarcoidosis or TB).

Daily calcium fluxes and homeostasis (Fig. 20.4)

The net dietary intake of calcium should be about 1000 mg per day, but is often less. The net intake from the gut is equal to the absorption (300 mg/day) minus the faecal excretion (125 mg/day). Bone contains more than 99% of the body's calcium (1000 g), of which 1% is rapidly exchangeable. In a state of metabolic balance, the net daily fluxes in and out of bone are about 500 mg. The extracellular fluid contains 900 mg of calcium. Each day the kidneys filter 10 000 mg of calcium, of which about 9825 mg is reabsorbed.

The mechanisms affecting the overall calcium balance are determined by the need to maintain plasma calcium concentration within a narrow band. The main effectors of change are PTH and 1,25-dihydroxy vitamin D.

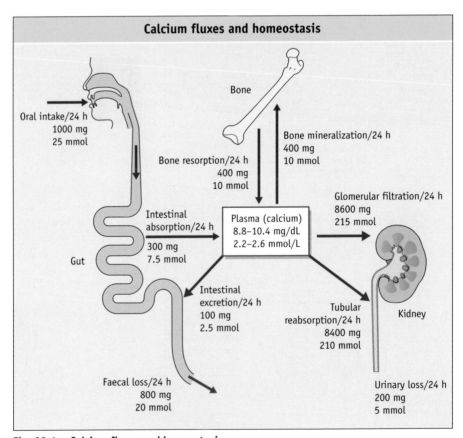

Fig. 20.4   Calcium fluxes and homeostasis.

Components of plasma calcium

Ionized calcium represents 50% of the total; this is the biologically important fraction, so it is highly regulated. The level of protein-bound calcium is variable, but is approximately 40% of the total. The remaining fraction (10%) is complexed with anions such as citrate, sulphate, or phosphate.

Measurement of plasma calcium concentration

- The standardized total calcium is a derived value, assuming the albumin concentration is 40 g/L. It is the measured total calcium concentration minus (measured albumin in g/L minus 40), multiplied by 0.02
- Acidaemia decreases plasma binding; for each 0.1 decrease in pH the plasma calcium concentration increases by 0.05 mmol/L
- 1 mmol/L calcium equals 4 mg/dl
- The normal total calcium concentration is 2.1–2.55 mmol/L (= 8.4–10.2 mg/dl)
- The normal ionized calcium concentration is 1.12–1.23 mmol/L (= 4.48–4.92 mg/dl)
- The calcium concentration multiplied by the phosphate concentration tends to be constant

PATHOGENESIS AND PATHOLOGY

HYPERCALCAEMIA

Hypercalcaemia occurs when the influx of calcium into the extracellular fluid exceeds the efflux. Limited renal excretion is the usual bottleneck, as the maximal renal calcium excretion is 1000 mg (25 mmol) per day, but this may be reduced in hypercalcaemia. The causes of this reduced excretion include enhanced tubular reabsorption resulting from hyperparathyroidism, malignancy or thiazides, or decreased filtration because of impaired renal function. Hypercalcaemia impairs the renal water concentration leading to dehydration, which increases the extracellular fluid calcium concentration.

Increased gut absorption also occurs with oral or parenteral vitamin D excess, whereas increased 1,25-dihydroxy vitamin D synthesis occurs in association with granulomas such as those due to sarcoidosis or TB. Cortisol deficiency enhances the sensitivity to vitamin D.

The third source of hypercalcaemia is increased bone resorption caused by PTH excess, or malignancy (with production of PTH-related protein (PTH-RP), 1,25-dihydroxy vitamin D or cytokine, or osteolytic metastases). Immobility in prolonged illness or exposure to low gravity, as happens with astronauts, also causes increased dissolution of bone calcium stores and can lead to hypercalcaemia, especially with increased bone turnover – as seen in Paget's disease and thyrotoxicosis, and in young persons.

The main causes of hypercalcaemia are:

- Hyperparathyroidism
- Malignancy – humoral, or metastasis with or without immobilization
- Granulomatous disease (e.g. sarcoidosis, TB)

In addition to these, a number of other causative factors may be involved, such as:

- Drugs – e.g. thiazides, lithium, vitamin D intoxication, calcipotriol, vitamin A, milk-alkali
- Immobilization – especially in the young, who have a high bone turnover
- Familial hypocalciuric hypercalcaemia
- Thyrotoxicosis
- Addison's disease
- Rhabdomyolysis – the recovery phase
- Renal transplant (tertiary hyperparathyroidism may occur after this – see below)

Hyperparathyroidism

This is subdivided into three groups:

Primary hyperparathyroidism   This is usually due to a single adenoma (of monoclonal origin), but the occurrence of two separate adenomas is not rare, especially in the older age groups. Alternatively, primary hyperparathyroidism may be due to four-gland hyperplasia, which may be sporadic or familial (see Ch. 23). It is almost invariably present in multiple endocrine neoplasia (MEN-1). Rare familial hyperparathyroidism (isolated) occurs, and may be associated with jaw tumours. Hyperparathyroidism is occasionally found in MEN-2a (but *not* in MEN-2b). Parathyroid carcinoma is extremely rare and may be a long-lasting indolent disease. It is important to distinguish hypocalciuric hypercalcaemia from primary hyperparathyroidism.

Secondary hyperparathyroidism   Renal failure is an important cause; it is largely due to increased phosphate. Osteomalacia due to dietary deficiency, or malabsorption such as in coeliac disease, also leads to secondary hyperparathyroidism.

Tertiary hyperparathyroidism   A transition to autonomous parathyroid secretion may occur after prolonged secondary hyperparathyroidism. It is particularly conspicuous when the underlying cause is treated; for example, it may occur after a renal transplant, or treated malabsorption conditions such as gluten exclusion in coeliac disease.

Malignancy-associated hypercalcaemia

This is usually due to tumoral production of PTH-RP and is especially associated with squamous cell carcinoma in the bronchus and kidney and renal tract. Breast cancer can lead to osteolytic metastases and PTH-RP production causing hypercalcaemia.

Myeloma leads to bone pain in 80% of cases and hypercalcaemia in 20–40%, which is cytokine related. T-cell lymphoma often leads to the production of PTH-RP, whereas other lymphomas produce 1,25-dihydroxy vitamin D. Osteolytic bone metastases may lead to hypercalcaemia, the commonest primary tumour sites being the breast and thyroid gland.

Granulomatous diseases and hypercalcaemia

Sarcoidosis occasionally causes hypercalciuria or hypercalcaemia, but especially with widespread disease. Macrophages in granulomas can lead to 1α-hydroxylation of circulating 25-hydroxy vitamin D produced in the liver. Unlike renal 1α-hydroxylase this reaction is not inhibited by its product, but rather by glucocorticoids. Glucocorticoids also antagonize the action of 1,25-dihydroxy vitamin D. TB-associated hypercalcaemia is often marked by concomitant decrease in albumin and may be missed, as the total plasma calcium may not be elevated. Other causes include silicone granulomas, berylliosis, leprosy and Wegener's vasculitis.

HYPOCALCAEMIA

The main causes of hypocalcaemia are:

- Hypoparathyroidism
- Pseudohypoparathyroidism
- Magnesium deficiency
- Chronic renal failure
- Vitamin D deficiency or resistance
- Acute pancreatitis
- Phosphate excess

In addition to the above, the following may be causative factors:
- Rhabdomyolysis
- Malignant disease – from osteoblastic metastases, or as a result of chemotherapy
- Endotoxic shock
- Post-thyroidectomy for thyrotoxicosis
- Constitutively activated calcium-sensing gene

Hypoparathyroidism

This most often occurs after neck surgery – when it is often transient, and is a feature of 'hungry bones', as in hyperparathyroidism and thyrotoxicosis. Autoimmune hypoparathyroidism may be isolated, or associated with Addison's disease, diabetes mellitus or premature ovarian failure, or more complex disorders including mucocutaneous candidiasis and alopecia with varying degrees of immune incompetence. Idiopathic hypoparathyroidism occurs especially in old age, when it may be associated with diabetes mellitus. The parathyroids are susceptible to iron overload, as seen in haemochromatosis and β-thalassaemia. Congenital parathyroid agenesis may occur either as an isolated phenomenon or as part of di George's and other syndromes (often arising from mutations on chromosome 22).

Pseudohypoparathyroidism

In pseudohypoparathyroidism (PHP) there is increased PTH secretion but resistance to its action, which leads to biochemical hypoparathyroidism. There are two main types of PHP.

Classification of pseudohypoparathyroidism

- *Type I*. This is due to a failure to generate cAMP and phosphaturia after exogenous PTH; there are several subtypes:
  - *Type Ia*. This is associated with Gsα mutations and often other hormone-resistant states. It may also be associated with Albright's hereditary osteodystrophy (AHO), the main features of which are short fourth and fifth metacarpals, a short stature and a round face. Pseudopseudohypoparathyroidism (pseudoPHP) is also found with AHO but normal PTH responses and bone biochemistry. Phenotypic variations including PHP-Ia and pseudoPHP may be found within the same family, which suggest these may be different expressions of the same genetic defect; they may sometimes be sex-linked and due to imprinting
  - *Type Ib*. This also exhibits an absence of cAMP response to PTH but there are normal Gsα levels and no AHO features
  - *Type Ic*. Here there is an absence of cAMP response to PTH, and normal Gsα G1 levels, but multiple hormone resistance
- *Type II*. In contrast to the type I variants, there is also reduced phosphaturic response to PTH but normal cAMP production; hence this type is due to downstream intracellular defects

Magnesium deficiency

Magnesium deficiency leads to impaired secretion of PTH. Magnesium repletion rapidly corrects hyposecretion of PTH. However, profound magnesium deficiency can impair PTH action.

Chronic renal failure and hypocalcaemia

Hyperphosphataemia is an early response to even mildly impaired glomerular filtration. Since, as mentioned earlier, the calcium concentration multiplied by the phosphate concentration is approximately constant, a decrease in calcium concentration follows this primary increase in phosphate concentration.

The increased phosphate results in secondary hyperparathyroidism, and the decreased renal function leads to impaired production of 1,25-dihydroxy vitamin D, and so there arises the full constellation comprising raised phosphate, low calcium, raised PTH and low 1,25-dihydroxy vitamin D, which characterizes chronic renal failure.

Vitamin D-related hypocalcaemia

Vitamin D-related hypocalcaemia may be privational, caused by dietary vitamin D deficiency, decreased skin exposure, or increased pigmentation. An alternative cause is malabsorption; this may be due to coeliac, hepatobiliary or Crohn's disease.

Renal disease may lead to decreased production of 1,25-dihydroxy vitamin D. Hepatic disease can lead to decreased 25-hydroxy vitamin D; this may also be caused by drugs such as anticonvulsants.

Vitamin-D-dependent rickets may also occur, of which there are two types (see Osteomalacia/rickets, p. 340).

Pancreatitis

In pancreatitis, the release of pancreatic lipase leads to the production of free fatty acids from omental or retroperitoneal fat. These free fatty acids chelate calcium avidly from the extracellular fluid, causing hypocalcaemia. There may also be hypomagnesaemia associated with a poor diet, or alcohol excess; this carries a poor prognosis.

Phosphate-excess induction of hypocalcaemia

In this there is often coexisting renal impairment (see above), especially if there is excess ingestion or parenteral administration of phosphate. It is also seen with tumour lysis during chemotherapy of neoplasms – for example acute lymphatic leukaemia in children – and in rhabdomyolysis during the oliguric phase.

METABOLIC BONE DISEASE

These constitute a vast collection of disorders, many of which are rare inherited disorders of unknown aetiology. Reference should be made to readily available texts on bone disorders.

Classification of widespread bone diseases

- Osteoporotic syndromes
- Osteomalacic syndromes
- Bone protein abnormalities
- Paget's disease

Osteoporosis

Osteoporosis is characterized by diminished bone mass accompanied by microarchitectural deterioration and increased fragility. Its clinical significance is that it increases the bone's vulnerability to fracture and the consequences of pain, deformity and disability. However, osteoporosis is not normally painful in the absence of fractures. The major cause of the increased bone fragility is loss of bone mineral, which provides about 80% of the mechanical strength of bone.

Bone mass increases during childhood and adolescence by linear and transverse growth. Epiphyseal fusion limits linear growth. After the peak bone mass is reached, a plateau follows in which bone turnover is in balance. Genetic and hormonal factors determine not only the sex differences in the peak values reached but also the rapidity of perimenopausal bone loss in women (**Fig. 20.5**). The consequence is that older women are particularly prone to osteoporosis-related fractures. However, these are also not uncommon in ageing men.

Bone consists of small structural units that constantly undergo a cycle of activity and remodelling (**Fig. 20.6**). This physiological pattern of activation–resorption–formation gives rise to two major patterns of bone loss:

Classification of bone turnover changes associated with osteoporosis

- *Type I.* Increased resorption
- *Type II.* Diminished bone formation

Compensatory increases in bone formation may be seen in type I but this is insufficient to prevent bone loss. The increased frequency of activation leading to increased bone turnover is associated with increased numbers of resorption cavities, and hence a diminishment of bone

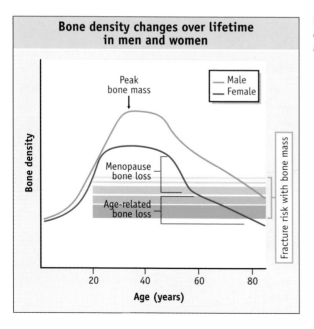

Bone density changes over lifetime in men and women

Peak bone mass

— Male
— Female

Menopause bone loss

Age-related bone loss

Bone density

Fracture risk with bone mass

Age (years)

20   40   60   80

Fig. 20.5 *Bone density changes over the lifetime in men and women.*

337

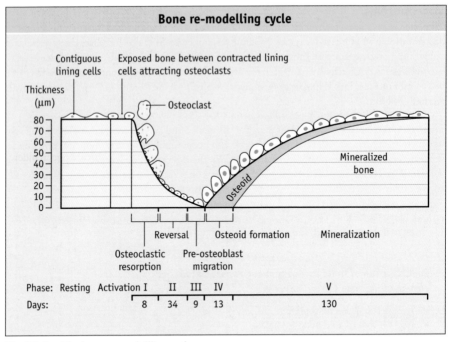

Fig. 20.6   *The bone-remodelling cycle.*

Fig. 20.7   *Cancellous bone structure.*

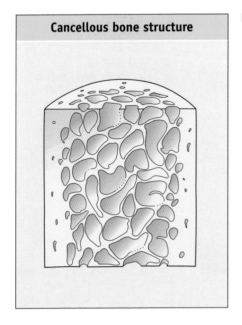

mass. Not infrequently enhanced resorption may coexist with and be exacerbated by reduced new bone growth (i.e. a hybrid of types I and II).

Two major types of bone are recognized:

1. *Cortical (also known as compact bone)*. This constitutes approximately 80% of bone mass especially the shafts of the long bones
2. *Cancellous (also known as trabecular or spongy bone)*. This constitutes approximately 20% of bone and is composed of rods and plates acting as lightweight struts (**Fig. 20.7**). Cancellous bone has a relatively much greater surface area and so it has a higher rate of metabolic activity (principally on the bone surfaces). Thinning of the plates and rods with ageing is initially potentially reversible, but if there is any perforation or fracture they can become disconnected and then the mechanical damage is irreversible.

Osteoporosis caused by states of increased resorption and high turnover particularly affect sites with a high proportion of cancellous bone – hence fractures are prone to occur at the distal radius and dorsal vertebrae. Type II osteoporosis usually affects cortical bone in older people, predisposing them to hip fractures (**Fig. 20.8**).

Risk factors for osteoporosis include:

- Genetic – this factor is responsible for 70–80% of the individual variability in bone mass. Inheritance is probably polygenic; candidates include vitamin D receptor polymorphism and collagen type I promoter polymorphism. Hence the family history is important
- Ethnic – there is a reduced risk in Afro-Caribbeans because of greater peak bone mass
- Oestrogen deficiency – including premature menopause (i.e. at an age less than 45 years), anorexia and amenorrhoea
- Previous fragility fractures
- Immobilization

Secondary osteoporosis:
- Myeloma
- Primary or secondary hypogonadism, including hyperprolactinaemia, male hypogonadism
- Thyrotoxicosis – this is largely reversible on treatment
- Cushing's syndrome
- Hyperparathyroidism – especially in postmenopausal women
- Malabsorption, chronic liver disease, postgastrectomy
- Rheumatoid arthritis (independent of drug side-effects)
- Osteogenesis imperfecta, Ehler's–Danlos syndrome, homocystinuria
- Mastocytosis
- Drugs – including corticosteroids (see below), heparin, cyclosporine, alcohol abuse

Steroid-induced osteoporosis Corticosteroids in pharmatological doses affect especially the cancellous bone, and increase the risk of vertebral crush. Rib and also hip fractures are the

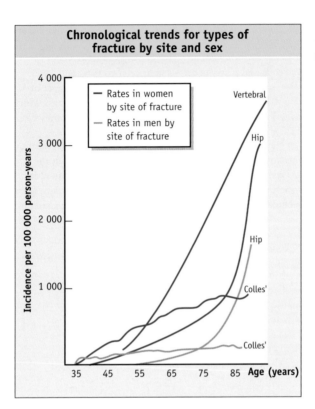

Fig. 20.8 *Chronological trends for fractures by site and sex.*

result. The majority of bone loss occurs in the first 6 months. It is generally held that the risk is increased by oral prednisolone (in a dosage of at least 7.5 mg daily, or the equivalent, for at least 6 months). Suggested mechanisms include a decrease in calcium absorption from the gut, and an increase in urinary calcium loss leading to secondary hyperparathyroidism and increased bone resorption. There is also a decrease in bone synthesis, which in part may be due to the induction of hypogonadotrophic hypogonadism in men on long-term oral corticosteroids.

Osteomalacia/rickets

These conditions are classically associated with abnormal supply, absorption, metabolism or response to vitamin D leading to failure of bone mineralization and often excess osteoid formation; hence there are soft (malacic) rather than fragile (porotic) bones as above.

There are two types of vitamin-D-dependent rickets:

Classification of vitamin-D-dependent rickets

- *Type I.* Due to deficiency of renal 1α-hydroxylase
- *Type II.* Due to receptor defects causing end-organ resistance to 1,25-dihydroxy vitamin D

The critical factors in the aetiology of both osteomalacia and rickets appear to be the concentrations of extracellular fluid calcium and phosphate at the osteoid surface. Factors leading to their depletion, notably hypophosphataemia, can cause failure of mineralization. Various drugs can also interfere with this – including large doses of etidronate, aluminium (especially in renal failure), or fluoride.

> - Note that the classical sharp distinction between osteoporosis and osteomalacia blurs in the elderly, and steroid-treated patients who predominantly display features of osteoporosis (see above) often also have features of vitamin D deficiency

Causes of osteomalacia/rickets include:
- Inadequate UVB light – for instance from being housebound, living at the higher latitudes in winter, wearing too much clothing, increased skin pigmentation, and use of sunscreen
- Inadequate dietary intake of vitamin D, calcium or phosphate, or binding due to agents such as phytate, aluminium hydroxide
- Malabsorption – such as seen postgastrectomy, and in coeliac disease, Crohn's disease, gut resection, scleroderma and TB
- Chronic pancreatitis, hepatobiliary disease, or the results of anticonvulsant use
- Hypophosphataemia – either congenital (which is generally due to an X-linked trait, but there may occasionally be other modes of inheritance – for instance as seen in neurofibromatosis) or acquired (for example as a result of oncogenic (mesenchymal) tumours or fibrous dysplasia)
- Fanconi syndromes – either congenital (occurring with or without cystinosis, and renal tubular acidosis) or acquired (for instance as a result of obstruction, gammopathies, amyloid, diabetes or heavy metal poisoning)

Bone protein abnormalities

Type I collagen composes over 85% of bone matrix protein and provides the basic building block of bone matrix fibre as a triple-helical coil of two α_1(I) and one α_2(I) chains. The repeated glycine–proline–modified-proline triplet content confers the major structural features of bone collagen fibres. Collagen molecules are packed end to end with short intervening gaps, and lie staggered side by side, each offset from its neighbour by about a quarter of a molecule length. The gene for α_1 (I) is on chromosome 17 and that for α_2 (I) on chromosome 7. Collagen is synthesized and secreted as propeptides, together with amino and carboxy propeptide extensions aiding fibril formation; these are then cleaved, some reaching the circulation in amounts correlating with bone formation rates. Post-translational changes include important cross-links forming pyridinolines with lysyl and hydroxylysyl residues. The pyridinolines are released during bone resorption and urinary measurements of these therefore quantify the level of resorptive activity.

Non-collagen proteins are much smaller but nevertheless constitute 50% of bone protein production on a molar basis.

> **Classification of major non-collagen bone proteins**
>
> - Proteoglycans – especially chondroitin sulphate and heparan sulphate
> - Growth-related proteins
> - Cell attachment proteins
> - γ-carboxylated proteins (gla) – e.g. osteocalcin

The function of the major osteoblast enzyme, alkaline phosphatase, remains unknown. Abnormalities of collagen type I give rise to the various forms of osteogenesis imperfecta.

Paget's disease

This is not primarily a metabolic disorder but may have distinctive biochemical effects. It is common, especially in Caucasian people of European descent, and geographical clustering is also recognized – in the UK it occurs particularly in northeast Lancashire. Electron microscopy reveals inclusion bodies like viral nucleocapsids, which suggests a possible aetiology from viruses such as measles, canine distemper and other paramyxoviruses.

Pagetic involvement occurs in separate bones; initially there is bone lysis but following this abnormal new woven bone is produced. Structurally abnormal osteoclasts (with up to 100 nuclei per cell) are present in increased numbers. Increased markers of bone turnover such as urinary pyridinoline and hydroxyproline are found. An increased level of bone-specific alkaline phosphatase is also characteristic – indicating that there is a secondary effect on the osteoblasts. Rarely, Paget's disease causes hypercalcaemia, especially if there is associated immobility, but there is also apparently a higher coincidence of primary hyperparathyroidism than would be expected.

INVESTIGATION AND DIAGNOSIS

HYPERCALCAEMIA

The following procedure may be used for investigating hypercalcaemia:

- First, confirm the hypercalcaemia: adjust for protein, avoid a tight tourniquet and preferably test while the patient is fasting
- Check the ionized calcium level if possible
- Check the PTH level (a two-site immunoradiometric assay is preferred) – if this is high then the hypercalcaemia is primary or tertiary hyperparathyroidism or hypocalciuric hypercalcaemia; if it is low then check for sarcoidosis by performing a chest X-ray and measuring ACE activity
- Look for features of malignancy, especially in the lung, breast, thyroid, and renal tract
- Check the phosphate and alkaline phosphatase levels
- Check the 24 hour urine calcium excretion
- Check the thyroid and adrenocortical functions
- Check the immunoglobulins, serum and urine protein electrophoresis (and check the Bence Jones protein reaction)

HYPERPARATHYROIDISM

A procedure for investigating hyperparathyroidism is:

- First assess the severity of hypercalcaemia
- Check for complications such as renal calcification, impairment, or stones
- If surgery is contemplated then decide whether imaging is indicated (it is often not appropriate for a first operation)
- Useful isotope scans include thallium–technetium subtraction (**Fig. 20.9**) and more recently sestamibi or tetrafosmin scans (**Fig. 20.10**)
- Perform neck ultrasound (if fine needle aspiration is performed then measure the PTH level in the aspirate)
- Exclude hypocalciuric hypercalcaemia
- If the hyperparathyroidism is the tertiary type, investigate a possible renal or gastrointestinal pathology as indicated

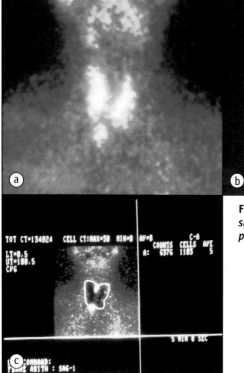

Fig. 20.9 *(a–c) Thallium–technetium subtraction scan for localization of parathyroid adenoma.*

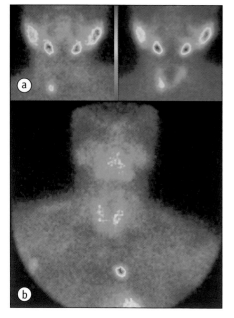

Fig. 20.10 *Sestamibi parathyroid scan (a) showing adenoma in the neck, (b) showing an ectopic mediastinal adenoma.*

- Look for features suggestive of MEN-1 or MEN-2a
- CT or MRI of the neck and mediastinum may help if previous neck exploration has failed

MULTIPLE MYELOMA

Multiple myeloma may be investigated as follows:
- First, quantify the plasma or urinary paraproteins, and β_2-microglobulin
- Assess the renal function
- Perform a skeletal survey
- Check the haematological status (with bone marrow examination)

HYPOCALCAEMIA

A procedure for investigating hypocalcaemia is as follows:
- First, confirm the hypocalcaemia: measure the proteins, and possibly check ionized calcium
- Check the phosphate and alkaline phosphatase levels (use an appropriate age-related range)
- If alkaline phosphatase is elevated then determine whether it is bony in origin (by electrophoresis, or heat stability)
- Check the PTH level (avoid any delay in transit to the laboratory)
- Check the 25-hydroxy vitamin D level (measurement of 1,25-dihydroxy vitamin D is rarely indicated, however)
- For PHP, perform the Ellsworth–Howard test to check urinary phosphate and cAMP responses to PTH injection
- Check the magnesium level
- Check the urinary calcium excretion
- X-ray the relevant bones (e.g. hands, wrists, pelvis, femora, tibiae, skull)
- Check the renal function, including tubular function and aminoaciduria if indicated

OSTEOPOROSIS

The following procedure may be used to investigate osteoporosis:
- Check the calcium, phosphate, alkaline phosphatase levels
- Check the renal and liver function
- Check the blood count, film, viscosity or sedimentation rate
- Check the immunoglobulins, using serum or urinary protein electrophoresis
- Check the gonadal status in all men, and if amenorrhoeic or after simple hysterectomy in women younger than 50 years
- In hypogonadotrophic hypogonadism, consider the possibility of pituitary disease, increased prolactin, or iron overload
- Consider Cushing's syndrome
- Take an X-ray of the dorsolumbar spine if there is backache, kyphosis, rib crowding, or a decrease in height of more than 5 cm
- Serum and urinary bone formation or turnover markers may also be clinically helpful
- Perform bone densitometry (see below)

Bone densitometry

This is a key investigation in the assessment of osteoporosis. The development of DEXA has revolutionized the field. It uses only safe, low dose radiation that is approximately equal to background levels. It is also simple and rapid to perform, and non-interventional. DEXA is accurate and precise, capable of measuring both the particular areas of interest, especially the lumbar spine and femoral neck, and also the whole body calcium and other aspects of body composition. It should be noted that models made by different manufacturers generate different absolute values for bone mean density (BMD), partly because of slight differences in the technology used. The measurements are usually expressed as the bone mineral content of the region or whole body, or more commonly as the bone density (actually the bone per unit area in g/cm²).

The measurement is interpreted by referring the measured value to the appropriate population mean (sex, age or race). Deviation from the mean is expressed as a number of standard deviations (σ), assuming a Poisson distribution. It is now recognized that for each 1 σ decrease there is approximately a two to three times increased risk of fracture – which underpins the use of DEXA in diagnosis, prognosis and monitoring (including response to therapy). The age-related σ score is referred to as the Z score.

Bone strength is directly related to the bone density. This has led to the WHO definition of osteoporosis in terms of the deviation of the measured value in σ from the young-normal mean (called the T score) (**Fig. 20.11**):

Classification of osteoporosis from the T score

- *Normal.* BMD T score less than 1 σ below the young-normal mean
- *Osteopenia.* BMD T score 1–2.5 σ below the young-normal mean
- *Osteoporosis.* BMD T score more than 2.5 σ below the young-normal mean
- *Severe/established osteoporosis.* Prevalent fracture(s) plus BMD more than 2.5 σ below the young-normal mean

---

Various ultrasound methodologies have also been developed that specifically measure the attenuation of the speed of sound through the os calcis. It has been suggested that this value provides information about the bone 'quality' as opposed to its mineral content.

PAGET'S DISEASE

A suggested procedure for investigating Paget's disease is:
- Measure the serum calcium, phosphate and alkaline phosphatase
- Consider also measuring markers of bone turnover such as urinary hydroxyproline or pyridolines
- Perform an isotope bone scan to identify the extent and sites of skeletal involvement (**Fig. 20.12**)
- Take an X-ray of the areas thus indicated as the radiological appearance is characteristic (**Fig. 20.13**)
- Perform MRI or CT scanning of areas in which there is neurological compression (e.g. the skull or spine) (**Fig. 20.14**)
- If there is any sudden new pain, consider a bone biopsy to identify possible malignancy

CLINICAL FEATURES AND MANAGEMENT

HYPERCALCAEMIA

Mild chronic hypercalcaemia (which is usually due to hyperparathyroidism) is often asymptomatic. Osmotic diuresis leads to polyuria, thirst and nocturia. There is often non-

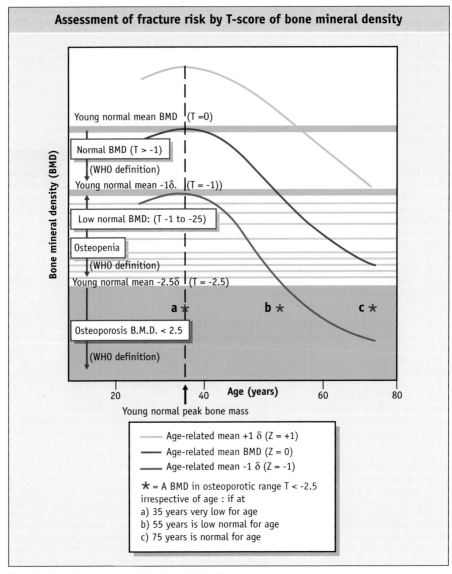

Assessment of fracture risk by T-score of bone mineral density

Young normal mean BMD (T =0)

Normal BMD (T > -1)

(WHO definition)

Young normal mean -1δ. (T = -1))

Low normal BMD: (T -1 to -25)

Osteopenia

(WHO definition)

Young normal mean -2.5δ (T = -2.5)

a ✳   b ✳   c ✳

Osteoporosis B.M.D. < 2.5

(WHO definition)

Bone mineral density (BMD)

20   40 Age (years) 60   80

Young normal peak bone mass

—— Age-related mean +1 δ (Z = +1)
—— Age-related mean BMD (Z = 0)
—— Age-related mean -1 δ (Z = -1)

✶ = A BMD in osteoporotic range T < -2.5
irrespective of age : if at
a) 35 years very low for age
b) 55 years is low normal for age
c) 75 years is normal for age

Fig. 20.11 *Assessment of fracture risk by T score.*

specific malaise, lethargy, depression, and 'foggy' impaired cerebration, which may only become apparent only retrospectively after correcting the hypercalcaemia. Abdominal pain due to increased gastric acidity, constipation and occasionally pancreatitis may occur, and nausea and vomiting may herald metabolic decompensation. Renal impairment can develop with or without nephrocalcinosis (**Fig. 20.15**) and may be associated with renal calculi leading to pain, especially when moving, haematuria and infection.

Hypercalcaemia and osteoporosis, especially when associated with myeloma or in postmenopausal women with hyperparathyroidism, may lead to bone pain – as may metastases (**Fig. 20.16**). Neuromuscular weakness and pain of neuromuscular origin may be found in hypercalcaemia, as may mental depression, confusion, dementia and even impaired

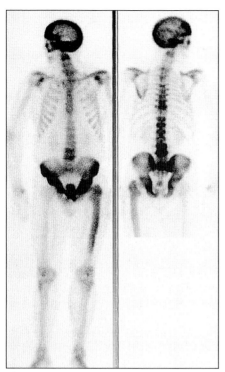

Fig. 20.12   *Isotope bone scan showing skeletal involvement with Paget's disease.*

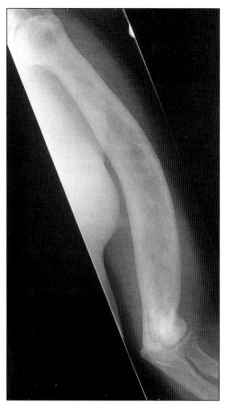

Fig. 20.13   *Typical radiological appearance of bone involved with Paget's disease.*

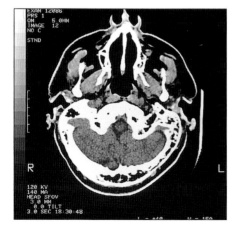

Fig. 20.14   *CT scan of pagetic bone in the skull causing platybasia.*

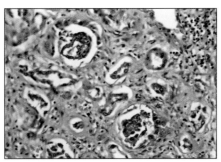

Fig. 20.15   *Nephrocalcinosis due to hypercalcaemia.*

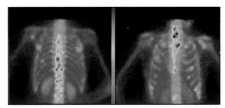

Fig. 20.16   *Bony metastases and hypercalcaemia.*

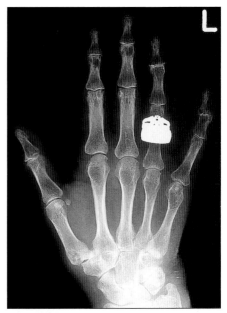

Fig. 20.17   *Chondrocalcinosis associated with pseudogout.*

consciousness in hypercalcaemic crisis. Pruritus is especially common if there is associated renal impairment. Pseudogout and chondrocalcinosis can also occur (**Fig. 20.17**).

Hyperparathyroidism

Mild degrees may be asymptomatic (though may lead to resistant osteoporosis). Symptoms of hypercalcaemia can occur (see above), up to severe hypercalcaemic crisis.

Clinical features

- *Corneal calcification*. This may be seen in long-standing hyperparathyroidism
- *Bone changes*. Now rare, these include subperiosteal erosions (**Fig. 20.18**) and brown tumours
- *Concomitant vitamin D deficiency*. Occult deficiency can occur with lower plasma calcium concentrations; it worsens bone disease

There are a number of indications for surgery:

- Marked hypercalcaemia: greater than 3 mmol/L (= 12 mg/dl)
- Marked hypercalciuria: greater than 10 mmol (= 400 mg) per 24 hours
- Renal calculi
- Worsening renal function
- Bone disease (if there is vitamin D deficiency, cautiously replenish preoperatively)
- Severe neuromuscular disease
- Possibly if there are severe psychiatric complications

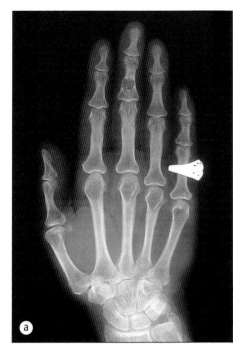

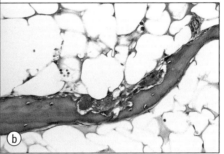

Fig. 20.18 *Subperiosteal erosions due to hyperparathyroidism (a) macroscopic, seen on hand X-ray (together with brown tumours), (b) microscopic with multinuclear osteoclasts.*

Management of surgery   The most important requirement for successful surgery is the surgeon's experience. In first-time neck surgery many surgeons do not attempt to localize tumours. A preoperative vocal cord check is often advocated. All four glands need identifying; if in doubt a small biopsy can be taken for immediate frozen section. If there are no obviously abnormal glands then mark all parathyroids found with a clip or stitch for future operation. A single adenoma is found in 80% of cases of primary hyperparathyroidism. The presence of two adenomas is not exceedingly rare, however, especially in older individuals. If four-gland hyperplasia is found, either remove all four (with or without subcutaneous implantation of half a gland in the forearm) or remove three and a half glands.

Postoperative hypocalcaemia is common for up to 48 hours after successful surgery. If severe then treat with intravenous calcium, and if prolonged treat with oral calcium supplements with or without alfacalcidol or calcitriol, as required.

Hypercalcaemia of malignancy

In patients who are often obviously ill, the site of the tumour may or may not be apparent with or without metastases. As breast cancer may not be palpable, it may be necessary to perform a mammogram. If there is lung cancer, it is generally of the squamous cell type, and frequently associated with clubbing (**Fig. 20.19**). Hypercalcaemia due to renal carcinoma may be occult or present with a mass or haematuria, or both. Multiple myeloma is typically associated with bone pain and pallor (anaemia/renal failure); also superficial deposits may be present (**Fig. 20.20**). A finding of increased calcium concentration after successfully treated cancer often represents coincidental hyperparathyroidism.

Management   For the acute management of hypercalcaemic crisis see Chapter 14. Subsequent palliation can be afforded by continued use of bisphosphonates such as high dose

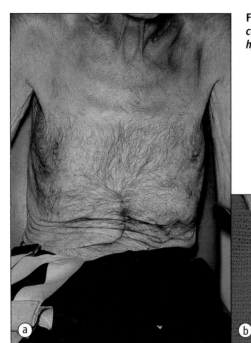

Fig. 20.19   *(a, b) Squamous cell lung cancer associated with clubbing and hypercalcaemia.*

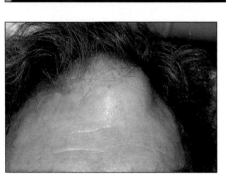

Fig. 20.20   *Myeloma deposition on the skull in a hypercalcaemic patient.*

oral clodronate, or repeated intravenous pamidronate infusions, which help bone pain as well as mitigating the hypercalcaemia. Salmon calcitonin may have additional analgesic as well as hypocalcaemic effects.

Sarcoidosis

In sarcoidosis, there is hypercalcaemia in only about 1–2% of cases. The following features are generally found in this condition:

Clinical features

- Florid manifestations – for instance in the lung, or erythema nodosum (**Fig. 20.21**)
- Hypercalciuria, which is common, and often precedes hypercalcaemia
- Bone cysts

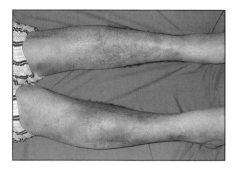

Fig. 20.21 *Erythema nodosum in sarcoidosis associated with hypercalcaemia.*

Management The main therapy is corticosteroids (starting, for instance, with a dosage of 40–60 mg prednisolone). However, long-term use of these may lead to osteoporosis.

HYPOCALCAEMIC AND OSTEOMALACIC DISORDERS

For emergency treatment of hypocalcaemia see Chapter 14.

Hypoparathyroidism

The long-standing hypocalcaemia may cause a presentation with refractory epilepsy, and also can lead to subcapsular cataracts and basal ganglia calcification. The hallmarks of hypocalcaemia, however, are the features of tetany such as perioral and acral tingling, carpopedal spasm and, most ominously, stridor leading to laryngeal spasm.

Signs of tetany

- *Chvostek's sign*. This is elicited by tapping over the facial nerve in front of the parotid. The sign is positive if an ipsilateral twitch follows (however, this is so common in normocalcaemia as to be of dubious diagnostic value)
- *Trousseau's sign*. This is more useful, and is obtained by occluding the arm at more than systolic pressure. This is positive if within 3 minutes there is *main d'accoucheur* (thumb adduction) (**Fig. 20.22**)

Autoimmune parathyroid damage may be part of the hypoparathyroid/ Addison's/moniliasis (HAM) syndrome or the wider range of disorders seen in polyglandular autoimmune type I syndrome.

Management Treatment of hypoparathyroidism consists of calcium supplements. The average dosage is 1 g/day (at least initially), plus alfacalcidol 0.5–2 μg or calcitriol 0.25–1 μg per day.

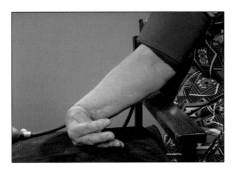

Fig. 20.22   *Trousseau's sign, produced by occlusion of arterial flow, producing main d'accoucheur.*

There should be lifelong monitoring (every 2–6 months) of both the calcium level and renal function. Also, as serum calcium increases there is relatively greater hypercalciuria; this may call for the use of thiazides.

In refractory hypoparathyroidism, consider hypomagnesaemia and treat if present.

Pseudohypoparathyroidism

Clinical features

- Short stature
- A round face (a typical AHO feature)
- Shortness of the thumb, and fourth and fifth metacarpals (**Fig. 20.23**)

Management   Treatment is with calcium and alfacalcidol or calcitriol, as in hypoparathyroidism. However, other replacement therapy – for instance of sex steroids, or thyroid hormone – may also be needed.

Osteomalacia and rickets

Clinical features   Consider the possibility that it may be a consequence of gastrectomy, malabsorption, or hepatobiliary or renal disease.

Clinical features of osteomalacia

- Bone pain and tenderness
- Fractures and pseudofractures (Looser's zones) (**Fig. 20.24**)
- Proximal myopathy leading to waddling gait

In rickets, the age at presentation determines the clinical picture: it is most prominent in fastest growing bone.

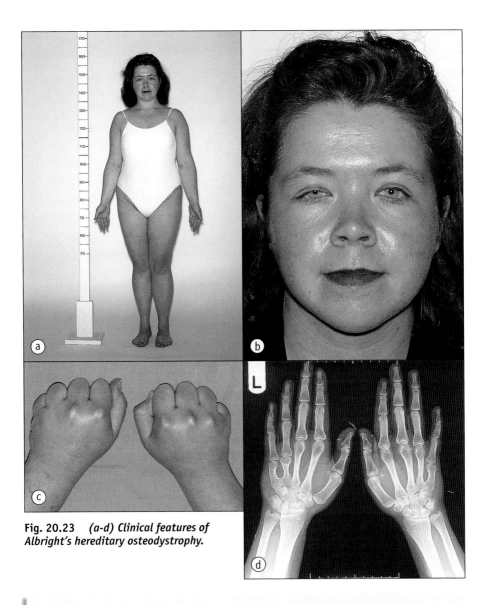

Fig. 20.23 *(a-d) Clinical features of Albright's hereditary osteodystrophy.*

Clinical features of rickets

- At birth – craniotabes of the skull
- In the first year – distortion of the wrist, rickety rosary (beads) at the costochondral junction, and Harrison's grooves on the thorax
- In toddlers – bow legs
- In later childhood – knock knees
- Myopathy leading to weakness and pain may prevent walking, limiting deformity
- Bony tenderness
- Tetany

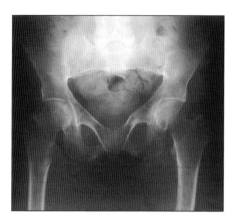

Fig. 20.24 *X-rays showing Looser's zones in osteomalacia.*

Hypophosphataemic rickets – Congenital hypophosphataemic rickets is X-linked, so females are less severely affected (there is random inactivation of the X chromosome).

It is important to diagnose this condition early to prevent deformities. It may be associated with deafness and spinal cord compression.

Acquired hypophosphataemic rickets may be due to mesenchymal tumour. This is usually benign, and often occult, but occasionally malignant (e.g. chondrosarcoma).

It may also be associated with neurofibromatosis, or with kappa light-chain nephrotoxic gammopathies.

Clinical features of hypophosphataemic rickets

- Bowing – which usually occurs in second year of life, and may be severe
- Absence of myopathy
- Dental root hypoplasia – which often leads to abscesses (the enamel is normal, but there are dentine deficiencies)
- Progressive calcification of paraspinal ligaments

Management   When the cause is dietary deficiency, the use of vitamin D_3 and calcium supplements leads to a rapid, marked increase in 1,25-dihydroxy vitamin D_3. In severe cases there may be some benefit from brief initial treatment with alfacalcidol or calcitriol. In the early stages, treatment may lead to increased pain and even a transient decrease in serum calcium; this is termed the 'stir-up' phenomenon.

Vitamin-D-resistant type I rickets responds to physiological levels of 1α-hydroxylated analogues, whereas vitamin-D-resistant type II requires pharmacological levels of 1α-hydroxylated analogues.

Hypophosphataemic rickets requires effervescent oral phosphate; this needs frequent dosing (1–2 tablets three to five times per day) and often leads to diarrhoea, which the use of loperamide or codeine phosphate improves so encouraging compliance with the phosphate therapy. Alfacalcidol or calcitriol is also required to mineralize the bone and decrease secondary hyperparathyroidism. Nephrotoxic gammopathy can be successfully treated with alfacalcidol and bendrofluazide.

Long-term untreated rickets may result in the need for osteotomy or spinal cord decompression.

In oncogenic osteomalacia, if the tumour is identified then successful resection restores biochemical normality.

OSTEOPOROSIS

Uncomplicated osteoporosis is asymptomatic. Decreased skin thickness may be measured with callipers over the dorsum of hand. In women a thickness of 1.5 mm or less suggests the likelihood of osteoporosis, whereas a thickness of at least 2.2 mm suggests that osteoporosis is unlikely. Thinning of skin with age occurs with osteoporosis, but not in individuals with maintained BMD (**Fig. 20.25**).

In established osteoporosis where there has been a previous fragility fracture, there is a markedly increased risk of further fractures. Vertebral crush fractures may be symptomatic or

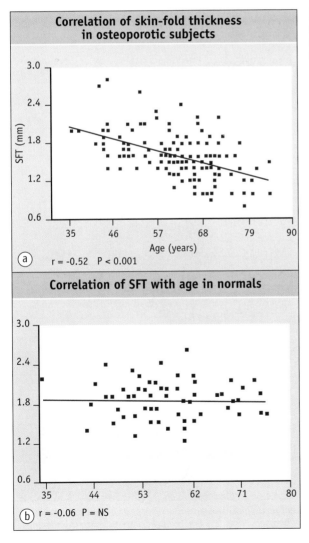

Fig. 20.25 *Skin thickness changes: (a) in osteoporotic subjects but not (b) normal subjects with age.*

asymptomatic. When symptomatic they are often of sudden onset with or without a detectable precipitant, and cause severe pain for up to 6 weeks, sometimes radiating with a root distribution. If the pain persists or worsens over a longer time then an investigation for suspected malignancy should be undertaken. Asymptomatic vertebral fracture may present with loss of height (note other possible causes such as multiple level disc degeneration). A positive family history is common but not invariable (**Fig. 20.26**). Kyphosis may occur from thoracic vertebral collapsed vertebrae (**Fig. 20.27**), or rib crowding from collapse of lumbar vertebrae (**Fig. 20.28**).

Clinical features of secondary osteoporosis

- *Steroid associated*. Cushingoid facies, very fragile ecchymotic skin (**Fig. 20.29**)
- *Hypogonadism in men*. Decreased facial and body hair, testicular atrophy, or fine facial creases
- *Anorexia nervosa, or excessive exercise*. There may be either primary or secondary amenorrhoea
- *Thyrotoxicosis*. This may be masked
- *Osteogenesis imperfecta tarda*. Blue sclerae are evident (**Fig. 20.30**)
- *Ehlers–Danlos syndrome* (**Fig. 20.31**)
- *Alcohol abuse*. There may be hepatic stigmata, neuropathy or ataxia leading to falls
- *Pregnancy-associated*. Rapid painful vertebral collapses; the scenario may be repeated with subsequent pregnancies
- *Mastocytosis*. This may present with urticaria

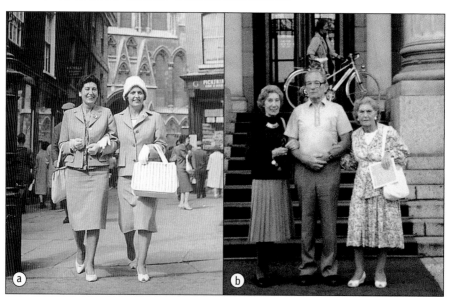

Fig. 20.26 *Sisters of initially similar height, but subsequent loss of height in one with osteoporosis (from Gosden 1996 Cheating Time. WH Freeman & Company, with permission).*

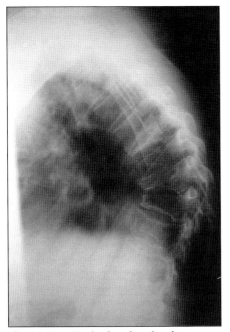

Fig. 20.27 *Kyphotic spine showing wedging and crushing of thoracic vertebrae.*

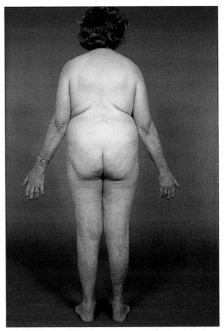

Fig. 20.28 *Rib crushing caused by lumbar vertebrae collapse – note the posterior creases.*

Fig. 20.29 *(a) Cushingoid facies and (b) fragile skin in steroid-induced osteoporosis.*

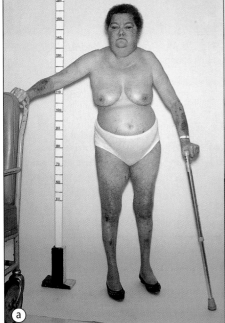

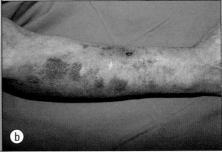

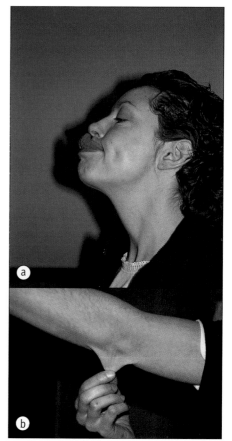

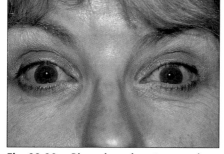

Fig. 20.30 *Blue sclerae in osteogenesis imperfecta tarda.*

Fig. 20.31 *(a, b) Osteoporosis associated with Ehlers–Danlos syndrome.*

Management   It is essential to ensure an adequate calcium intake (more than 1 g daily), though calcium supplements alone retard but do not abolish bone loss. In postmenopausal women nocturnal administration of oral calcium is best retained. Bisphosphonates have low oral bioavailability so it is necessary to avoid a further decrease with concomitant food or drug supplementation. Available treatments include etidronate sodium 400 mg/day for 2 weeks every 3 months, in between calcium supplementation (0.5–1.5 g for 11 weeks).

Alendronate and risedronate are more powerful, taken daily or weekly whilst fasting and with water half an hour before food or other tablets. With alendronate or risedronate it is best to use calcium supplements of at least 500 mg per day, taken at a different time. Care in taking these drugs according to protocol is advised so as to minimize upper gastrointestinal side-effects. Patients with severe oesophageal problems may benefit from intermittent infusions of pamidronate. Salmon calcitonin increases bone density and decreases fracture risk. When salmon calcitonin is given by injection it frequently causes flushing or nausea. If taken in an inhaled form it is much better tolerated. Both routes of administration produce analgesia, which can be of value in patients with acute spinal crush fractures.

Hypogonadal males require testosterone replacement (see Ch. 19). HRT (see below) is indicated in primary or secondary amenorrhoea and also in premature menopause.

When osteoporosis is steroid induced, use of bisphosphonates together with calcium and vitamin D supplements is recommended. Treatment with calcitriol 0.25 µg twice daily treatment is well tolerated, but of poorly documented benefit. It is essential to monitor serum calcium and renal function regularly when patients are treated with calcitriol. In the institutionalized or housebound elderly it has been shown that the ingestion of 1 g calcium and 800 IU vitamin D per day decreases the hip fracture rate – a safe and cost-effective regimen.

Osteoporosis associated with thyrotoxicosis tends to improve with treatment. That caused by Ehler's Danlos syndrome tends to improve with age. Pregnancy-associated osteoporosis tends to reverse postpartum, but calcitonin, calcium and vitamin D may help. Mastocytosis may be caused by release of heparin, or cytokines, so heparin therapy may be useful.

An algorithm for treatment is shown in **Fig. 20.32**, and one for the use of bone densitometry is shown in **Fig. 20.33**.

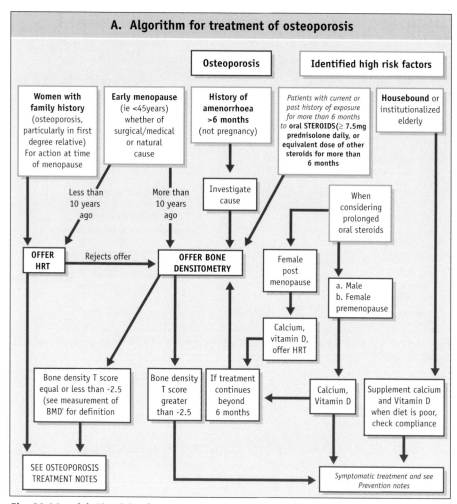

Fig. 20.32 *(a) Algorithm for treatment of osteoporosis (© Leeds Teaching Hospitals NHS Trust).*

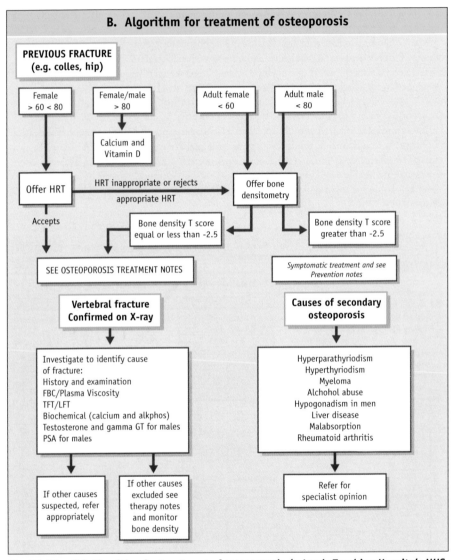

Fig. 20.32   (b) Algorithm for treatment of osteoporosis (© Leeds Teaching Hospitals NHS Trust).

Hormone replacement therapy – HRT benefits current users, but the effects are dissipated by 5 years after stopping. This limitation applies to protection both against osteoporosis and against ischaemic heart disease. There is a small increased risk of breast cancer detectable after 10 years, so this possibility should be monitored by regular palpation and mammograms (the recommended interval is every 18–24 months). There is also an increased risk of venous thromboembolism in first 3 months, but with a very small incidence.

The average bone-sparing doses are: conjugated oestrogen 0.625 mg, estradiol valerate 2 mg, and estradiol patches 50 µg. Selective oestrogen receptor modulators (SERMS) such

Algorithm for use of bone densitometry

Confirm diagnosis (Bone Densitometry,DEXA) if it will alter management or clinically indicated (see also 'identified high risk factor' in Fig.20.32)

INDICATION FOR BMD	PURPOSE OF BMD
Women with menopause < 45 (including surgical) if it is now > 10 years since menpause or secondary amenorrhea > 6 months	If HRT contraindicated and or woman uncertain or does not wish HRT
Risk factors for osteoporosis (see Fig.20.32) at menopause	If woman uncertain and does not wish HRT, to assess future fracture risk
Patients with possible secondary osteoporosis	Patients uncertain and does not wish HRT, to assess future fracture risk
Previous low impact fracture	If uncertainty about diagnosis
Height loss > 2 cm	If uncertainty about diagnosis
X-ray evidence of osteopenia	If uncertainty about diagnosis
Patients with ongoing or planned oral corticosteroid therapy for more than 6 months (≥ 7.5 mg prednisolone or equivalent)	Monitor therapy

Bone densitometry (DEXA T score > -1.0)

Low bone mass (DEXA Tscore -1.0 to -2.5	Lifestyle advice
Low bone mass (DEXA Tscore -1.0 to -2.5	Lifestyle advice Calcium and vitamin D supplements Treat as for prevention
Osteoporosis (DEXA T score < -2.5)	Lifestyle advice Pain relief Exclude secondary causes Calcium and vitamin D supplements Treatment Consider referral

Fig. 20.33 *Algorithm for use of bone densitometry (© Leeds Teaching Hospitals NHS Trust).*

as Raloxifene 60 mg daily are of proven value in the prevention or treatment of vertebral osteoporosis, with beneficial effects also on the breasts and uterus, but none on hot flushes.

- Side-effects of HRT include: mastalgia, nausea and calf tenderness, especially in the initial 3 months
- Low dose HRT decreases side-effects; combine with 1 g calcium supplements to augments the effects on bone
- Relative contraindications include: otosclerosis, migraine, hepatobiliary disease, breast cancer, melanoma and endometriosis
- Neither hypertension (if controlled) nor continued smoking contraindicates HRT

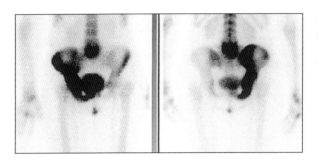

Fig. 20.34   *Paget's disease of the pelvis.*

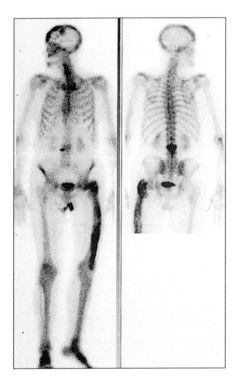

Fig. 20.35   *Paget's disease of the femur.*

Lifestyle influences on bone mass/fracture prevention – Bone mass can be increased by weight-bearing exercise. However gross excess exercise should be avoided premenopausally as it can lead to secondary amenorrhoea.

If there is cognitive impairment or an increased tendency to fall, the home can be modified, and hip protectors used.

Dietary calcium intake should be 1 g premenopausal, or postmenopausal with HRT, increasing to 1.5 g after the menopause. Ensure there is also adequate vitamin D intake from the diet or exposure to sunlight.

The following lifestyle advice is also pertinent:

- Avoid drugs leading to orthostatic hypotension
- Avoid excessive weight reduction: especially prior to peak bone mass
- Stop smoking
- Avoid excessive alcohol intake
- Avoid excessive caffeine consumption

HYPOPHOSPHATASIA

This is a rare condition characterized by low levels of alkaline phosphatase (not the bone-specific isoform). It presents with various degrees of severity ranging from death in utero to only dental manifestations. There is an accumulation of phospho compounds including phosphoethanolamine, pyrophosphate and pyridoxal phosphate. Adults may have osteopenia, chondrocalcinosis, or proximal femoral fractures. Often bone biochemistry includes calcium levels in blood and urine that are normal/high, especially in children, and

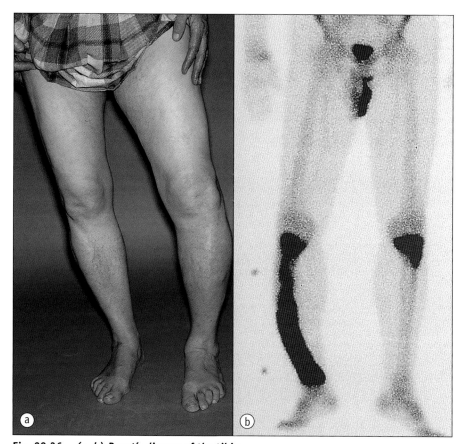

Fig. 20.36 *(a, b) Paget's disease of the tibia.*

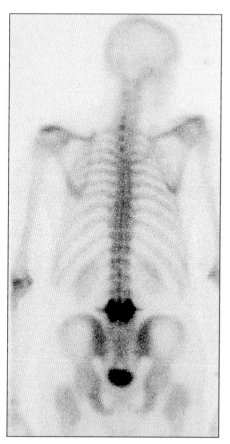

Fig. 20.37   Paget's disease of the vertebrae.

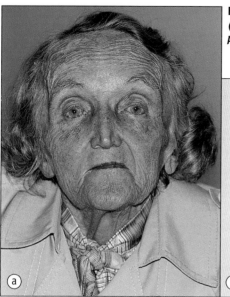

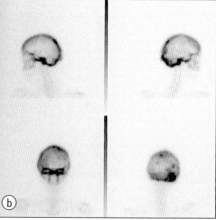

Fig. 20.38   (a) Paget's disease of the skull (b) with isotope bone scan of the same patient's skull.

phosphate levels that are high-normal or higher than the normal range. It is best to avoid treating with vitamin D metabolites or minerals. The bone has the histological appearance of osteomalacia.

Renal osteodystrophy is a specialized topic (refer to standard texts on nephrology).

PAGET'S DISEASE

Paget's disease is commonly asymptomatic and is often discovered incidentally on finding raised alkaline phosphatase. It may, however, cause bone pain, which may be localized and boring in nature. Bone with long-standing changes of Paget's disease often develops a distorted architecture leading to secondary osteoarthritic changes. The most commonly affected bones are the pelvis (**Fig. 20.34**), femur (**Fig. 20.35**), fibula (**Fig. 20.36**) vertebrae (**Fig. 20.37**) and skull (**Fig. 20.38**). Compression syndromes lead to deafness (common), spinal cord compression and blindness. Platybasia may lead to brainstem and pyramidal compression. When multiple bones are involved this can lead to high output cardiac failure due to an arteriovenous shunting effect through the vascular affected bone. Affected bones are often warm, hyperaemic and may have an audible bruit. Pagetic bone is prone to develop painful microfractures and occasionally transverse fractures of long bones. Sarcomatous transformation is very rare: it carries a poor prognosis despite radical surgery. Hypercalcaemia and hypercalciuria may develop during prolonged immobilization.

Management A procedure for treatment is as follows:
- The main standby is bisphosphonates
- With etidronate sodium, use a high dose intermittently to avoid mineralization defect
- Pamidronate is used at a dose of 60 mg i.v. in 250–500 ml saline over 4 hours; give between one and four infusions as needed
- The first infusions (but rarely later ones) may cause transient, influenza-like symptoms
- Biochemical improvement or normalization is to be expected
- Remission may be for any period from months to permanent
- Calcitonin or plicamycin (mithramycin) are rarely required
- Newer orally active bisphosphonates used in Paget's disease include tiludronate, alendronate and risedronate

chapter 21

Hypoglycaemia

INTRODUCTION

Blood glucose is maintained within close limits (3.3–5.6 mmol/L) in normal individuals, including postprandially, for up to several days of fasting. The need to avoid low blood sugar levels largely derives from the absolute necessity for nervous tissue metabolism, especially within the cerebral cortex. The transport across the nerve cell membrane is dependent on the concentration gradient of glucose and is independent of insulin action. Cerebral metabolism is impaired when the plasma glucose falls below 3.0 mmol/l. A range of counter-regulatory mechanisms is activated at different thresholds above the level that causes neuroglycopenia and is strikingly effective in healthy people.

PATHOGENESIS AND PATHOLOGY

Hypoglycaemia occurs entirely as a result of the action of inappropriately secreted insulin (and more rarely that of non-insulin hypoglycaemic agents), or failure of hepatic glucose release (glycogenolysis and gluconeogenesis) or of counter-regulatory mechanisms (glucagon, adrenaline (epinephrine), cortisol and GH).

Classification of hyperinsulinaemic conditions

- Insulinoma
- Diffuse islet cell hyperplasia:
  — infant – nesidioblastosis
  — adult
- Exogenous insulin administration:
  — accidental/inappropriate
  — factitious/felonious
- Sulfonylurea drugs:
  — accidental/inappropriate
  — factitious/felonious
- Autoimmune insulin antibodies (seen especially in Japanese individuals)
- Non-islet cell hypersecretion of insulin (very rare)
- Tumoral (non-islet-cell hypoglycaemia)

Hypoglycaemia may be associated with non-islet-cell tumours secreting hypoglycaemia-inducing growth factors, especially IGF-II. These are consistently large tumours, and were previously thought to act mainly by increased glucose utilization by the tumour. Most are now considered to act by secreting incompletely processed IGF-II, which although larger than mature IGF-II does not circulate in the ternary complex with IGF-BP3 and the acid-labile subunit. Rather it occurs as a smaller complex that is more biologically active at the liver, inhibiting glucose production and skeletal muscle, enhancing glucose uptake.

Several types of tumour are associated with hypoglycaemia including mesenchymal (e.g. fibrosarcomas, mesotheliomas, leiomyosarcomas and haemangiopericytomas), epithelial (e.g. hepatomas, gastric, pancreatic exocrine and lung carcinomas) and haematopoietic types.

Miscellaneous causes of hypoglycaemia include:

- *Drugs.* Examples include ethanol, salicyclates, quinine, quinidine, haloperidol, pentamidine, β-adrenergic blockers, and ackee fruit poisoning
- *Infancy.* Examples are small-for-dates babies, Beckwith–Wiedemann syndrome, erythroblastosis fetalis and maternal diabetes
- *Metabolic disorders.* These include glycogen storage disease, defects in amino acid or fatty acid metabolism, Reye's disease, galactosaemia, fructose intolerance and carnitine deficiency
- *Endocrinopathy.* Examples include hypopituitarism, isolated GH deficiency, isolated ACTH deficiency and Addison's disease
- *Organ failure.* This may be due to sepsis, liver disease, renal failure, lactic acidosis, or shock

INVESTIGATION AND DIAGNOSIS

Hypoglycaemia may be difficult to diagnose because:
- It is relatively rare
- It is usually intermittent
- It is often suspected by patients claiming symptoms relieved by food or sugar
- Venous plasma glucose may fall below 2.5 mmol/L in fasting normal women
- Self-measurement by reflectance meters is unreliable in the low range of plasma glucose

The time of occurrence and the relationship to food as well as the nature of symptoms are unreliable guides to the underlying cause, despite long-held convictions to the contrary.

The initial step is to establish the fact of true hypoglycaemic episodes, defined as arterial or arterialized capillary plasma (not venous – see above) glucose less than 3.0 mmol/L. This can be definitely established only by laboratory measurement but can be performed on specimens collected by the patient into fluoride/heparin capillary tubes or on appropriately prepared filter paper. Since the majority of episodes occur in the fasting state, depending on the strength of suspicion about the validity of the condition one can arrange for the patient to attend at hospital on three mornings after fasting for 16 hours for measurement of plasma glucose. At the same time, adequate serum should be collected and sent rapidly to the laboratory for measuring insulin and C peptide (and sometimes proinsulin and hydroxybutyrate) if the glucose level is less than 3.0 mmol/L.

Alternatively if the index of suspicion is high it is advisable to arrange admission for a formal 72 hour fast. Essential features of this include strict exclusion of any caloric intake, including in drinks, elimination of all medication where possible, avoidance of caffeine and maintenance of physical activity in the waking hours. Blood is drawn every 6 hours for glucose and saved for insulin, C peptide and proinsulin measurement. When the glucose level falls below 3.3 mmol/L sampling should be performed every 1–2 hours until the plasma glucose falls below 2.5 mmol/L *and* the patient has symptoms. It is essential that all measurements are laboratory generated. The fast should continue wherever possible, despite symptoms, until biochemical confirmation is obtained.

If serious features such as coma or fits mandate immediate correction of possible hypoglycaemia then it is imperative that proper and full blood samples are properly taken prior to the administration of glucose. When plasma glucose levels are low without concomitant clinical features the fast should continue for the full 72 hours. When the fast ends, samples should be taken as previously, and a sulfonylurea drug screen added, with measurements of β-hydroxybutyrate, IGF-I and IGF-II (whether the duration is the full 72 hours or circumstances dictate its truncation). If applicable, one should also measure cortisol and GH or check the glucose response at 10, 20 and 30 minutes after administration of glucagon (1 mg i.v.).

Classification of hypoglycaemia

- Normal (pseudohypoglycaemia)
- Hyperinsulinaemic
- Non-hyperinsulinaemic

A pragmatic clinical approach to investigating hypoglycaemia is:
- First, check whether patient looks ill; if so, suspect a tumour or metabolic consequences of severe illness such as multiple organ failure
- In young females with paramedical connections episodes are often spurious, and sometimes factitious

ENDOGENOUS HYPERINSULINAEMIA

Insulinomas are usually benign, and often small; fewer than 10% are multiple, or associated with MEN-1. The characteristic biochemical findings when blood is sampled with a plasma glucose level of less than 2.8 mmol/L are:

Biochemical findings with insulinoma:
- Insulin > 30 pmol/L
- C-peptide > 300 pmol/L
- Proinsulin > 20 pmol/L

Biochemical findings in factitious hyperinsulinism due to exogenous insulin:
- C peptide < 100 pmol/L
- Proinsulin < 20 pmol/L

Biochemical findings in sulfonylurea drug overdose:
- Insulin > 30 pmol/L
- C peptide >100 pmol/L
- Proinsulin low

The rare autoimmune syndrome is difficult to identify, though other autoimmune conditions may coexist. It appears to be relatively common in Japan. The presence of hypoglycaemia postprandially may be associated with inappropriate insulin secretion in the late-developing dumping syndrome. It may also occur in patients with diffuse changes in islet cell structure and function in the adult counterpart of nesidioblastosis. There is no role for the 5 hour glucose tolerance test in the diagnosis of 'reactive' hypoglycaemia.

Localization of insulinoma

Often the most sensitive approach is for an experienced surgeon's hands to palpate the pancreas. However, it is desirable to try and localize the source of insulin preoperatively. This can be attempted using dynamic CT or MR scanning, which though imperfect may be useful in experienced hands.

Transhepatic portal venous sampling is invasive but can be very helpful. Intra-arterial calcium injected selectively into the major pancreatic arteries restricts the source to a small area of pancreas, provided only one injection provokes a rapid release of insulin into a draining hepatic vein. Alternatively it may elicit responses from all injections if there is diffuse islet disease.

Endoscopic ultrasonography can be useful, especially if the source is near the head of pancreas. Results from an octreotide scan are often disappointing as positive somatostatin receptors are found in only half or less of insulinomas examined. On the other hand, peroperative ultrasonography is highly valuable.

CLINICAL FEATURES AND MANAGEMENT

Symptoms of hypoglycaemia may be subdivided into:
- Autonomic symptoms
- Neuroglycopenic symptoms (due to cerebral insufficiency of glucose)

Investigators have failed to reach agreement for the precise allocation of some symptoms, including, surprisingly, such features as hunger, blurred vision, drowsiness and weakness. Features vary with circumstances, cause and age.

Common features of hypoglycaemia in patients with insulinomas

- In 85% – a combination of diplopia and blurred vision, sweating, palpitations and weakness
- In 80% – confused or abnormal behaviour
- In 53% – unconsciousness or coma
- In 12% – generalized seizures

There is marked variation in symptoms experienced by various people but consistency between episodes for any single individual. The common presumption that autonomic features precede neuroglycopenic symptoms is not invariably true and indeed neuroglycopenia may occur alone.

The protean presentations of hypoglycaemia require verification by 'Whipple's triad'. This comprises:

- Biochemically proven hypoglycaemia (defined as arterialized blood glucose less than 3.0 mmol/L
- During spontaneously occurring symptoms
- Which are specifically reversed when the low blood sugar level is corrected

MANAGEMENT

The immediate management of hypoglycaemia includes its acute correction by the use of intravenous glucose injection using a 50% solution. One must be wary of excess dosage, which can lead to serious, even fatal, cerebral oedema. Intramuscular glucagon may also be of great value in the acute situation. Subsequent treatment is directed to the underlying cause as determined by the investigative protocols previously discussed.

Insulinomas require surgical extirpation, the main problem being localization of small tumours. There is also an increasing use of peroperative endoscopy to supplement the skilled surgeon's palpation. If multiple tumours are present or there is diffuse disease (nesidioblastosis) a decision is required about the amount of pancreatic resection needed, balancing the crises of recurrent hypoglycaemia against those of exocrine pancreatic insufficiency and diabetes mellitus. Malignant insulinomas are relatively rare but may continue to cause hypoglycaemia postoperatively, which can be addressed by use of diazoxide (in combination with a thiazide diuretic to deal with the ensuing sodium retention). Hypertrichosis is a distressing side-effect, especially in women, which may be caused by diazoxide after long-term use. Streptozotocin is an antimitotic agent with the potential for specific destruction of pancreatic islet beta cells. In about half of insulinomas there is sufficient density of somatostatin receptors to provide a therapeutically useful response from the use of long-acting analogues of somatostatin such as octreotide or lanreotide.

In tumoral hypoglycaemia the main focus of treatment is surgical debulking of these often large tumours, followed sometimes by chemotherapy and radiotherapy. Occasionally GH therapy has been useful in ameliorating intractable hypoglycaemia due to such tumours. In many seriously ill patients with sepsis, multiorgan failure or both, the hypoglycaemia is more of an epiphenomenon, but if severe it nevertheless requires appropriate glucose administration pending possible correction of the underlying causes. In the case of long-standing late dumping syndrome, octreotide is of considerable value, albeit often associated with frequent side-effects especially abdominal bloating and steatorrhoea.

chapter 22

Gastrointestinal Hormones

INTRODUCTION

The first hormone to be described, secretin, was isolated from the gastrointestinal tract in 1902 (by Bayliss and Starling). Despite this, the endocrine function of the gut remains incompletely understood. The endocrine cells of the gut are not grouped together, but rather scattered throughout its length (**Fig. 22.1**). The peptide hormones produced act mostly as paracrine agents, acting on neighbouring cells, or as neurotransmitters within the myenteric plexi rather than as circulating hormones. Interestingly, many of these peptides also function as neurotransmitters within the central nervous system, particularly in control of appetite.

Clinical disorders associated with gastrointestinal hormones are very rare. There are no recognized consequences of gut hormone deficiency, but syndromes of excess are found in association with gastroenteropancreatic (GEP) tumours (also called gastrointestinal neuroendocrine or gut hormone tumours).

PATHOPHYSIOLOGY

The endocrine cells of the gastrointestinal tract produce a large number of peptides, whose functions are only partly understood (**Fig. 22.2**). There are a number of features of these endocrine cells and their peptide products that have implications for the behaviour of GEP tumours:

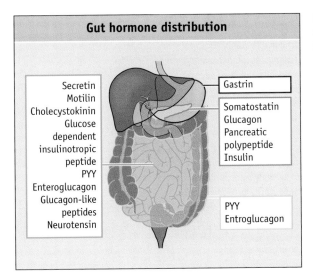

Gut hormone distribution

Secretin
Motilin
Cholecystokinin
Glucose dependent insulinotropic peptide
PYY
Enteroglucagon
Glucagon-like peptides
Neurotensin

Gastrin

Somatostatin
Glucagon
Pancreatic polypeptide
Insulin

PYY
Entroglucagon

Fig. 22.1 *Distribution of hormones through the gastrointestinal tract.*

Fig. 22.2   Functions of common gastrointestinal hormones

Hormone	Function
Gastrin	Gastric acid secretion
Cholecystokinin	Pancreatic enzyme secretion
	Gall bladder contraction
	Pancreatic growth
Secretin	Alkaline pancreatic secretions
Glucose-dependent insulinotropic peptide (GIP)	Insulin secretion
Enteroglucagon	Gut growth
Glucagon-like peptide 1 (GLP-1)	Insulin secretion
	Inhibition of gastric acid secretion
Peptide-tyrosine-tyrosine (PYY)	Delays gastric emptying
	Inhibition of gastric acid secretion
Motilin	Contraction of gastrointestinal smooth muscle
Somatostatin	Inhibition of:
	• Gastric acid secretion
	• Gastric emptying
	• Gall bladder contraction
	• Gastrointestinal mobility
	• Secretion of insulin and glucagon
	• Pancreatic enzymes secretion
Vasoactive intestinal polypeptide (VIP)	Inhibition of gastric acid secretion
	Relaxation of biliary and intestinal smooth muscle
	Insulin secretion

- They are pluripotential with respect to peptide hormone production, having the capability to produce different peptides under different circumstances; therefore a tumour associated with excess of one gastrointestinal hormone may secrete excessive amounts of another hormone, causing a secondary tumour syndrome as it evolves
- The peptide hormones are derived from larger precursor propeptides, which can be processed in alternative ways to produce different peptides with various biological effects (**Fig. 22.3**)
- There may be molecular heterogeneity of peptide hormones; for example, somatostatin can occur in forms containing 14 or 29 amino acids, excess of the former causing hyperglycaemia and that of the latter causing hypoglycaemia, owing to differential inhibition of other peptide hormone actions

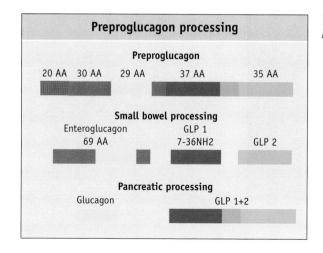

Fig. 22.3 *Processing of preproglucagon.*

Gastrointestinal diseases, such as inflammatory bowel disease, malabsorption and diarrhoea, are associated with characteristic changes in gastrointestinal hormone levels. However, the clinical significance of these changes remains unclear.

Tumours associated with gastrointestinal hormone excess are rare (see **Fig 22.5**). They usually arise sporadically but can occur in association with MEN-1 (see Ch. 23), when they are invariably multiple.

CLINICAL FEATURES AND INVESTIGATION

CARCINOID TUMOURS

Carcinoid tumours can be derived from the following embryonic tissues:

- *Foregut.* Bronchus, stomach and pancreas
- *Midgut.* Small intestine and ascending colon
- *Hindgut.* Distal colon and rectum

Rarely they may arise in the gonads.

They have an annual incidence of 1 in 150 000, the commonest sites being the appendix (40%), small bowel (25%), rectum (15%) and bronchus (10%).

Carcinoid syndrome

The carcinoid syndrome (**Fig. 22.4**) occurs in about 10% of patients with carcinoid tumours. It results from the secretion of a variety of peptide products by the tumour, but particularly serotonin, bradykinins, histamine and substance P. However, most carcinoid tumours drain into the liver, and their peptide products are degraded there so that they do not exert any clinical effect. Only if the tumours metastasize to the liver (as do small bowel tumours commonly, but not tumours of the appendix or rectum), or drain directly into the systemic circulation (as do bronchial carcinoids), does the carcinoid syndrome occur.

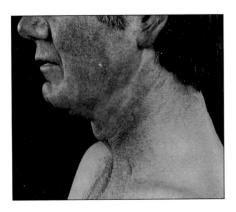

Fig. 22.4 *Flushing in the carcinoid syndrome.*

Clinical features of carcinoid syndrome

- Flushing (95%)
- Secretory diarrhoea (75%)
- Bronchospasm
- Endocardial fibrosis (50%)
- Tricuspid incompetence (90%)
- Pulmonary valve lesions (50%)
- Pellagra (10%)
- Cachexia
- Carcinoid crises
- Circulatory collapse with flushing and diarrhoea
- Pleural fibrosis
- Arthropathy
- Myopathy

Diagnosis

The diagnosis of a carcinoid tumour is based on the histological appearance, particularly the presence of neuroendocrine markers and the effect of staining with silver.

The carcinoid syndrome is usually confirmed by the finding of elevated levels of 5-hydroxyindoleacetic acid (5HIAA), a metabolite of serotonin (5-hydroxytryptamine, or 5HT), in a 24 hour urine collection.

GASTROENTEROPANCREATIC TUMOURS

The different syndromes of gastrointestinal excess have their own characteristic features (**Fig. 22.5**). Among these are glucagonoma syndrome rash, necrolytic migratory erythema (**Fig. 22.6**), and the multiple ulcers (often in atypical sites such as the oesophagus or small bowel) seen in the gastrinoma syndrome (**Fig. 22.7**).

Diagnosis

Once the suspicion has been raised the diagnosis is based on the finding of elevated levels of the particular hormone on a fasting gut hormone screen. In the case of the gastrinoma

Fig. 22.5 Features of the gut hormone tumour syndromes

Gut hormone tumour	Clinical features
Gastrinoma (annual incidence 1:1 000 000)	Peptic ulceration: • Multiple • Atypical sites e.g. jejunum, Oesophagus • Complications e.g. perforation, haemorrhage Diarrhoea/steatorrhoea
VIPoma (annual incidence 1:10 000 000)	Secretory diarrhoea: • Usually > 3 L per day • Weakness, dehydration Hypokalaemic acidosis
Glucagonoma (annual incidence 1:20 000 000)	Necrolytic migratory erythema Impaired glucose tolerance Venous thrombosis, possibly life-threatening Weight loss
Somatostatinoma (annual incidence 1:50 000 000)	Impaired carbohydrate metabolism • Hyperglycaemia • Hypoglycaemia Steatorrhoea Gall bladder disease

syndrome, confirmatory evidence of increased basal acid secretion is needed, since gastrin levels are usually increased in patients on drugs to reduce gastric acid secretion and in people with achlorhydria.

Patients more commonly present with a pancreatic neuroendocrine tumour that appears to be non-functioning. In these patients the diagnosis is made either on the histological appearance or after the tumour has followed a more indolent course than that expected of a pancreatic adenocarcinoma. Also the pancreatic polypeptide levels are usually elevated and other hormones, such as somatostatin or neurotensin, may be found in excess. Immunocytochemistry may demonstrate that tumours have the capability to synthesize a number of different peptide hormones, even if they are not found in excess in the circulation.

TUMOUR IMAGING

Most GEP and carcinoid tumours are large at the time of diagnosis, usually with hepatic metastases, and are easily identified by ultrasound or cross-sectional imaging (CT or MRI – Fig. 22.8). In contrast, gastrinomas, insulinomas (see Ch. 21) and bronchial carcinoids are usually very small, just a few millimeters in diameter, and so can be difficult to identify. Although bronchial carcinoids are almost always identified by a combination of plain radiographs and cross-sectional imaging, gastrinomas and insulinomas may require a combination of methods. These include:

Radiolabelled octreotide (somatostatin analogue) scanning may also be helpful in identifying the extent of metastatic disease, particularly from carcinoid tumours (Fig. 22.10).

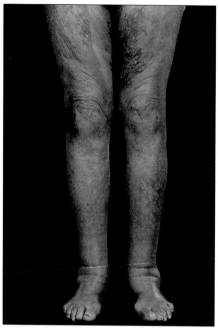

Fig. 22.6 *Necrolytic migratory erythema – the pathognomonic feature of the glucagonoma syndrome.*

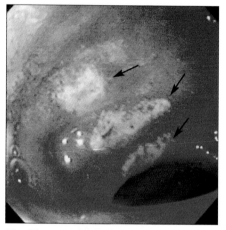

Fig. 22.7 *Multiple duodenal ulcers in a patient with the gastrinoma syndrome.*

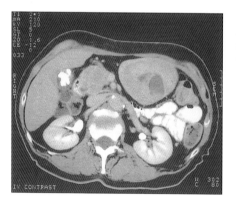

Fig. 22.8 *CT scan of a patient with a metastatic glucagonoma showing a large calcified primary lesion in the pancreas and hepatic metastases.*

Identification of all tumours in patients with MEN-1 may require various imaging modalities, as multiple duodenal gastrinomas are a frequent occurrence (see **Fig. 22.9**).

MANAGEMENT

Where possible, curative surgical resection is indicated. This is most commonly an option for insulinomas and small gastrinomas. Where the tumour has not been localized preoperatively then consideration should be given to perioperative localization by palpation and intraoperative ultrasound.

- *Highly selective visceral angiography* (**Fig. 22.9**)
- *Endoscopic ultrasound.* This is good for small lesions of the pancreatic head
- *Radiolabelled octreotide (somatostatin analogue) scanning.* This is useful if tumours are somatostatin receptor positive (this is less common with insulinomas) and has good resolution if there is a high receptor density (**Fig. 22.10**)
- *Venous sampling after selective arterial injection of secretagogue.* Secretin is injected for gastrinomas, and calcium for insulinomas; the method allows regionalization of the tumour to an arterial bed

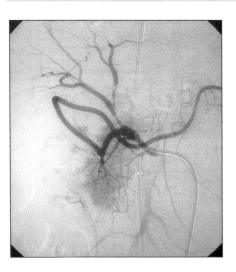

Fig. 22.9   Highly selective visceral angiography showing multiple blushes in the duodenum from microgastrinomas associated with MEN-1.

In the case of other tumours where metastases have already occurred, occasional patients may be cured by excision of the primary tumour and liver with all metastases followed by hepatic transplantation. For the majority, however, the options are to reduce symptoms from tumour bulk and hormone excess by:

- Surgical debulking of tumour metastases
- Hepatic embolization of hepatic metastases
- Chemotherapy or immunotherapy:
  — 5-fluorouracil, streptozotocin and/or doxorubicin for GEP tumours, with response rates of 60–70%
  — Interferon α for carcinoid tumours with response rates of around 75%
- Somatostatin analogues such as octreotide, which reduce hormone secretion and possibly tumour bulk when tumours carry analogue-binding receptors

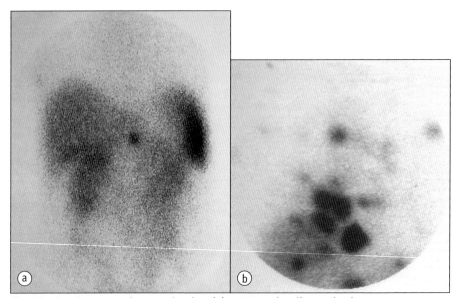

Fig. 22.10 *Octreoscan images showing (a) a 1.5 cm insulinoma in the pancreas; (b) soft tissue and bone metastases from a carcinoid tumour.*

Patients with metastatic gastrinoma or unlocalized primary gastrinoma should be treated with omeprazole to reduce gastric acid secretion, the dose being titrated upwards until symptoms are relieved.

PROGNOSIS

The behaviour of carcinoid and other GEP tumours is very hard to predict. The original patient with gastrinoma syndrome described in 1955 (by Zollinger and Ellison) was still alive 40 years later despite having metastases at the time of diagnosis. Rarely, however, the tumours are much more aggressive and rapidly metastasize so proving fatal. In the majority of cases, the course of the disease is more indolent than for adenocarcinomas, with median survival rates in excess of 5 years.

chapter 23

Plurihormonal, Genetic and Ectopic Hormone Syndromes

INTRODUCTION

This chapter encompasses the following heterogeneous group of disorders:

- Multiple endocrine neoplasia – familial
  – sporadic
- Other familial endocrine neoplastic syndromes
- Somatic mutations in endocrine disorders
- Ectopic hormone secretion

The unifying premise tying these disparate scenarios together is that all somatic cells share the same genetic complement in any individual, which is differentially expressed to allow cellular differentiation and phenotypic expression. The degree to which genes for different hormones are expressed in different tissues other than the classical glands varies. Some groups appear together more often than do others, which accounts for the prevalence of some syndromes.

PATHOGENESIS AND PATHOLOGY

The dysregulation of hormone secretion underlying all these disorders does not directly involve the genes involved in the hormone production – hence the hormones produced are in themselves essentially normal. However, differences from the authentic glandular products may arise from abnormalities in hormone processing. This is seen, for instance, with POMC, which may not cleave fully into equimolar fragments including ACTH and β endorphin. Other hormonal differences can arise post-translationally, resulting for example from changes in the degrees of glycosylation and methylation.

MULTIPLE ENDOCRINE NEOPLASIA

Two major varieties of MEN are recognized:

- Multiple endocrine neoplasia type 1 (MEN-1)
- Multiple endocrine neoplasia type 2 (MEN-2)

Both of these can display various subtypes, and both can also occur either sporadically or as familial forms.

Familial forms

The familial types have been linked to point mutations in tumour suppressor genes. The gene for MEN-1 is located on chromosome 11 (11q13) and its protein product is called menin. The gene for MEN-2 is located on chromosome 10 (10q11.2) and has been identified as the *RET* proto-oncogene, which encodes a receptor tyrosine kinase expressed in neural crest-derived tissue.

The mutations in the *MEN-1* gene found in different families appear scattered throughout the gene. In contrast, mutations of the *MEN-2* gene are associated with particular phenotypes (**Fig. 23.1**). MEN-2a is most commonly the result of mutation at codon 634 in exon 11. Other mutations in the adjacent exon 10, part of the extracellular cysteine-rich region, are more commonly associated with familial medullary carcinoma of thyroid (MCT), as are several mutations in the intracellular tyrosine kinase domain. The *RET* proto-oncogene is of particular interest, as it appears to have two separate functions: that of encoding receptor tyrosine kinase, as mentioned above, and an activating role in the

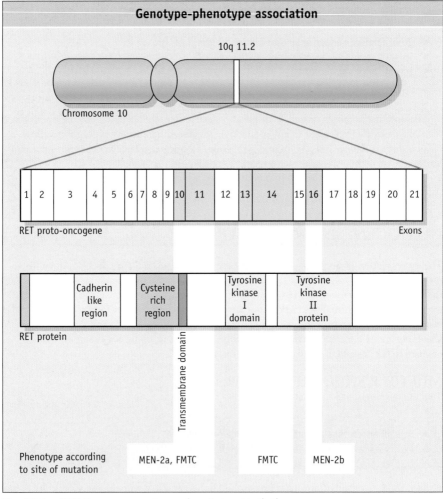

Fig. 23.1 *MEN-2a gene: genotype–phenotype association.*

development of Meissner's and Auerbach's plexuses in the intestine. Mutations causing loss of the latter function have led to Hirschsprung's disease in several families. These mutations were found to be on codons 618 and 620, whereas the MEN-2b phenotype (which is associated with ganglioneuromatosis but virtually never hyperparathyroidism) is predominantly associated with mis-sense mutations in codon 918 largely derived from the paternal chromosome.

Germline mutations are associated with familial syndromes. In MEN-1 it appears that the two-hit hypothesis (proposed by Knudsen) is applicable – that is, the inherited mutation on one allele requires a second somatic mutation in the normal dominant allele in order to have a deleterious effect on the phenotype. In MEN-2, in contrast, the associated mis-sense mutations are activating – hence only a single allele needs to be affected to cause disease (Fig. 23.2).

Sporadic forms

Sporadic MEN-1 and MEN-2 syndromes result from somatic mutations (see below). As mentioned above, about a third of MEN-2 cases have mutations in the *RET* proto-oncogene, particularly at codon 918.

APUDOMA THEORY

Many endocrine tumours display characteristic features. These have been the basis of the APUD (amine precursor uptake and decarboxylase) hypothesis (of Pearse). According to this hypothesis there is an embryological origin in the neural crest for cells ultimately giving rise to such tumours. An elegant transplant experiment involving chick and quail chimaeras (by

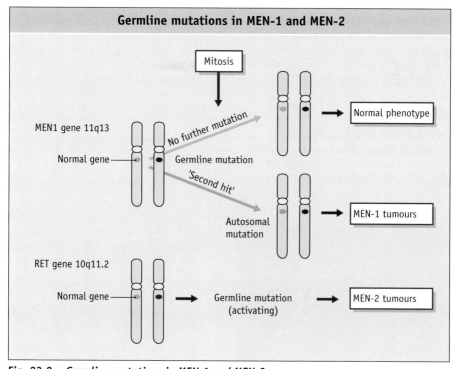

Fig. 23.2 *Germline mutations in MEN-1 and MEN-2.*

Le Douarin and colleagues) lent support for it with regard to C cells of the thyroid. However, the theory is not an adequate explanation for the origin of all cells displaying APUD characteristics.

Features characterizing APUD tissue include:

Features of APUD tissue

- 5-hydroxytryptophan uptake
- Fluorogenic amine content
- α glycerophosphate
- Esterase or cholinesterase, or both
- Amino acid decarboxylase activity
- Chromogranin
- Dense core secretory granules
- Membrane-bound secretory vesicles
- Rough endoplasmic reticulum
- Smooth endoplasmic reticulum
- Free ribosomes

MEDULLARY CELL CARCINOMA OF THYROID

These tumours are often a presenting feature of MEN-2. They may be difficult to differentiate from other thyroid tumours. They commonly (in 60–80% of cases) contain amyloid, which stains with Congo red (**Fig.23.3**). The characteristic finding, however, is immunostaining with calcitonin antiserum (**Fig. 23.4a,b**). The premalignant phase of MEN-2 displays C-cell hyperplasia, but this may be difficult to assess; various quantitative criteria are used such as 'greater than 50 C cells in each of at least three high power fields'. Sporadic cases showing C-cell hyperplasia in the thyroid outside the area of frank carcinoma raise the question of undiagnosed familial disease, so necessitating genetic and hormone screening.

SOMATIC MUTATIONS

Somatic mutations (the *Gsp* oncogene) may cause constitutive activation of Gs protein. These can occur in single or multiple tissues, and have been associated with endocrine and non-endocrine disorders, especially:

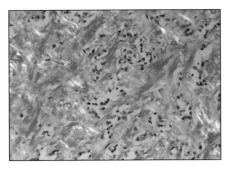

Fig. 23.3   *MCT: amyloid tissue stained with Congo red.*

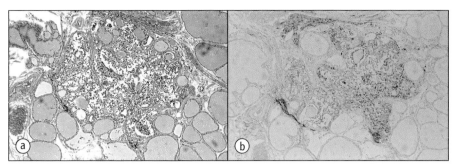

Fig. 23.4 *(a, b) MCT: immunostaining with calcitonin antiserum*

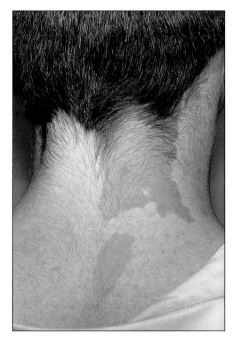

Fig. 23.5 *McCune-Albright syndrome.*

- McCune–Albright syndrome (**Fig. 23.5**)
- Acromegaly
- Toxic thyroid adenoma

INVESTIGATION AND DIAGNOSIS

MEN

MEN-1

Hyperparathyroidism is present in 95% of cases. The presence of hyperparathyroidism should be confirmed biochemically, and a sestamibi scan considered. MEN-1 should also always be suspected if concomitant pituitary or pancreatic disease is present. Watch out also for other features such as carcinoids, or adrenal cortical disorders.

If there is a known positive family history then consider examining the *MEN-1* gene for mutation.

Also check the following:
- The fasting glucose and gut hormone profile (i.e. gastrin, glucagon and pancreatic polypeptide)
- PRL levels (and those of GH if acromegaly is suspected)
- The pituitary, with a MRI or CT scan

MEN-2a

First check the calcitonin level if there is a suspicious fine needle aspirate, or a positive family history. If the calcitonin is borderline then consider a pentagastrin stimulation test.

If the calcitonin is positive then check for lymph node, lung and adrenal metastases.

If there is a positive history then investigate a possible *RET* proto-oncogene mutation.

Check the following:
- 24 urine catecholamine excretion every 1–2 years
- The adrenals, with a CT or MRI scan
- The calcium and PTH levels
- CEA, as an increase in this suggests a poor prognosis

Also watch out for diarrhoeal or ectopic ACTH syndromes.

MEN-2b

The procedure for this is as above, except that hyperparathyroidism is not seen. Also, it is necessary to screen or act earlier because of the more aggressive behaviour of this type.

Check for hypertrophy of the corneal nerves by slit-lamp examination.

Note any marfanoid features (see **Fig. 23.10**, p. 393) and symptoms of ganglioneuromatosis, in the gut and bladder.

OTHER SYNDROMES
von Hippel–Lindau syndrome

Investigate the possibility of a mutation in gene located at chromosome 3p24-25. Also, a phaeochromocytoma is sometimes seen, especially with a mutation at codon 238.

Check for the following tumours:
- Pancreatic tumour – which is rarely endocrinologically active
- Renal carcinoma, cerebellar and retinal lesions

Neurofibromatosis type I

Check for phaeochromocytoma if there are any suggestive clinical features.

Polyposis coli/Gardener's syndrome

If there are any concomitant thyroid nodules then perform a fine needle aspiration.

ECTOPIC HORMONE PRODUCTION
Ectopic ACTH production

Localize the possible source of production with a CT scan of the thorax. Consider also other possible sites including the pancreas, thyroid (medullary cell carcinoma), adrenals (phaeochromocytoma), liver and ovaries.

Assess the potassium and acid/base status, and blood sugar. Also check the following:

- Urinary cortisol excretion
- Plasma ACTH levels (and if the diagnosis is uncertain then check for POMC precursors)
- Dexamethasone suppressibility (See Ch. 18)
  CRH or desmopressin tests, or both, may also be useful.

Ectopic ADH secretion

Check the thorax with a CT scan if a plain chest X-ray is inconclusive. Consider also other possible sites, including the duodenum, pancreas, ureter, bladder and prostate.

Possible causes include:

- Thymoma
- Mesothelioma
- Ewing's sarcoma

Pancreatic islet tumours (see Ch. 22)

Check first for coincidental hyperparathyroidism. There may also be multiple hormone production, especially gastrin, VIP, pancreatic polypeptide, glucagon, ACTH, somatostatin and GHRH. Also check the PRL level.

There may be multiple sites; metastases occur especially with Zollinger–Ellison syndrome.

Malignant hypercalcaemia

Check for PTH (which is usually undetectable), and consider measuring PTH-related hormone.

Investigate for malignancy using chest X-ray, CT scan, bronchoscopy or cytology as appropriate. Consider the possibility of:

- Renal, bladder, oesophagus, head and neck squamous carcinomas
- Thyroid and breast cancer
  Look for bony metastases, using an isotope scan plus X-rays as indicated

Check also for haematological malignancy especially myeloma, using serum and urine protein electrophoresis, tests for Bence Jones protein, and β2 microglobulin. If haematological malignancy is found then check the blood count and bone marrow, and take a CT scan of the chest and abdomen.

CLINICAL FEATURES AND MANAGEMENT

MEN-1 SYNDROME

There is almost invariably hyperparathyroidism. However, the presenting complaint is often due to a pancreatic islet cell tumour, which occurs in only 30–80% of patients with the syndrome. This can be partly explained by the usually striking clinical features of the pancreatic lesion in contrast to the hypercalcaemia due to the hyperparathyroidism.

Note that within the large population of presumed sporadic hyperparathyroidism patients is a subset of clinically unrecognized MEN-1 patients.

Gastrinoma (Zollinger–Ellison syndrome) (see also Ch. 22)

This is the commonest pancreatic lesion, forming more then 50% of such lesions. The lesions are frequently multiple, often metastatic to the liver, and may be extrapancreatic. The clinical features include:

Clinical features of gastrinoma

- Recurrent severe peptic ulceration
- Raised fasting gastrin secretion and gastric acid production
- Frequent steatorrhoea and diarrhoea
- Possibly other associated tumour products, e.g. ACTH, glucagon and pancreatic polypeptide

Management (see also Ch. 22)
- Localization includes dynamic CT and MRI scanning; endoscopic/intraoperative ultrasound (**Fig. 23.6**) can be useful
- Octreotide scanning can demonstrate distant metastases
- In difficult cases, demonstrate post-secretin gastrin secretion
- Use selective intra-arterial calcium injections as a gastrin secretagogue; this is measured in the hepatic vein
- If the tumour is localized then remove by surgical resection (laparoscopic methods are available). If lesions are multiple then consider partial resection
- Incompletely treated tumours require a high dose proton pump blocker, e.g. omeprazole. In metastatic disease, consider streptozotocin, 5-fluorouracil, octreotide, hepatic artery embolization, interferon or radical surgery
- Total gastrectomy is infrequently indicated nowadays, unless there is poor drug compliance
- Postoperative management may entail the use of insulin or pancreatic exocrine supplements

Insulinoma
This accounts for 30% of pancreatic tumours in MEN-1. (See Ch. 21 for details.)

Glucagonoma (see also Ch. 22)
This is a rare, α-cell islet tumour. Fifty per cent of such tumours are malignant (surgically incurable) at the time of presentation. The clinical features include:

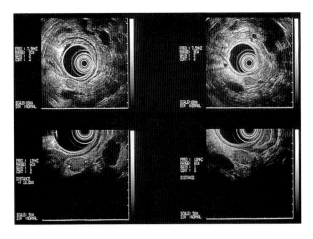

Fig. 23.6 *Endoscopic ultrasound showing multiple gastrinoma in MEN-2a.*

Clinical features of glucagonoma

- High plasma glucagon and glucose intolerance
- Variable presence of necrolytic migratory erythematous rash
- Weight loss
- Stomatitis
- Anaemia
- Possibly concomitant production of other ectopic hormones such as ACTH or gastrin

Management
- The first-line treatment is surgery; the tumour is usually in the tail of the pancreas
- This may not remove all of the tumour, because of secondary spread
- Adjuvant medical therapy may therefore be required, involving octreotide or streptozotocin

VIP-oma
This rare tumour usually occurs as part of the MEN-1 complex. Its clinical features include:

Clinical features of VIP-oma

- Watery diarrhoea, hypokalaemia and achlorhydria – which may be metabolically devastating
- Tumours, largely in the tail of the pancreas

Management
- Octreotide may bring about a dramatic reduction in symptoms
- Chemotherapy is also strikingly effective for VIP-oma compared with other pancreatic syndromes
- In some cases surgery may prove curative
- In long-term follow-up any relapses may respond to high dose corticosteroid given for up to 6 months

Follow-up of pancreatic tumours
It is evident with long-term follow-up that a progression in hormone production and hence clinical features occurs, the most significant of which is the late appearance of hypergastrinaemia. Hence it is recommended that the follow-up includes repeat full gut hormone profile measurements at approximately 6–12 month intervals.

Hyperparathyroidism
(For the clinical features of hyperparathyroidism, see Ch. 20.)
Management of hyperparathyroidism in MEN-1
- Surgery is the only currently available therapy
- Even if adenomas are present and removed, all four glands are affected
- There is a high recurrence rate of hypercalcaemia after subtotal surgery

- Total parathyroidectomy leads to hypoparathyroidism
- Autotransplantation of parathyroid tissue into the forearm is performed in some centres

Pituitary tumours

(For the clinical features and management of pituitary tumours, see Ch. 15.)
Other rare manifestations of MEN-1 include the following.

Carcinoid tumours (see also Ch. 22)

Carcinoid tumours are capable of producing several peptides as well as 5HT and related compounds. Localization should be performed with an octreotide scan (**Fig. 23.7**), CT and MR scanning, and a small bowel enema. Carcinoid syndrome (see below) is usually seen in midgut lesions with multiple hepatic metastases.

The clinical features include:

Clinical features of carcinoid tumours

- Carcinoid syndrome: flushing, diarrhoea, wheezing and right heart valvular disorder
- 24 hour urinary 5HIAA levels are usually raised
- Carcinoids of foregut origin may secrete 5-hydroxytryptophan and various peptides such as ACTH, CRH, GHRH or histamine
- Massive release of vasoactive compounds occurs in carcinoid crisis, e.g. in surgery

---

Management
- Surgery is often but not invariably indicated; debulking is beneficial
- Hepatic metastases may be embolized or resected; a hepatic transplant may be required
- Octreotide may ameliorate flushing and diarrhoea, and lower 5HIAA levels
- Octreotide pretreatment perioperatively minimizes the risk of crisis
- Long-term benefit may occur in selected patients with chemotherapy using 5-fluorouracil, or interferon α

Adrenocortical lesions

These lesions are usually non-functional. (For their management see Ch. 18.)

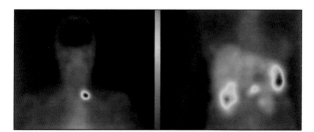

Fig. 23.7   *Octreotide scan of carcinoid tumour.*

MEN-2A SYNDROME

The earliest presentation of this syndrome is usually with MCT as this chronologically usually precedes phaeochromocytoma and is expressed more often (**Fig. 23.8**). It usually appears as a solitary mass in the upper or mid thyroid. There may also be the following suspicious or tumoral features:

Clinical features

- Hardness or lymphadenopathy
- Flushing, diarrhoea or wheezing
- Rarely ectopic ACTH secretion

There are also less common features of the MEN-2a syndrome, including pruritic and pigmented papular lesions of the skin on the upper back, a form of lichen amyloidosis (notalgia, **Fig. 23.9**), which often occurs early. Primary hyperparathyroidism occurs in 10–25% of MEN-2a carriers and is normally mild, occurring late in cases with codon 634 mutations. Early stages involve parathyroid hyperplasia, progressing to one or more adenomas with increasing age.

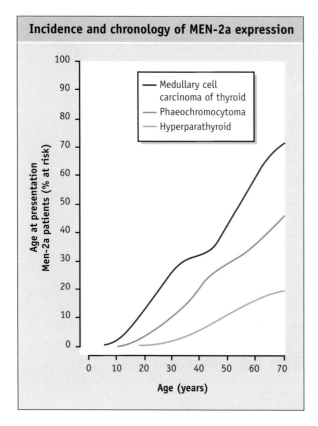

Fig. 23.8 *Incidence and chronology of phenotypic expression of MEN-2a.*

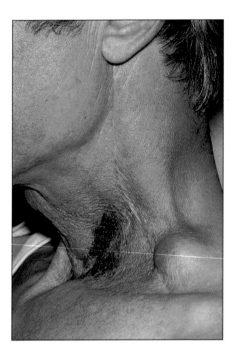

Fig. 23.9   Skin pigmentation (notalgia) in MEN-2a.

Phaeochromocytoma generally presents later clinically than MCT but of course may be picked up on screening such patients (see below). The lesion is bilateral in 50% of cases. (For its clinical features and management see Ch. 18.)

MEN-2B SYNDROME

Clinical features

- Marfanoid features
- Thickened lips
- MTC, phaeochromocytomas
- Thickened corneal nerves, skeletal manifestations
- Subfertility

This syndrome is characterized by marfanoid features (**Fig. 23.10**), thickened lips due to neuromas at the mucocutaneous junction, early and aggressive MCT, and phaeochromocytomas but not parathyroid disorders. Slit-lamp examination may demonstrate thickened corneal nerves. Other skeletal manifestations include pectus excavatum and slipped femoral epiphyses. Intrinsic subfertility seems likely, which with other features means familial occurrence is rare. Most cases are new mutations.

SCREENING FOR FAMILIAL ENDOCRINE SYNDROMES

The identification of specific genes responsible for many heritable conditions has greatly improved the scope for screening, which previously depended on detecting the late and variable phenotypic markers – usually biochemical or hormonal.

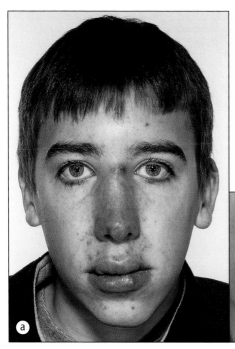
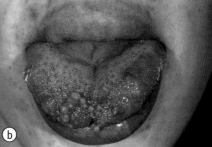

Fig. 23.10 *(a) Marfanoid facies and (b) labial and lingual neuromas of patient with MEN-2b.*

MEN-2a provides the clearest situation as specific mutations in the *RET* proto-oncogene can be identified in 95% of familial cases (see above). Gene carriers born to an affected parent are known to display C-cell hyperplasia prior to malignant transformation and prophylactic total thyroidectomy by skilled paediatric endocrine surgeons is commonly offered at a much earlier age (usually about 6 years) than when identification relied on detecting pentagastrin-releasable calcitonin. This is because rare cases of frank carcinoma have been found at such early times. The detection of phaeochromocytoma requires regular biochemical screening, commonly 24 hour urinary catecholamines measured every 2 years. Rising adrenaline levels often indicate prodromal adrenomedullary hyperplasia. A potential new marker in this syndrome is plasma normetanephrine and metanephrine. Annual measurements of calcium are indicated.

In contrast, the mutations associated with MEN-1 are scattered throughout the gene and are more often not identified. Biochemical screening, including measurement of calcium, PRL and gut hormones, therefore remains important.

Von Hippel–Lindau mutation analysis is useful for screening especially if phaeochromocytoma occurs in the family. As above, the measurement of plasma of normetanephrine and metanephrine has been advocated.

The incidence of phaeochromocytoma in neurofibromatosis type I is probably too low to warrant screening in the absence of any suggestive clinical features.

ECTOPIC HORMONE SECRETION
Management of ectopic ACTH secretion (see also Ch. 18)
- Block cortisol synthesis; if complete give dexamethasone 0.25–0.5 mg
- If the source is identified then remove this surgically (**Fig. 23.11**)

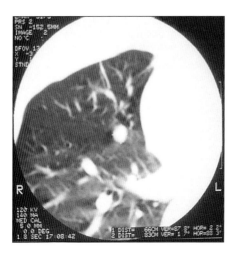

Fig. 23.11 *8 mm diameter bronchial carcinoid in right lower lobe causing ectopic ACTH syndrome.*

- Replace corticosteroids and gradually reduce to permit normal activity of the hypothalamo-pituitary axis (HPA)

Management of ectopic ADH secretion (see also Ch. 14)
- If there is acute hyponatraemia leading to fits or coma, partly correct this with 2N saline
- Restrict fluid input to 500 ml/day
- Monitor plasma and urinary electrolytes and osmolality
- Operate and remove any obvious resectable solitary tumour
- In chronic symptomatic hyponatraemia, use demeclocycline

MALIGNANT HYPERCALCAEMIA (see also Ch. 14)

Management
- The key feature is rehydration with saline
- First-line drug therapy is with intravenous pamidronate
- Alternatives include plicamycin, calcitonin and corticosteroids

MISCELLANEOUS GENETIC SYNDROMES

Carney's syndrome

This syndrome has an autosomal dominant inheritance. The gene causing it has been mapped to chromosome 2 (2p11). The clinical features are:

Clinical features

- Myxomas of the heart, skin or breast
- Spotted pigmentation of the skin
- Testicular, adrenal or pituitary tumours, or peripheral nerve schwannomas

---

Cowden's syndrome

The gene causing this has been mapped to chromosome 10. The clinical features are:

Clinical features

- Multiple hamartomas of the skin, mucous
  membranes, breast, thyroid or colon
- Facial trichilemmomas
- Breast cancer
- Papillary thyroid cancer

Klinefelter's syndrome
(See Ch. 19.)

Turner's syndrome
(See Ch. 19.)

chapter 24

Obesity

INTRODUCTION

Obesity is an excess of body fat. It results from an imbalance between energy expenditure and caloric intake. It is classified on the basis of the body mass index, or BMI (**Fig. 24.1**), which correlates closely with total body fat mass. In the USA 55% of people are overweight, and in the UK the figure is 40%; about 20% are obese in both populations. This prevalence is increasing, mainly because of an excessive intake of high fat food and a lack of physical activity, although a number of different factors play a lesser role in the development of obesity (**Fig. 24.2**).

Fig. 24.1 Classification of obesity by BMI

Body mass index = (weight in kg)/(height in metres)^2 (or $704.5 \times lb/in^2$)

Underweight	< 18
Normal	18–25
Overweight	25–30
Obese	30–40
Morbid obese	> 40

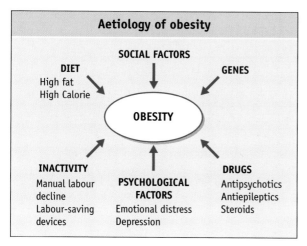

Aetiology of obesity

SOCIAL FACTORS

DIET
High fat
High Calorie

GENES

OBESITY

INACTIVITY
Manual labour decline
Labour-saving devices

PSYCHOLOGICAL FACTORS
Emotional distress
Depression

DRUGS
Antipsychotics
Antiepileptics
Steroids

Fig. 24.2 *Factors influencing the development of obesity.*

PATHOPHYSIOLOGY

The mass of body fat is determined by the balance between energy expenditure and caloric intake.

Energy expenditure is largely determined by the resting energy expenditure (REE, **Fig. 24.3**). A lesser contribution is made by the thermic response to food, and physical activity contributes about 15% to the total energy expenditure. Contrary to popular belief, there is no evidence that obese people have a lower REE (or basal metabolic rate, BMR) than lean individuals; indeed, the REE increases as fat mass increases. However, there is some evidence that, at any given weight, an obese individual has a lower REE than a lean individual of the same weight; this difference is possibly due to a variation in the activity of the sympathetic nervous system. Futile cycles, in which energy expenditure is uncoupled from any useful physiological function, appear to have a role in energy balance in animals. They occur principally in brown adipose tissue, but this is not found in adult humans, and these cycles are probably not important in human energy balance.

Caloric intake is determined both by the total food intake and by the balance of nutrients (**Fig. 24.4**). In the 'Western diet' more than 30% of calories are derived from fat. Fat has a higher calorific content per unit mass than either carbohydrate or protein, is more palatable and has less impact on satiety.

REGULATION OF APPETITE

The appetite is regulated by the hypothalamus. Afferent impulses from the gastrointestinal tract and circulating satiety factors from adipose tissue influence the levels of hypothalamic peptides and neurotransmitters that control the appetite, including stimulants such as neuropeptide Y (NPY) and suppressants such as leptin (**Fig. 24.5**). NPY is the most potent

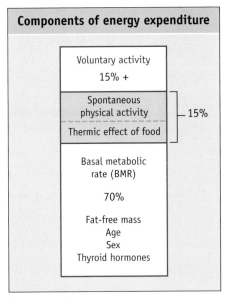

Components of energy expenditure

Voluntary activity
15% +

Spontaneous physical activity
Thermic effect of food
— 15%

Basal metabolic rate (BMR)

70%

Fat-free mass
Age
Sex
Thyroid hormones

Fig. 24.3   Components of energy expenditure.

Fig. 24.4   Calorific content of nutrients

Nutrient	Cal/g
Fat	9
Alcohol	7
Protein	4
Carbohydrate	4

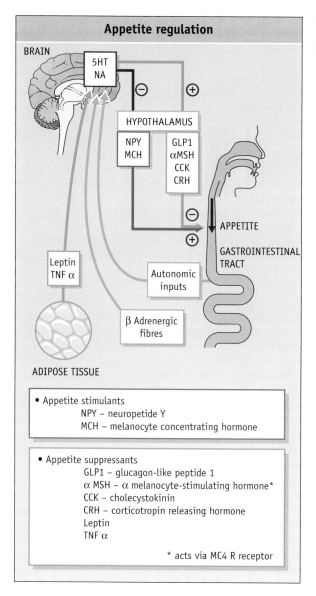

Fig. 24.5 *Factors implicated in human appetite regulation.*

Appetite regulation

BRAIN

5HT
NA

HYPOTHALAMUS

NPY
MCH

GLP1
αMSH
CCK
CRH

APPETITE

GASTROINTESTINAL TRACT

Leptin
TNF α

Autonomic
inputs

β Adrenergic
fibres

ADIPOSE TISSUE

- Appetite stimulants
  NPY – neuropetide Y
  MCH – melanocyte concentrating hormone

- Appetite suppressants
  GLP1 – glucagon-like peptide 1
  α MSH – α melanocyte-stimulating hormone*
  CCK – cholecystokinin
  CRH – corticotropin releasing hormone
  Leptin
  TNF α

  * acts via MC4 R receptor

appetite stimulant so far identified. The peptide hormone leptin was discovered because of its absence in various rodent models of obesity, such as the *ob ob* mouse. It is a potent adipose-tissue-derived satiety factor. However, in obese humans the leptin levels are almost always elevated owing to the increased mass of fat. Mutations in leptin and its receptor, and other related regulatory peptides or their receptors, have been identified in familial cases of obesity, but such cases are extremely rare (**Fig. 24.6**). Leptin has also been found to regulate reproductive function, which is a protective mechanism making procreation less likely in times of starvation.

Fig. 24.6   Causes of obesity in humans

Specific gene mutations	• Leptin • Leptin receptor • Melanocortin-4 (MC-4) receptor • POMC processing • Prohormone convertase-1 (PC-1) • PPAR γ
Dysmorphic syndromes	• Prader–Willi • Bardet–Biedl • Simpson–Golabi–Behmel • Cohen • Carpenter • Alstrom • Lipodystrophy
Endocrine causes	• Hypothalamic damage – associated with abnormalities in thermoregulation, thirst and pituitary function • GH deficiency • Cushing's syndrome • Hypothyroidism • PCOS – cause or effect?
Drugs	• Glucocorticoids • Oral contraceptive • Progestins • Sodium valproate • Antipsychotics • Amitriptyline • Hypoglycaemic agents, including insulin

SPECIFIC CAUSES OF OBESITY

Specific causes of obesity (**Fig. 24.6**) are uncommon. In most cases the development of obesity is an interplay between genetic and environmental factors. Genetic factors are estimated to contribute about one-third of the variance in adult weight through differences in REE, thermic responses to food and spontaneous physical activity. Development of obesity relates to both overeating and lack of physical activity, whilst maintenance of obesity relates mainly to excessive food intake. Partitioning, the distribution of fat mass, is determined by other factors such as hormones, particularly sex hormones, and intrauterine growth, a small fetus being more likely to develop central adiposity.

Risk factors for the development of obesity include:

- Age: childhood, puberty, early adulthood (25–35 years), pregnancy, menopause
- Recent weight loss
- Mother with gestational diabetes
- Overweight parents: if both, the offspring have a two- to threefold increased risk
- Family history of depression, substance abuse or sexual abuse

CLINICAL FEATURES AND INVESTIGATION

Investigation of the obese individual involves:
- Amount and distribution of body fat
- Identification of any secondary causes of obesity
- Presence of obesity-related morbidity
- Risk of complications of obesity
- Potential for weight loss

In the history there are four areas of particular emphasis. First, a note should be made of any previous attempts at weight loss, as these may demonstrate the potential for future attempts. Secondly, the minimum and maximum adult weight should be recorded, and changes in weight. Frequent weight cycling is associated with more resistant obesity. Other relevant factors include smoking, and alcohol and drug usage. Finally, the degree of motivation is significant.

ASSESSMENT OF BODY FAT

The amount of body fat is best assessed using the BMI, as defined previously. There are a variety of other clinical and investigational techniques for assessment of fat mass, but there is no evidence that they have any greater clinical value than the BMI. These other methods include:

- Skinfold thickness
- Plethysmography
- Immersion
- Isotope methods:
  — heavy water: deuterium or tritium
  — potassium
- Conductivity/impedance
- Fat-soluble gas
- Imaging:
  — ultrasound
  — CT
  — MRI
  — DEXA

The BMI correlates closely with morbidity and mortality from obesity, but fat distribution is also important. The central abdominal pattern of fat distribution (android) confers a greater risk of cardiovascular and metabolic disease than the gluteofemoral (gynoid) distribution (Fig. 24.7). This distribution can be assessed using the waist:hip ratio, but the abdominal circumference is a better measure of abdominal fat. Increased risk of morbidity is associated with an abdominal circumference of greater than:
- 102 cm (44") for males
- 88 cm (38") for females

OBESITY-RELATED DISEASES

Obesity is associated with an increased morbidity and mortality. A BMI of greater than 40 is associated with an increased risk of sudden death and an approximately 2.5-fold excess mortality rate.

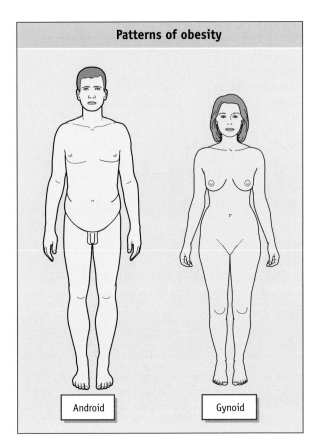

Fig. 24.7 *Android and gynoid patterns of obesity.*

Obesity is also implicated in a variety of disorders, including cancers (largely hormone-related ones), cardiovascular disease and vascular and metabolic disturbances (**Fig. 24.8**). A BMI of greater than 29 is associated with a fourfold increased risk of coronary heart disease, whilst the risk of developing diabetes is increased between 40- and 90-fold when the BMI exceeds 35, depending on the ethnic population.

The only investigations needed in the obese patient are to determine potential consequences, such as dyslipidaemia, fatty liver or polycythaemia, or to exclude possible secondary causes where indicated, such as hypothyroidism or Cushing's disease.

There are a number of endocrine abnormalities associated with obesity. These features include:

Endocrine features associated with obesity

- Elevated serum cortisol levels, which are suppressed with administration of dexamethasone
- Diminished basal and stimulated GH secretion
- Increased estrone:estradiol ratio, and testosterone and adrenal androgen levels in women; increased oestrogen and decreased testosterone levels in men; decreased SHBG levels in both sexes

Fig. 24.8   Conditions associated with obesity

Vascular and metabolic disease	Malignancies	Others
Hypertension*	Endometrium	Osteoarthritis
Dyslipidaemia	Ovary	Obstructive
Diabetes type 2*	Breast	sleep apnoea*
Coronary heart	Prostate	Respiratory
disease*	Colon	compromise
Stroke*	Biliary tree	Gall bladder disease
		Gastro-oesophageal reflux
		Venous stasis
		Stress incontinence

* Coexisting disease associated with particularly high risk.

MANAGEMENT

The best strategy for managing obesity is a public health one aimed at preventing its development. The key elements are the promotion of a healthy diet and an increase in levels of physical activity.

Treatment of obesity should be considered when:

- BMI exceeds 30
- BMI is between 25 and 30 *and* there are at least two other risk factors, such as coexisting disease (see high risk conditions in **Fig. 24.8**), smoking or a family history of coronary heart disease
- BMI is between 25 and 30 *and* the abdominal circumference is excessive

The three components of management are dietary change to reduce the calorie intake, increased physical activity and behavioural therapy to maintain motivation and increase compliance. The aim of treatment should be to reduce body weight by about 10% in 3–6 months and, most importantly, to maintain the weight reduction over the longer term. Rarely, more rapid weight loss is justified in particularly high risk individuals. The goal of therapy must be realistic, however; in individuals with a strong family history of obesity it is unrealistic to aim for a normal body weight.

DIET

Reduction of caloric intake is the most effective way of ensuring weight reduction. The initially reduction in caloric intake should be:

- 300 to 500 kcal per day for patients with a BMI of between 25 and 35
- 500 to 1000 kcal per day for patients with a BMI of greater than 35

A rough estimate of the optimal caloric intake can be obtained by using the individual's desirable weight (based on a weight for height table), multiplying by 30 to 35 kcal/kg for men and 25 to 30 kcal/kg for women. Alternatively the individual's REE can be calculated and the appropriate intake for the necessary caloric reduction derived from this.

Reduction of calorie intake is best achieved by reduction of the fat intake, because of its high calorific value per unit mass and poor satiation potential compared with carbohydrate. The dietary fat intake should ideally represent less than 30% of the calorie intake. There should be a particular emphasis on reducing the saturated fat intake, as this will improve lipid profiles by reducing the amount of LDL cholesterol.

Various diets are available, many of them commercially. The most appropriate is a low calorie diet (LCD) providing at least 800 kcal/day with the recommended nutrient balance. Alterations in nutrient balance, as seen in diets low in carbohydrate, high in protein or comprising single nutrients, are potentially dangerous. Note that it is important to maintain ample water intake whichever diet is used.

Very low calorie diets (VLCD), providing 400 to 800 kcal/day, may be used to achieve rapid weight loss in individuals at very high risk, although the long-term outcome for these is no different than for LCD. A VCLD is often provided in the form of diet drinks enhanced with appropriate vitamins and minerals. There is a greater risk of side-effects with VLCD, including electrolyte disturbance, deranged liver function and gall stones.

There is no indication for the use of ultra low calorie diets (200 to 400 kcal/day), or starvation diets (less than 200 kcal/day).

PHYSICAL ACTIVITY

The initial increase in physical activity should involve a low level of intensity, for example slow walking, for around 30 minutes on 3 days each week. This should be increased to a higher level of intensity, for example brisk walking, for around 45 minutes on 5 days each week. This regimen will contribute an energy expenditure of around 100 to 200 kcal/day.

Loss of weight through an increase in aerobic activity has several effects. First, it lowers BP. Secondly, it has a beneficial effect on lipid profiles, reducing levels of triglycerides and increasing the level of HDL cholesterol. Thirdly, it lowers both the fasting insulin and blood glucose levels.

BEHAVIOUR THERAPY

A number of specific interventions may be helpful in modifying behaviour, including group settings to reinforce achievements in weight reduction. Attention should be given to the following behavioural considerations:

- Nutritional principles, such as meal replacement, portion control and weighing of food
- Stimulus avoidance or control, to address the circumstances under which excessive intake occurs
- Use of motivational aids, such as log books and food diaries, which help to maintain compliance
- Relaxation and stress management

There is evidence that if obese individuals change their eating pattern, so that they eat less food but more often, there are similar benefits to those seen with increased activity in terms of weight reduction, better lipid profiles and lower blood glucose levels.

Smoking cessation

Smoking cessation is crucial for lowering the cardiovascular risk in this high risk group of patients and should be strongly encouraged. However, it must be understood that an associated weight gain, of on average 2–3 kg (4.5–7 lb), is almost inevitable despite interventions aimed at preventing this increase.

If these interventions fail to produce the intended weight reduction then consideration should be given to drug therapy or surgery.

DRUG THERAPY

Currently available drug therapies target nutrient absorption or satiety. Future targets of drug development include modulating the appetite, particularly by altering the circulating leptin levels.

Drug therapy should be used in conjunction with lifestyle changes. If weight loss cannot be achieved at all with diet then drug therapy is unlikely to be of value. One-third of obese individuals fails to respond to pharmaceutical agents.

Drugs that have been used to treat obesity include:
- Noradrenergic agents, such as benzphetamine and phentermine
- Dopaminergic agents, such as bupropion
- Serotoninergic agents, such as fenfluramine and dexfenfluramine

The noradrenergic and domapinergic agents are suitable only for short-term use and are therefore of limited value. Furthermore the noradrenergic agents have amphetamine-like side-effects. The serotoninergic agents have been withdrawn following concerns about an excess risk of valvular heart disease and pulmonary hypertension in past users.

- The use of drugs is contraindicated during pregnancy and lactation, and in those with unstable hypertension or coronary heart disease

Currently two drugs are widely available to assist with weight reduction:
- Orlistat is a non-systemic lipase inhibitor that blocks dietary fat absorption, reducing it by about 30%. However, if too much fat is ingested then the unpleasant side-effects of oily leakage or steatorrhoea may occur. There may also be a reduction in the absorption of fat-soluble vitamins, particularly D and E, so these may need supplementing
- Sibutramine is a selective serotonin and noradrenaline (norepinephrine) reuptake inhibitor that increases sympathetic nervous system activity, thereby inducing satiety

- The use of Sibutramine is contraindicated in patients with hypertension, coronary heart disease or cerebrovascular disease, as its side-effects include an increase in blood pressure and heart rate

The use of these drugs to facilitate weight loss is recommended for 12 months, although they may be helpful in the longer term for weight maintenance.

SURGERY

Surgical procedures to treat obesity (bariatric surgery) are recommended in the following situations:

- If the BMI is greater than 40, *or*
- If the BMI is greater than 35 with comorbidities, such as diabetes, hypertension or severe cardiorespiratory disease, *and*
- Medical therapy has failed

Jejunoileal bypass has been used in the past, but it results in significant complications. The currently favoured procedures are gastroplasty with or without gastric bypass (**Fig. 24.9**). Note, however, that the more extensive the procedure the higher is the rate of complications, which include particularly a sense of fullness, dumping and vitamin deficiencies.

Surgical treatments are usually associated with a sustained 50% loss in excess body weight at 5–10 years. There is also a reduction in comorbidity. For example, in some centres 80% of those with diabetes had normal blood glucose levels after bariatric surgery.

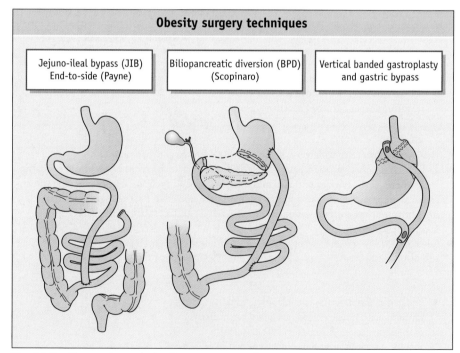

Obesity surgery techniques

| Jejuno-ileal bypass (JIB) End-to-side (Payne) | Biliopancreatic diversion (BPD) (Scopinaro) | Vertical banded gastroplasty and gastric bypass |

Fig. 24.9   *Commonly used obesity surgery procedures.*

PROGNOSIS

The most difficult part of obesity treatment is maintenance of weight reduction. After weight reduction has been achieved continued observation, monitoring and encouragement are needed to maintain success. It is important to emphasize that the REE will be reduced to a level appropriate to the new body weight for that individual and therefore a reduced calorie intake must be maintained in the long term. If there is no weight maintenance programme, allowing indefinite contact as needed, then almost all individuals will regain the weight lost within 5 years.

Index